Basic Pediatr
Intensive Care

Third Edition

Basic Pediatric Intensive Care

Third Edition

Sunit Singhi
MBBS, MD, FIAP, FAMS,
Professor
Head, Department of Pediatrics
Head, Emergency and Intensive Care Units
Advanced Pediatrics Centre
Postgraduate Institute of Medical Education and Research
Chandigarh (India)

Foreword by
BNS Walia

PEEPEE
PUBLISHERS AND DISTRIBUTORS (P) LTD.

Basic Pediatric Intensive Care

Published by
Pawaninder P. Vij
Peepee Publishers and Distributors (P) Ltd.
Head Office: 160, Shakti Vihar, Pitam Pura, Delhi-110 034
Correspondence Address:
7/31, First Floor, Ansari Road, Daryaganj, Post Box-7243
New Delhi-110002 (India)
Ph: 65195868, 23246245, 9811156083
e-mail: peepee160@yahoo.co.in
e-mail: peepee160@rediffmail.com
e-mail: peepee160@gmail.com
www.peepeepub.com

First Edition: **2005**
Second Edition: **2007**
Third Edition: 2009

ISBN: 81-8445-053-2

Printed at
Lordson, C-5/19, Rana Pratap Bagh, Delhi-110 007

To my parents

Whose nurturing during early years taught me human values

To my wife – Pratibha

Whose unending love enriched my life,

and her support and encouragement are my strength

To my wife's parents

Who gave me their trust and encouraged me to set higher goals

Foreword

Are children born to die a premature death, should they continue to die of potentially treatable or curable disease? Should all this waste of human resource be allowed to go on when the appropriate knowledge and skills are available to the medical profession? The administrators will continue to harp on the tune of financial constraints. But it is not often realized that non-availability of intensive care units in adequate numbers in the country not only leads to loss of precious lives, but also denies an opportunity to young medical graduates to learn the essential skills for saving lives and thus sets up a self perpetuating cycle. All intensive care is expensive so is pediatric intensive care. But is it more expensive than human life? Medical educators and administrators need to rethink their priorities, because a pediatric intensive care unit can add to the life of an admitted child a good seventy years, whereas the average predicted survival period for a coronary unit care is 20 years.

Not to speak of postgraduate training, even the training of a medical graduate in the 21st century cannot be considered complete without training in intensive care. At postgraduate level, the trainee must be provided good grounding in pediatric intensive care to be able to discharge his responsibilities effectively. Hence the need for establishment of Pediatric Intensive Care units in all medical colleges and tertiary care hospitals.

Prof. Sunit Singhi has put together an excellent book on Pediatric Intensive Care. The method adopted by him of elucidating the physiological alterations and then their correction are the key to the success in any life-threatening situation. The management evolves according to the situation that develops and for the purpose; the instructions are precise and sequential.

The book is the fruition of years of experience of Prof Singhi in patient management and training of residents in Pediatric Intensive Care. This compact volume covers all aspects of Pediatric Intensive Care, from who requires intensive care to the planning of such a unit; from basics of resuscitation to the complex aspects of mechanical ventilation. The book reflects not only what is relevant but also what is practical in a developing country, without too many frills added. In fact the author has avoided those details, which though can be considered ideal, but may not be practical with the existing facilities and circumstances. The book is resolutely clinical and deals mainly with the underlying problems that warrant intensive care –for example shock, respiratory failure, seizures, fluid and electrolyte imbalance—their early recognition and appropriate management irrespective of the specific disease process in which they may occur. An understanding of the fundamental principles can help apply these in virtually any setting for the care of seriously sick children. A chapter on organization of PICU would be extremely helpful for pediatricians embarking on this challenging venture. The chapter on procedures would be useful in honing practical skills. All in all, the book provides a straightforward, rationalised and updated approach to the management of a critically ill child. It is a virtual goldmine of practical information and shall be of immense value to all students and practitioners who deal with critically ill children.

BNS Walia

MD, FRCPCH (London), FAMS

Emeritus Professor of Pediatrics

Former Director

Postgraduate Institute of Medical Education & Research, Chandigarh

Preface to the Third Edition

It is very satisfying to see that simplified approach presented in previous editions of **Basic Pediatric Intensive Care** found favors with the young residents and general pediatricians. Their enthusiastic response to second edition and rapid stride and changes in our knowledge and practice were good enough reasons to prepare a new edition of this book in a short span of four years. The book continues to maintain its basic format and simplicity and addresses the issues that are relevant to our patients, feasible in our health care setup and manageable within available resources. Very expensive and rarely used forms of therapies and monitoring (such as ECMO, high frequency oscillations etc.) do not find mention in the book.

In our country the prevalence of critically ill patients is disproportionately high, but intensive care coverage remains incomplete and uncertain, especially in rural area and small cities and towns. To improve availability of pediatric intensive care to every child we need to take the lead and foster the development of critical care within the country and the region. One of the cost effective ways to do so is to enable general pediatricians, and health professionals to learn principles of critically care management. Intensive care may be viewed as provision of life saving therapies, supported by proactive monitoring to evaluate response to various therapeutic measures and detect complications. An intensive care unit (ICU) is the place where these principles are applied to management of critically ill patients under one roof. However, application of these management principles to critically ill patients outside an ICU in our country remains slow, perhaps because of the mindset, economic constraints and logistics.

I believe that it is feasible to extend principles of intensive care management at all levels of health care without a formal ICU in a graded manner even if the facilities in these units may be the most basic ones. Two good examples are treating respiratory failure caused by pneumonia with oxygen by nasal catheter, and treat hypovolemia caused by diarrhea with rapid administration of fluids. Color of the patient, respiratory rate, pulse, BP, urine flow etc are monitored manually to assess the response and to determine need for next therapeutic step. There are several such therapies and monitoring, which has been successfully used at primary care level by non-specialist doctors, by general pediatricians in a small hospital setting and by specialists in emergency department but have not found widespread use because of lack of appropriate protocols. Good intensive care does not necessarily mean expensive equipment and high cost care, but can also be provided in more basic settings with less cost inputs, yet achieving gratifying results. I hope that the material presented in this book will continue to help students and pediatricians to easily comprehend and effectively apply principles of intensive care for preserving children's lives and translate them into services for everyone who needs them within given resources at primary care, small hospital, at district (secondary level) hospital, and not just in a formal PICU.

In the revised edition new material is added on several subjects *viz.* respiratory failure, weaning from ventilation, monitoring, antibiotics, acid base disorders, sedation and analgesia, general care (electrolyte disturbances) and ARDS. Some sections particularly in chapter on Shock have been rewritten to incorporate newer recommendations. New chapters are added on Acute Heart Failure. Fever in PICU and Critical Care Neuromuscular Weakness. New section on accidental HIV exposure and management, and oral and GI decontamination are added in the appendix. I hope that the students and pediatricians will find this useful.

Sunit Singhi

Preface to the First Edition

Pediatric Intensive Care has a profound impact on the survival and quality of life of children with critical illnesses. The need for child-specific intensive care units is being increasingly appreciated. In 1993 I was asked to write a chapter on Pediatric Intensive Care. It was at that time that the seeds for this book were sown. I felt that there was a need for a text which could form the framework for guiding the 'in-training' Pediatric residents as well as young enthusiastic pediatricians who wanted to practice this challenging speciality but did not feel confident to do so. I therefore decided to write a book that covered the basic concepts of Pediatric Intensive Care in an easy to understand format that would be helpful to Pediatric residents and Pediatricians when they start working in the PICU for the first time. This book is intended for them.

The progress and development of the book went through several stages of maturation, from initial handouts to a spiral bound course book, over the last ten years. During these years voluminous amount of new information kept pouring, some of the concepts changed, and the practice of pediatric critical care medicine matured dramatically. However, the constancy of my teaching and training the residents over the years helped in ensuring that these got incorporated . The focus of the book is on fundamental principles of critical care which are applicable to all critically ill children irrespective of primary disease. Moreover, these principles are not confined to care of patients in an Intensive Care Unit but are applicable to care of all sick children whether they are being cared for in an emergency room, a general ward, or a nursing home. Application of these principles to care of sick children to the extent that it is feasible in a given set-up may help to improve their outcome. I have specifically tried to deal with important clinical matters or issues, where confusion and doubts usually prevail among inexperienced care providers. The emphasis is on systematic approach to management rather than care of specific diseases. Priority has been given to details of intensive care therapies and monitoring; relevant pathophysiology has been dealt with briefly. Descriptions of individual diseases, differential diagnosis and specialized aspects of care for specific diseases and conditions which are available in standard pediatric textbooks have been intentionally omitted. While recent advances have been mentioned, it has been my effort to present the information in a concise and non-controversial manner. A chapter detailing guidelines for organization, administrative structure, personnel, facilities and services, drugs and equipment requirement in setting up a Pediatric ICU has been included with a hope that it will help in creating more well-organized Pediatric ICUs over the country.

An appendix is specially included to give practical details of some common procedures that are required in an ICU and the scoring systems applicable to pediatric patients. It has been my endeavor to present the current information as objectively as possible. However, it is inevitable that personal opinions and biases occasionally surface at places in a book written by one person. I trust that these are far and few.

I hope that the book will help Pediatric trainees as well as trained Pediatricians in developing a strong foundation for the care of critically ill children. Even for those who are practising Pediatrics but not necessarily in Intensive Care, the information should be helpful in early recognition and optimal stabilization of critically ill children before they are sent to a referral center.

Sunit Singhi

Acknowledgements

This book owes its existence to many individuals who contributed to it directly or indirectly. I may not be able to name all of them. First, I wish to express my gratitude to Prof. B.N.S. Walia, who gave me the privilege to work at this prestigious Institute and persuaded me to take this fascinating field of Pediatric Critical Care as a career after almost 10 years of Pediatrics practice. He helped in setting up the unit. I am grateful to Prof. O.N. Bhakoo who supported all the efforts that went into developing Pediatric Emergency and Intensive Care services at PGIMER. I also express my gratitude to Prof. Ashok Sarnaik, Director, Pediatric Intensive Care, Michigan Children's Hospital, Detroit, U.S.A. who gave me the opportunity to learn ABC of Pediatric Intensive Care in his unit.

I sincerely acknowledge Dr. N. Jankiraman and all my dear colleagues from India and abroad. I had the privilege of their friendship, their involvement in our 'in depth' discussions on various aspects of Pediatric Intensive Care which helped me to assimilate various perspectives. All of this is reflected in the book at places in various ways. I also acknowledge contribution of all the Pediatricians and Pediatric residents whose enquiry and appreciation of the early forms of this book as well as of the basic intensive care courses that we organized at Chandigarh, Delhi, Kanpur, Surat and other places, which spurred me to finally write a text which could answer most of their questions.

I remain indebted to my wife Pratibha and daughter Samata for allowing extended hours in office and late nights while working on the book. Finally, I wish to thank my secretary Mr. Jatinder K. Karkara who has worked with me with enthusiasm in preparing the manuscript, and Mr. Pawaninder P. Vij, Director, PEEPEE Publishers and Distributors (P) Ltd., New Delhi who with gentle reminders, enthusiasm and hard work ensured timely publication of the book.

Contents

Chapter one

Pediatric Intensive Care

INTRODUCTION

With progress in medical science, it is now possible to offer to children with complex life threatening illnesses and unstable vital system functions, therapeutic measures to support and stabilize vital functions, and sustain life till the underlying primary illness is treated. Intensive care aims to provide this advanced care in an organized manner. Monitoring of the seriously ill patients for early detection of life threatening events and for ongoing assessment of response to therapeutic measures is an essential ingredient of intensive care.

Intensive care thus consists of provision of life sustaining therapeutic measures and intensive continuous monitoring to detect and correct life threatening events. This book discusses basics of therapeutic modalities available for pediatric intensive care, monitoring of critically ill children, and practical aspects about providing these facilities in a Pediatric Intensive Care Unit (PICU). Details of the management of specific diseases have been omitted from this book.

Who Needs Intensive Care

Patients with potentially recoverable diseases who need organ system support and who can benefit from closer observation, with or without more invasive monitoring than is normally available on a pediatric ward are the most need of intensive care. They have either impending or established organ system failure arising as the result of an acute illness.

Certain pediatric conditions are more likely to require complex intensive care (Table 1.1). Need for intensive care should be carefully considered in patients with these conditions at the time of initial evaluation. However, admission to PICU should be restricted to those critically ill children who have potentially recoverable disease. Priority must be given to those who need artificial support to one or more vital systems and uninterrupted monitoring.

Table 1.1: Common conditions requiring intensive care

Shock	Hypovolemic, Septic Shock, Severe burns, cardiogenic
Acute respiratory failure	Severe pneumonia, Severe asthma, Upper airways obstruction: Diphtheria, Near drowning, Guillain-Barré Syndrome
CNS conditions	Raised intracranial pressure Acute meningitis Severe head injury Hypoxic encephalopathy Intracranial haemorrhage Encephalitis and Reye's syndrome
Acute hepatic failure	Fulminant Viral hepatitis Metabolic disorders (e.g. Wilson's disease)
Poisonings	Paracetamol, Iron, Alphos Organophosphate poisoning
Acute renal failure	Haemolytic-uraemic syndrome Acute tubular necrosis
Fulminant metabolic disease	Unexplained metabolic acidosis Diabetic ketoacidosis
Bites and envenomations	Snake bite and scorpion sting

A number of 'procedures' are conventionally recognized as being 'intensive care dependent' meaning that under normal circumstances it would be unacceptable to perform these procedures outside a critical care environment (Table 1.2).

Table 1.2: Procedures that are conventionally recognized as being intensive care dependent

1.	Endotracheal intubation, and care of Intubated patient
2.	Continuous positive airway pressure (CPAP)
3.	Artificial/ mechanical ventilation
4.	Continuous invasive cardiovascular monitoring
5.	Use of antiarrhythmic, inotropic or vasoactive drug infusions
6.	Acute renal support (haemodialysis, haemofiltration, plasmafiltration and peritoneal dialysis)
7.	Cardioversion or DC countershock
8.	Acute or external cardiac pacing
9.	Intracranial pressure monitoring
10.	Complex intravenous nutrition
11.	Complex anticonvulsant therapy
12.	Active or forced diuresis
13.	Pericardiocentesis
14.	Mechanical circulatory support

Children should be referred to a PICU if:

- There is a reasonable anticipation of the immediate or imminent need for an intensive care dependent procedure.
- They have the potential to develop airway compromise.
- They have symptoms or evidence of shock (tachycardia, confusion/anxiety, cold clammy skin, poor capillary refill, poor urine output), respiratory distress or respiratory depression.
- Have an unexplained deteriorating level of consciousness, repeated or prolonged seizures.
- Have required or are in need of some form of continuing resuscitation.
- Have received a significant injury.
- Have undergone prolonged surgery or any major surgical procedures.
- Have potential or actual severe metabolic derangement, fluid or electrolyte imbalance.
- Have an acute organ (or organ/system) failure.
- Have (or organ/system failure) and experience a severe acute clinical deterioration in an established chronic disease.
- Require one-to-one nursing because of the severity of an acute illness.
- Decision to refer a patient to PICU should be made by most senior member of the team.

When to Admit

It is important to realize that benefits of intensive care can only be achieved if optimal management is instituted early, before permanent damage such as cerebral ischemia has occurred. The best of intensive care cannot reverse the effect of even short periods of cerebral hypoxia. Pediatricians therefore should be familiar with critical complications of childhood illnesses. Anticipation and early recognition of critical problems is key to successful intensive care before irreversible damage occurs.

Patients should be admitted to intensive care before their condition reaches a point from which recovery is impossible. Clear criteria may help to identify those at risk. Early referral improves the chances of recovery, reduces the potential for organ dysfunction, may reduce length of stay in intensive care and hospital, and may reduce the costs of intensive care.

Stabilization of Patient before Transfer to ICU

A pediatrician must appreciate the need for prompt resuscitation and stabilization of the sick children before transferring the patient to a PICU. Many of the conditions that require intensive care need stabilization. These measures should include assessment of vital signs (Table 1.3) and if abnormal provision of the airway, breathing, circulation, control of seizures and raised intracranial pressure, correction of arrhythmia. Correction of hypoglycemia and initiation of broad spectrum antibiotics, if specific situation demands, nasogastric tube to decompress stomach, gastric lavage/emesis/skin wash etc. as needed for specific poisonings should also be undertaken before transfer to PICU.

Table 1.3: Normal range of vital signs

Age Group	*Heart rate (per min)*	*Resp. rate (per min)*	*Systolic BP (mmHg)*	*Diastolic BP (mmHg)*
Newborn	90-205	30-55	60-100	40
1mo-2yrs	70-190	20-40	80-110	50
2-8 yrs	70-140	20-30	85-120	60
> 8 yrs	60-110	16-20	85-130	70

Once patients are stabilized they should be transferred to the intensive care unit by experienced intensive care staff with appropriate transfer equipment.

All patients transferred to PICU must receive similar attention before proceeding to specific specialized care.

Initial Treatment

In critical illness, at least initially, the need to support the patient's functions should take priority over establishing a precise diagnosis. Patients with life threatening shock or respiratory failure need immediate treatment to support failing vital organ functions rather than diagnosis of the cause, as the principles of management are the same . The actual later management may differ depending on the cause but the principles of treating life threatening organ failures do not depend on precise diagnosis.

Approach to Critical Care Delivery

1. **Formulate clinical hypothesis** including data base from history, bedside examination, laboratory values, and radiologic findings.
2. **Define therapeutic goals** and seek the least intervention in achieving each goal. Judgement of the success of therapy cannot be made if the goals have not been set. For example in a patient in shock.
   a. Goal of pharmacologic support is to ensure adequate perfusion.
   b. Recognize that there is risk benefit ratio to these goals–eg. prolonged administration of vasoactive drugs at high levels may lead to tissue hypoperfusion.
3. **Do no harm.** *Always assess the cost of any intervention or action to be sure that the benefit outweighs the risks.* An example is adding positive end expiratory pressure (PEEP) to help improve oxygenation. While there is often an improvement in oxygenation, there may also be a reduction in venous return a fall in cardiac output and a reduction in oxygen delivery.
4. **Liberate patients from drugs and interventions** as early as possible so that treatments do not outnumber diagnoses. Daily assessment for continuing or discontinuing the following should be conducted:
   a. Is ongoing sedation necessary?
   b. Can the patient undergo a spontaneous breathing trial?
   c. If the patient can breathe spontaneously, can they move forward to extubation?
   d. Can the following devices be discontinued to facilitate comfort, reduce need for analgesics and sedatives and reduce risk of infection?
      - Central lines
      - Chest tubes
      - Nasogastric tubes.

Chapter two

Cardiopulmonary Resuscitation

Pediatric cardiopulmonary resuscitation (CPR) includes the knowledge of sequential assessments and skills to restore effective ventilation and circulation to the child in cardiorespiratory or respiratory arrest. CPR consists of measures for establishing and maintaining the airway, controlling breathing and providing adequate circulation. These measures are commonly known as the 'ABC', signifying airway, breathing and circulation, the goal of which is to maintain oxygenated blood flow to the brain and other vital organs.

Every pediatrician should have the expertise in performing CPR. In addition, the pediatrician should assume leadership to train nursing staff and paramedics for administering basic life support measures.

Basic Life Support (BLS) includes sequential assessments and skills designed to restore and support effective ventilation and circulation in the child with respiratory or cardio-respiratory arrest. BLS CPR requires skills, but no adjunct or equipment and can be performed even outside the hospital.

Pediatric advanced life support (PALS) comprises BLS alongwith use of other adjunctive equipment and special techniques to assess and support the pulmonary and circulatory function and may not be optimally performed outside the hospital.

Illnesses that commonly result in a need for CPR in children are follows:

1. *Respiratory:* upper airway obstruction (viral laryngotracheitis, diphtheria, foreign body etc.), lower airway diseases such as pneumonia and bronchiolitis.
2. Severe infections.
3. Shock - all forms.
4. Accidental injury and trauma.
5. Poisoning with narcotics and sedatives.
6. *Environmental causes:* near drowning smoke inhalation, envenomation and bites.

Cardio-respiratory arrest in children is often secondary to a primary respiratory failure causing hypoxemia. It can often be anticipated in situations of respiratory distress or paralysis. Early intervention can prevent progressive deterioration of respiratory and circulatory status.

BEGINNING CARDIOPULMONARY RESUSCITATION: BASIC LIFE SUPPORT

At the beginning assess the level of responsiveness of the child and determine the need for airway, breathing and ventilation, and circulation (Table 2.1).

Table 2.1: Primary survey

Airway
- Open the airway
- Head tilt with chin lift/Jaw thrust

Breathing
- Check breathing
- Two initial breaths

Circulation
- Check pulse
- Perform chest compressions

1. **Determine unresponsiveness:** The level of responsiveness is determined by tapping the shoulders of the child and making a loud call to elicit a response.

Positioning: If the patient is unconscious position him on a firm flat surface and determine the state and adequacy of ventilation immediately.

2. **Airway:**

Open the airway: The most important step in CPR is to open the airway and restore breathing. In an unconscious child, tongue generally falls back and obstruct the airway. The following maneuvers to open airway are geared to relieve this obstruction:

i. *Head Tilt-Chin Lift*: To perform this technique: tilt the head gently back into a neutral position by placing one hand on the child's forehead and slightly extended the neck. Then lift the mandible upward and outward by placing fingers (not the thumb) of the other hand under the bony part of the lower jaw at the chin. One should be careful not to close the mouth or push on the soft tissues under the chin.

ii. *Jaw thrust:* This technique without head tilt is used in patients with suspected neck or cervical spine injury. For this lift the jaw upward and outward by placing three fingers under each side of the lower jaw at its angle.

3. **Breathing:**

Check for presence of breathing by any of the following methods:

- Look for a rise and fall of the chest and abdomen
- Listen for exhaled air
- Feel for exhaled air

If spontaneous breathing is present, a patent airway must be maintained.

Rescue breathing: Rescue breaths are the most important support for a child who is not breathing. The correct volume of each breath is the volume that causes the chest to rise. Pausing between the breaths maximizes the oxygen content and minimizes carbon dioxide concentration in the delivered breaths.

If no spontaneous breathing is detected, mouth to mouth or mouth to nose rescue breathing is initiated while a patent airway is maintained by a chin lift or jaw thrust. If the patient is an infant (<1 year old), place your mouth over the infant's nose and mouth, creating a seal. In older children (1-8 years old) pinch the nose tightly with the thumb and forefinger of the hand maintaining head tilt and make a mouth to mouth seal. Give two slow breaths (one to one and half second per breath), pausing after the first breath to take a breath.

Rescue breaths should be delivered slowly: If performed rapidly it may cause gastric distension. If two rescuers are present, the second rescuer may provide cricoid pressure to compress esophagus against the vertebral column. This maneuver may prevent gastric distension and reduce the likelihood of regurgitation. Attempts at relieving gastric distension during CPR by pressure on the abdomen should be avoided because it will cause aspiration of gastric contents.

If there is difficulty in achieving an effective breath i.e. a rise in chest, the airway may be obstructed. Following actions should then be taken:

i. Child's mouth is rechecked and any obstruction is removed.
ii. Head tilt and chin lift is readjusted.
iii. Rescue breaths are repeated upto 5 times (at least 2 times) with slightly greater volume or pressure.

If still unsuccessful, **obstruction by a foreign body must be suspected.** It should also be suspected in when a child presents with choking, stridor and cyanosis. If foreign body is suspected in an infant, deliver five back blows with heel of the hand between shoulder blades and subsequent five chest thrust. In a child over one year of age perform Heimlich maneuver. Blind finger sweep must be avoided since the foreign body may be pushed further down into the airway (see Procedure Section for Sequence of Actions for Foreign-Body Airway Obstruction).

4. **Circulation:**

Once the airway is opened adequately and two rescue breaths have been provided, check the pulse to determine the need for chest compression. Pulse check in infants is done by palpation of brachial or femoral artery and in older children by palpation of the carotid artery. Absence of a pulse in the large arteries in an unconscious child who is not breathing is defined as a cardiopulmonary arrest.

If a pulse is present but breathing is absent provide rescue breathing alone at a rate of 20 breaths per minute until spontaneous breathing resumes. For this count `one and two and' and at the count three and deliver breath. After giving approximately 20 breaths, make arrangement for ventilation with self-inflating bag and mask. If prolonged ventilation is anticipated secure tracheal airway and ventilate with self-inflating bag.

If no pulse is palpable or **heart rate is less than 60** per minute and signs of poor systemic perfusion are present: **begin chest compressions** at the rate of 100 per minute. Coordinate compressions and ventilation in a 15:2 ratio (30:2 if only one rescuer). Serial rhythmic compressions of the chest wall make the blood to circulate until further help is available. Chest compressions must always be accompanied by ventilation. To achieve optimal compressions the child should be supine on a hard flat surface. For a young infant the palm of the rescuer supporting the back of infant is good enough (See Procedure Section).

ADVANCED LIFE SUPPORT

Following basic life support, more sophisticated measures can be introduced to stabilize airway breathing and circulation. Critical step in escalating from basic to advanced life support occurs when 100% oxygen can be delivered by positive pressure ventilation through a secure airway. **Try to secure vascular access**, if help is available within the first minutes of resuscitation, for administration of drugs and fluid. **Or secure endotracheal airway and administer medications** through endotracheal route at the end of one minute if no help is available. Adrenaline, atropine, naloxone and lignocaine can be delivered through endotracheal route.

Oxygen

100% oxygen should be started as soon as CPR is initiated. Many factors lead to hypoxemia and inadequate tissue oxygenation during cardiopulmonary arrest. It is further compounded by low cardiac output; it is about one-third of normal during CPR even with the optimal technique. This leads to anaerobic metabolism and lactic acidosis, which impairs cardiac contractility and tissue response to drugs and attempts at defibrillation.

Ventilation

Bag-valve, Mask Ventilation

Ventilation face mask is selected to provide an airtight seal. It should extend from the bridge of the nose to the cleft of the chin, enveloping the nose and mouth but avoiding compression of the eyes. The mask is held on the face with one hand as a head tilt-chin lift maneuver is performed. The other hand compresses the ventilation bag. During mask ventilation position the head and neck for optimum airway patency. For infants and toddlers a neutral sniffing position without hyperextension of head is appropriate. In children older than 2 years this may be achieved by placing a folded towel under the neck and head.

Effective ventilation is determined by adequate chest movement. If effective ventilation is not achieved (i.e. chest does not rise) take following steps:

- Reposition the head
- Ensure that the mask is fitted snugly against the face
- Lift the jaw
- Consider suctioning the airway and
- Ensure that the bag and gas source are functioning properly.

A self-inflating bag-valve device delivers room air (21% oxygen) unless supplemental oxygen is provided. A reservoir bag is needed to give 100% oxygen. The bag-valve device used should be appropriate to patient size. The administered tidal volume is approximately 10 to 12 ml/kg. Neonatal size (200-250 ml) and Pediatric size (450 ml) bags are sufficient for routine resuscitations. Many self-inflating bags are equipped with a pressure limited pop-off valve set at 35 to 45 cm H_2O.

Endotracheal Intubation

(For details see chapter on Airway management and Procedure section).

Endotracheal intubation should be attempted soon after the initiation of bag and mask ventilation. It is the most effective and reliable method of assisted ventilation, protects the airway and provides avenue for higher oxygen delivery.

Indications for endotracheal intubation during CPR are:

1. Loss of protective airway reflexes
2. Administration of drugs
3. Need for mechanical ventilatory support
4. If patient needs to be transported.

Intubation attempts must not take more than 20 seconds. *Ventilation should never be interrupted for more than 30 seconds. If intubation is unsuccessful within 20 seconds or if the patient develops significant hypoxemia, cyanosis, pallor or a decreased heart rate during the procedure it must be interrupted.* The patient should be immediately ventilated using bag and mask, preferably with 100% oxygen before another attempt.

Following intubation, careful visualization of chest movements and auscultation of the lungs should be done to confirm proper tube placement. The most common mistake is to 'shove' the endotracheal tube as far as one can go—usually ending up in the right main bronchus and leaving left lung unventilated. Following confirmation of the tube placement tape and secure the tube in place. Failure to do so has often been the reason for ETT to fall out in the middle of CPR.

FLUIDS AND MEDICATION

Objectives

1. To correct hypoxemia.
2. To correct metabolic acidosis.
3. To increase perfusion pressure during chest compression.
4. To initiate spontaneous and/or more powerful cardiac contraction.
5. To accelerate heart rate.
6. To improve blood pressure and perfusion pressure.
7. To suppress abnormal ventricular activity.
8. To improve cerebral perfusion pressure.

Establishment of reliable vascular access within the first minutes of resuscitation is essential for infusion of fluid and medications possible. This is crucial for a successful CPR. However, during CPR, rapid establishment of IV access can be very difficult. In these situations, emergency administration of some medications may be achieved through endotracheal route. Intravenous or intraosseous route however, is preferred for drug delivery and is mandatory for the infusion of large volumes fluids. Fluid administration is extremely important for a successful CPR, especially when cardiac arrest results from trauma and sepsis.

Endotracheal Administration of Drugs (Table 2.2)

The endotracheal route is used for drug administration when vascular access is limited. Absorption rates and physiologic and pharmacologic effects compare favorably with intravenous route for adrenaline and atropine. To be absorbed, endotracheal medications must be delivered beyond the tracheal tube into the tracheobronchial tree. This is achieved by diluting the medication to a volume of 3 to 5 ml of normal saline and instilling into the tube, followed by several positive-pressure ventilations using a resuscitation bag.

Table 2.2: Drugs administered through endotracheal route

Drug	Dose
1. Adrenaline	0.1mg/kg (0.1ml/kg, 1:1000 solution)
2. Atropine	0.01 to 0.02 mg/kg
3. Naloxone	0.1mg per kg if <5 years or <20 kg 2.0mg per kg if >5 years or >20 kg

Venous Access

General Principles

1. Choose the largest, most accessible vein for venous cannulation when peripheral veins can be readily seen or palpated below the skin surface.
2. If veins are collapsed, select veins those are relatively constant with respect to anatomic location, e.g. femoral vein, medial cubital vein at elbow or long saphenous vein at the ankle.
3. Avoid cannulation of scalp veins because the veins are extremely small and attempts at cannulation may interfere with control of the airway and ventilation.
4. Intraosseous route is a reliable alternative to the intravenous route and should be attempted if intravenous route cannot be achieved. The main contraindication to intraosseous infusion is the presence of a fracture in the pelvis or extremity proximal to or in the bone chosen for intraosseous needle insertion.

Priorities of Vascular Access

Time should not be wasted in futile attempts to achieve peripheral or central venous cannulation and the resuscitation team should have a protocol for establishment of venous access. During CPR in children up to 6 years of age intraosseous cannulation should be attempted if reliable venous access cannot be achieved within three attempts or 90 seconds, whichever comes earlier.

Intracardiac administration of drugs should never be attempted. It may cause coronary artery laceration, cardiac tamponade, and pneumothorax. It does not result in more rapid circulation of drugs than intravenous route and it requires interruption of chest compression and ventilation.

Fluids

Administration of a crystalloid (normal saline or Ringer's lactate solution) bolus of 20 ml/kg over 2-5 minutes should be considered during CPR if child fails to respond to adequate oxygenation, ventilation, chest compression and adrenaline. A rapid bolus is for volume expansion is justified in virtually every pediatric arrest. Intravenous fluids are needed to restore normal circulating volume during resuscitation and to expand blood volume after cardiac arrest because of venous pooling, vasodilatation and capillary leakage. In a setting of hypovolemia or septic shock bolus administration of crystalloids 20 ml/kg may be repeated up to 60 ml/kg, while monitoring the response—the pulse, breath sounds, liver size, capillary refill, skin color, and peripheral edema. If hypovolemia was caused by blood loss, blood should be used.

Drugs

Drugs most commonly required during resuscitation are as follows:

Epinephrine

Epinephrine is both an alpha and beta receptor agonist, but the benefit in using this drug during CPR is primarily due to its alpha effects—namely on increase in myocardial and CNS blood flow during ventilation and chest compression. The value and safety of epinephrine's beta adrenergic effects is controversial. Some believe that it may actually be harmful because the beta adrenergic effect increases myocardial work.

Indications: Asystole, sinus or junctional bradycardia, fine ventricular fibrillation.

Dose: 0.1 ml/kg of a 1: 10,000 solution, if unsuccessful increase the dose upto 1 ml/kg of 1: 10,000 solution or 0.1 ml of 1:1000 solution.

Route: IV, endotracheal, intraosseous

Continuous infusion: 0.1–1.0 μg/kg/minute

Complications: intense peripheral vasoconstriction.

Dopamine

It is a chemical precursor of norepinephrine, has dopaminergic, beta and alpha adrenergic effects, depending on dose.

Dose: dopaminergic - 2-4 μg/kg/minute, beta - 5-10 μg/kg/minute, alpha -> 11 μg/kg/minute.

Route: Large peripheral or central vein.

Complications: arrhythmias, severe sloughs if it extravasates, treat with : local infiltration with phentolamine (alpha blocker).

Dobutamine

It is a synthetic catecholamine, and a potent inotropic agent useful in the treatment of heart failure. It produces an increase in myocardial contractility and mild peripheral vasodilation.

Dose: Continuous infusion 2.5 to 20 μg/ minute.

Route: Large peripheral or central vein.

Atropine Sulfate

It is a parasympatholytic drug that reduces cardiac vagal tone and enhances the rate of discharge to the sinus node and facilitates AV conduction.

Indication: treatment of sinus or junctional bradycardia accompanied by hemodynamic compromise, has sometimes been used in asystole.

Dose: 0.02 mg/kg/dose.

Total dose should not to be less than 0.1 mg (lesser dose may worsen bradycardia) and not to exceed 1.0 mg in children and 2 mg in adolescents (complete vagolytic dose).

Route: IV, endotracheal, intraosseous.

Adverse effect: Increases myocardial oxygen demand.

Lidocaine

Lidocaine suppresses ectopic ventricular activity by decreasing automaticity by slowing the rate of phase 4 diastolic depolarization. It also terminates arrhythmias by slowing conduction in reentrant pathways.

Indication: Ventricular fibrillation.

Dose: 1 mg/kg/bolus, followed by continuous infusion : 20-50 μg/kg/minute.

Route: Bolus may be given intravenously or intraosseous; continuous infusion intravenous only.

Adverse reactions: hypotension, seizures have been reported.

Amiodarone

Amiodarone is used to treat atrial and ventricular arrhythmia in children, including supraventricular and ventricular tacycardia. Amiodarone inhibits alpha and beta receptors, produces vasodilation, AV nodal delay slowing ventricular conduction and QT prolongation.

Dose: 5 mg/kg, IV, over 20 minutes. Repeat dose of 5 mg/kg may be given up to a maximum of 15 mg/kg.

Adverse reactions: Hypotension. Amiodarone should not routinely be administered with other agents, which prolong QT interval.

Sodium Bicarbonate

Sodium bicarbonate administration during CPR has not been shown to improve survival. Acidosis detected during resuscitation is ideally corrected through restoration of effective ventilation and systemic perfusion. It should only be considered in documented severe acidosis (pH <7.15) associated with prolonged cardiac arrest, hyperkalemia or tricyclic anti-depressant overdose.

Caution: Ventilation should be established before sodium bicarbonate administration.

Potential adverse effects: Hypernatremia, hyperosmolality, myocardial depression, paradoxical intracellular acidosis and shift of O_2—dissociation curve to left thereby reducing O_2 delivery to tissues.

Calcium

Calcium is not recommended for the treatment of asystole. Administration of calcium during cardiac arrest may cause cellular injury.

Indication: Documented hypocalcemia, hyperkalemia, hypermagnesemia.

Dose: 20 mg/kg of calcium chloride, 0.2 ml/kg of 10% solution IV.

Vasopressin:

There is limited data on use of vasopressin to recommend its use in resuscitation.

Medications for Hemodynamic Stabilization

First restore adequate circulating volume and correct hypoxemia.

If patient is hypotensive after fluid bolus start adrenaline infusion (0.1 µg/kg/min to 1.0 µg/kg/min).

If patient is normotensive after fluid bolus start dopamine (2-20 µg/kg/min) or dobutamine (2-20 µg/kg/min) continuous infusion.

Value of Blood Gases

Venous blood is more likely to represent oxygenation and acid-base status of peripheral tissues than the arterial blood. During CPR the arterial blood can show a respiratory alkalosis while venous blood shows a metabolic acidosis. The common practice of monitoring arterial blood gases during CPR should therefore be abandoned in favor of monitoring venous blood gases during CPR (or in any low-flow state).

How Long to Continue: Termination of CPR

There are no reliable predictors to guide termination of CPR. The goal of prolonged CPR is to increase the chance for survival, but this is not a desirable goal if the survivor is mentally impaired. The risk of functional impairment in any of the major organs is directly related to the duration of the ischemic insult. The ischemic time following cardiac arrest includes the time from onset of the arrest to onset of CPR (arrest time) and the duration of resuscitation effort (CPR time). Among adult patients who did not regain consciousness in the first hour following successful CPR, half of the survivors had a satisfactory neurological recovery if the arrest time was less than 6 minutes and the CPR time did not exceed 30 minutes. However, if the arrest time exceeded 6 minutes, more than 15 minutes of CPR always produced neurologic impairment in the survivors. Thus, in witnessed cardiac arrest in adults (when arrest time can be accurately determined) CPR can be continued for 30 minutes if the arrest time is less than 6 minutes, but if the arrest time is longer than 6 minutes, CPR should be terminated after 15 minutes.

Endtidal CO_2 during resuscitation

The tendency of the end-tidal PCO_2 to rise during CPR can be a valuable prognostic marker. When end-tidal PCO_2 does not rise above 10 mm Hg after a resuscitation time of 15 to 20 minutes, the resuscitative effort is unlikely to be successful.

However, at present there is no agreed specific criteria for ceasing CPR in children. The decision to terminate CPR may be taken by the physician after trial of adequate resuscitation and establishing cardiovascular unresponsiveness to acceptable resuscitative techniques.

POSTRESUSCITATION CARE AND OUTCOME

When CPR is successful in restoring spontaneous circulation, two concerns deserve attention in the early post-resuscitation period. The first is the potential for continued and progressive multiorgan damage (i.e. post-resuscitation injury). The second is the likelihood of neurologic recovery in patients who do not regain consciousness immediately after CPR. Therefore after successful resuscitative efforts, the child should be transferred to a pediatric intensive care unit, for repeated and regular cardiopulmonary assessments and appropriate interventions.

The problems that may occur in survivors following a cardio-pulmonary arrest includes:

- Myocardial ischemia–Cardiogenic shock, hypotension and acidosis.
- Hypoxic ischaemic encephalopathy–altered mental status and seizures.
- ARDS : refractory hypoxemia.
- Hepatic dysfunction.
- Renal failure secondary to tubular/necrosis.
- Coagulopathy.
- Mesentric ischaemia with intestinal bleeds.
- Metabolic: hypo/hyperglycaemia, metabolic acidosis, hypocalcemia.

The Management aim at early identification of these problems and minimized permanent injury. The management includes the following:

- *Hemodynamic stabilization and Inotropic support:* Consider fluid bolus 5-10 ml/kg if poor perfusion. Failure to initiate inotropes may lead to a repeat arrest after initial resuscitation. If the patient is hypotensive, commence adrenaline infusion (0.1 μg/kg/min) (dobutamine may be added after BP stable). In a normotensive patient, dobutamine or dopamine may be used.
- *Ventilatory support:* It should be continued until patient is neurologically improved with intact protective airway reflexes, hemodynamically stable and respiratory gas exchange is satisfactory.
- *Neurological support:* Control of seiures, optimization of cerebral perfusion, avoidance of hyperpyrexia and hyperglycaemia. Fever should be treated with paracetamol 15 mg/kg/dose.
- *Other supportive and renal replacement therapy as indicated:*Early enteral feeding: Mesentric ischemia can result in intestinal mucosal sloughing with diarrhoea and intestinal bleeds, hence enteral feeds must be given with caution. Usually, enteral feeds are started after 48 hours.
- Psychosocial support to the family.

Post-resuscitation injury: Is usually seen after prolonged ischemic times, and it is characterized by progressive multiple organ dysfunction. The condition is often fatal. There is no effective therapy at present. This is attributed to persistent vasoconstriction (i.e., the no-reflow phenomenon) and the release of toxic metabolic mediators produced during the period of ischemia and reperfusion.

Neurologic Recovery

Neurologic impairment is common in cardiac arrest patients who are successfully resuscitated. Many survivors do not regain consciousness immediately after CPR. Some prognostic factors may help to identify patients who are unlikely to awaken or achieve a satisfactory neurologic recovery. These are duration of coma, coma score and brain stem reflexes. Failure to regain consciousness in the first few hours after CPR is not a harbinger of prolonged or permanent neurologic impairment. Adult data shows that coma that persists longer than 4 hours after CPR carries a poor prognosis for full neurologic recovery. In an adult study it was found that after 1 day of persistent coma, only 10% of the patient achieved a satisfactory neurologic recovery. The recovery rate drops below 5% when the coma lasts 1 week, and no patient recovers neurologic function when the coma persists for 2 weeks. However, the actual time selected for informing families of a poor prognosis is a matter of individual preference. Glasgow Coma Scale (GCS) can also provide valuable prognostic information. A GCS score below 5 on the third day of persistent coma is almost always associated with a poor outcome. Absence of the pupillary light reflex after one or more days of coma indicates little or no chance for neurologic recovery. This reflex has no prognostic value in the first 6 hours after CPR because it can be transiently lost and then reappear.

A successful CPR outcome is the discharge from the hospital of a functioning patient with intact central nervous system, likelihood of which is increased when CPR is begun early and pursued systematically and expeditiously in accordance with the above guidelines.

Chapter three

Recognition and Stabilization of the Critically Ill Child

Early recognition of a critical illness is crucial to institution of life saving measures. This is especially true for children, because they have very little reserve and give very little time before lapsing into irreversible organ system damage. However, most pediatricians, unlike physicians for adults, are not well tuned to respond to an acute life threatening illness when faced with a seriously ill child. Guided by classical medical school teaching we endeavor to localize the disease and diagnose with help of history, physical examination, laboratory tests etc. before intervening. However, progress in our understanding of disease processes and technology has augmented our ability to intervene even before arriving at a precise etiological diagnosis of a potentially life threatening illness. In such situations, one must often make decision regarding therapeutic intervention based on recognition of key life threatening physiological derangements, so as to stabilize and restore vital functions and sustain life.

Who is Critically Ill?

As defined by Society of Critical Care Medicine a critical illness exists—"When impending or existing organ malfunction threatens or interferes with viability or cellular function". This may be an end result of any severe illness. The physician should be alerted to the possibility of a critical illness in the presence of any of the following conditions (this list is not complete or exhaustive).

1. Accident/trauma-with loss of consciousness, or bleeding, blunt abdominal/chest trauma, burns, fire-smoke inhalation, near-drowning.
2. Fever with altered consciousness/behaviour, toxicity, body temperature >40°C, hypothermia.
3. Unconsciousness, sudden paralysis.
4. Respiratory distress, slow/irregular breathing, stridor-obstructed airway.
5. Severe diarrhea and/or vomiting.
6. Suspected poisoning, snake bite, scorpion and other stings.
7. Acute bleeding.
8. Post-operative—after major surgery.
9. Sudden worsening of a previously known illness.

Critical Illness: Functional Impairments

The body is a network of homeostatic systems in which function is designed to optimize cardiac output and maintain oxygen delivery to various vital organs. In a healthy child all autonomic and hormonal responses are designed to meet these goals. Any condition that impairs the normal respiratory function, circulation, integrity of CNS, and metabolism disturbs homeostatic balance. Identification of physiologic impairment(s) that the illness might have caused is crucial to recognition of critical illness.

In the recognition of a critical illness, it is therefore essential to focus on identification of functional impairment of organ systems so as to direct the intervention(s) to make up for child's inability to compensate physiologically.

RAPID ASSESSMENT: PHYSICAL EXAMINATION

Critical care is generally equated with high technology and equipment. However, the recognition of critical illness and provision of early care, paradoxical as it may appear, depend entirely on the use of eyes, ears and hands. It is directed at assessment of the following ABCs:

A- Airway—to assess ventilation
B- Breathing—to assess oxygenation
C- Circulation—to assess adequacy of tissue perfusion
C- CNS status—to assess integrity of central neuronal control of all vital functions.

Airway/Breathing Examination

It is directed at the following:

1. *Airway:* Is it clear and breathing comfortable. Or any sign of airway obstruction (stridor), secretions!
2. *Breathing effort:* Is work of breathing increased (rocky or 'see-saw' breathing, grunting, head-bobbing), stridor?
3. *Respiratory rate:* Whether very slow, very fast (>60/min), or irregular.
4. *Chest movements:* Is the expansion with each inspiration adequate? Air entry on auscultation good and equal?
5. *Colour:* Normal pink, or blue-gray or ashen, which indicates cyanosis and poor oxygenation.
6. *Oxygen saturation:* If a pulse oximeter is available oxygen saturation (SaO_2) is a very useful parameter. A saturation of <92% suggests inadequate oxygenation.

Assessment of Circulation

The circulation is designed to meet body's need for oxygen and nutrient supply. Adequacy of circulation depends on cardiac output and blood pressure. Cardiac output in turn is determined by stroke volume and heart rate; stroke volume depends on myocardial contractility, preload (volume of blood coming to right side of heart) and after load (resistance to forward flow of blood).

Assessment of adequacy of circulation can be made from:

1. Peripheral perfusion—capillary refill, skin colour and temperature.
2. Central and peripheral pulses volume.
3. Heart rate.
4. Blood pressure.
5. Urine output in preceding few hours.

Palpation of Pulse

This is the most important part of assessment of circulation. This should be done over carotid (central) and brachial pulse. A good pulse examination can give all the information about stroke volume, blood pressure, systemic vascular resistance and of course, heart rate. Weak or absent carotid pulse indicates poor cardiac output/stroke volume, requiring immediate intervention. A poor peripheral pulse volume is an early sign of hypovolemia than hypotension and suggests critical loss of vital organ perfusion.

Heart Rate

Heart rate (HR) is an important determinant of cardiac output (CO) as CO= Heart rate × Stroke volume. Tachycardia suggests a compensatory effort to meet circulatory needs. It is an early and sensitive indicator of impending circulatory decompensation. It may not be possible to remember norms for HR at various age groups but following cut off limits should be memorized and interpreted as tachycardia:

- HR > 160 per minute, in children >5 years, as sinus tachycardia.
- HR > 180 per minute in children 1-5 years and HR > 200 per minute in infants may indicate supraventricular tachycardia.

- Bradycardia (HR < 60/min in infants, < 40/min after infancy) may be associated with low cardiac output.
- A very fast pulse rate (>200-220/min), irregular or absent pulse must be evaluated further using a ECG.

Peripheral Perfusion

The following signs indicate poor peripheral perfusion:

1. *Capillary refill >2 seconds*. This assesss rapidity of filling of cutaneous capillary bed and is estimated as the time taken for normal pink colour to return, after blanching the skin of distal extremity (foot/hand) with pressure of examiner's thumb. The extremity must be lifted slightly above the level of heart to ensure proper assessment.
2. *Cool or clammy extremities*: When cardiac output decreases, cooling of skin begins from peripheries (fingers to toes) and extends proximally.
3. Low toe temperature.
4. *Pale, blue or mottled skin:* Pallor indicates ischemia. Cyanosis suggests slow flow through skin or hypoxemia.

Blood Pressure (BP)

Blood pressure is dependent on cardiac output and systemic vascular resistance. A fall in BP therefore reflects decreased cardiac output. However, normal blood pressure may be maintained in spite of a fall in cardiac output because of compensatory vasoconstriction and tachycardia. Hypotension, therefore, is a late sign of circulatory decompensation. Even mild hypotension must be treated quickly and with vigour because it signals decompensation and imminent cardiopulmonary arrest. Normal systolic blood pressure for children >1 year is equal to 90 mm Hg + (2 x age in years) and the lowest normal limit is 70 mmHg + (2 × age in years).

CNS Function Assessment

The important components include assessment of level of Consciousness. This may be categorized as:

i. Alert
ii. Sleepy-or combative/agitated
iii. Fails to recognize parents (early coma)
iv. Comatose: dose not respond to pain.

The Glasgow coma scale helps in a more objective assessment of the level of consciousness. Infant's scale is useful for children upto 3 years of age; for older children adult scale is used (Table 3.1). A score <8 corresponds to deep coma.

Sudden cerebral hypoperfusion/ischemia causes complete loss of consciousness whereas gradual loss/alteration of consciousness level suggests insidious onset of circulatory impairment and cortical hypoperfusion. Patients with impaired consciousness should be assessed further for the following:

1. Integrity of brain stem.
2. Signs of raised intracranial pressure (ICP).
3. Ongoing seizure activity (Status epilepticus).

Integrity of Brain Stem

May be assessed from:

i. Examination of pupils: Size, reaction to light
ii. Brainstem reflexes: Doll's eye maneuver, Cold-caloric test
iii. Respiratory pattern
iv. Motor response and posture.

Table 3.2 shows signs typically seen with brain stem involvement at different levels.

Evaluation of Physiological Status

At the end of rapid cardiopulmonary assessment, and evaluation of CNS, it is possible to arrive at a reasonable assessment of the patient's status which may be categorized as follows:

1. Stable—normal airway, breathing and circulation.

Table 3.1: Glasgow coma scale for children

Eye Opening	**Best Motor Response**
4 Spontaneous	6 Obeys verbal command (> 2 years)
3. To verbal command	5 Localizes pain
2 To pain	4 Flexion withdrawal (> 6 months)
1 No opening	3 Flexion-decorticate (< 6 months)
	2 Extension-decerebrate
	1 No response
Best Verbal Response	
≤ 3 years	≥ 4 years
5 Smile, interacts	5 Oriented, converses
4 Crying, consolable	4 Disoriented, converses—Words
3 Inconsistently consolable	3 Inappropriate words – Vocal sounds
2 Inconsolable, restless	2 Incomprehensible speech
1 No response	1 No response

Table 3.2: Critical neurologic findings associated with brainstem injury at different levels

CNS level	*Pupil*	*Doll's eye*	*Respiratory pattern*	*Motor response*
Thalamus	Small reactive	Variable	Cheyne-stokes	Normal response
Midbrain	Midposition fixed	Absent	Hyper ventilation	Decorticate increased
PONS	Pinpoint fixed	Absent	Apneustic	Decerebrate, flaccid
Medulla	Small reactive	Present	Ataxic	No posturing, flaccid

2. Early respiratory failure—in respiratory distress.
3. Respiratory failure—cyanosis, gasping.
4. Shock—poor perfusion/ Decompensated shock-hypotension.
5. Poor cardiac function/irregular heart rate.
6. CNS problems—increased ICP, impaired consciousness or coma, uncontrolled seizures—status epilepticus.

STABILIZATION MEASURES

Depending on the physiological status following stabilization measures can be undertaken:

1. *Airway:* Opening the airway, endotracheal intubation.
2. *Respiratory support:* Oxygenation and bag ventilation.
3. *Circulatory support:* Vascular access-IV or intraosseous, Volume expansion using fluid bolus and Vasoactive drugs infusion.
4. *CNS protection:* Seizure control, control of ICP.
5. Correction of metabolic impairment.

Airway Stabilization

If airway is unstable i.e. if its patency cannot be maintained, or if there are excessive secretions—jaw-lift and head tilt to 15°, suction, and an oropharyngeal airway is needed.

If patient is in respiratory distress or is hypoxic 100% oxygen should be started.

If breathing efforts are not good and or chest expansion is inadequate, use of bag and mask for ventilation and 100% oxygen should be followed by tracheal intubation and bag ventilation.

Indication for endotracheal intubation in a critically ill child:

1. Functional/anatomic airway obstruction.
2. Loss of protective airway reflex-aspiration

is a risk (Coma, Glasgow coma scale score <8).
3. Inadequate CNS control of ventilation.
4. Excessive work of breathing.
5. Prolonged respiratory support is anticipated.

One should go ahead with a tracheostomy or a cricothyrotomy if any of the following indications are present:
1. Upper airway obstruction—Diphtheria.
2. Vocal cord paralysis.
3. Facial/upper airway burns, trauma.
4. Endotracheal intubation is difficult or the tube patency is difficult to maintain because of secretions, infection or bleeding.

Circulatory Support

If tachycardia and poor perfusion (compensated shock) or hypotension (decompensated shock) are present following measures are needed:
1. Establishment of a vascular access using a large peripheral vein. Often IV line may take time to establish because of collapsed veins. Intraosseous route may be used.
2. *Volume expansion*: 20 ml/kg N Saline or Ringer's lactate boluses as fast as possible till pulse is good volume followed by 10 ml/kg blood if shock is due to blood loss.
3. Administration of vasoactive drugs such as dopamine (5-20 μg/kg/min), and dobutamine (5-20 μg/kg/min) by intravenous infusion.

The immediate goal of therapy is to achieve a palpable peripheral pulse good capillary refill and correction of hypotension.

Urgent Arrhythmia Management

It is required in all patients with arrhythmia who are in shock. A defibrillator is required for it, hence it must be available in all emergency units.
1. Ventricular tachycardia—if pulse is palpable Cardioversion (0.5-1 joule/kg), Lidocaine 1 mg/kg IV or by endotracheal route. If pulse is not palpable defibrillate (2 joules/kg).
2. Ventricular fibrillation—Defibrillate (2 joules/kg).
3. Supraventricular tachycardia—Cardioversion (0.5-1.0 joules/kg) or adenosine 0.1 mg/kg IV (See Chapter on Arrhythmia).
4. Bradycardia, asystole—Epinephrine, Atropine 0.02 mg/kg, IV, and if needed external pacemaker.

CNS Protection

If coma, seizures, or increased ICP are present the stabilization should proceed as follows:
1. Ensure adequate airway and breathing, manage circulatory impairment and hypotension. If Glasgow coma scale score is <8 endotracheal intubation is indicated.
2. Seizure Control: Diazepam 0.2-0.3 mg/kg IV, may repeat every 5 minutes for 3 doses together with phenytoin 20 mg/kg IV.
3. Control ICP to maintain cerebral perfusion
   i. Head-up with forward tilt
   ii. Hyperventilate with bag–at a rate double of normal respiratory rate for age for about 10-20 minutes
   iii. Mannitol 0.25-0.5 g/kg (1.25-2.5 ml/kg of 20% solution) IV stat.
4. Give glucose (25% soln) 0.5 g/kg IV stat.

Further management and stabilization will need ancillary studies such as blood gases, hemoglobin estimation, oxyen saturation and capnography, chest X-ray, etc.

Chapter four

Acute Respiratory Failure

Components of respiration are ventilation and oxygenation. Ventilation deals with movement of gas in and out of lungs and oxygenation deals with uptake of oxygen at alveolar level. The lungs have two major metabolic functions—to provide oxygenation for tissue and to eliminate of CO_2.

Acute respiratory failure (ARF) is present when the ***respiration is no longer able to meet the metabolic needs of the body***. There are two basic types of respiratory failure: hypoxemic and hypercapnic.

Hypoxemic respiratory failure is defined as a room air PaO_2 of less than 60 torr.

Hypercapnic respiratory failure is defined as a $PaCO_2$ of more than 45 torr.

ARF may occur in a person without previous lung disease or may be superimposed on chronic respiratory failure.

Hypoxia refers to inadequate tissue oxygenation. It depends on tissue oxygen delivery (DO_2).

DO_2 = Cardiac output × arterial oxygen content (CaO_2).

$CaO_2 = 1.39 \times \text{oxygen saturation} \times [Hb] + .0031 \times PaO_2$.

PATHOPHYSIOLOGY

The normal process of respiration is a net function of the following:

i. Mechanical work of breathing i.e. contraction of diaphrgm and intercostal muscles and generation of negative intrapleural pressure.
ii. Expansion of lungs-alveolar ventilation.
iii. Gas exchange between alveolar air and pulmonary capillary blood through diffusion across alveolo-capillary membane.
iv. Transport of oxygen through blood to tissues and oxyen delivery.
v. Cell and tissue respiration.

In a healthy child, coordinated action of muscles of respiration and movements of chest wall, patent airways, complaints lungs, open alveoli and adequate perfusion of ventilated alveoli by circulating blood with a normal central control mechanisms ensure effective respiratory functions. Impairment of any of the above functions can lead to inefficient respiration, and cause respiratory failure (Table 4.1).Causes

Respiratory failure may result from primary airway or pulmonary insults and from other systemic non-pulmonary disorder. Hypoxemic respiratory failure is seen in patients with acute lung injury or acute pulmonary edema. These disorders primarily interfere with the lungs' ability to adequately oxygenate the blood. Hypercapnic respiratory failure is seen in patients with severe airflow obstruction, central respiratory failure, or neuromuscular respiratory failure. In neonates, surfactant deficiency and ineffective chest bellows may contribute to atelectasis (Table 4.1).

Table 4.1: Mechanisms and common causes of acute respiratory failure

• Upper airway obstruction	Diphtheria, Laryngotracheitis, Vocal cord paralysis
• Lower airway obstruction	Acute asthma, Bronchiolitis
• Alveolar air space disease	Pneumonia, interstitial lung disease, ARDS, other forms of pulmonary edema. Near drowning, Trauma, pulmonary hemorrhage
• Respiratory pump failure- (CNS, nerve, muscle disease)	Coma, Raised ICP, Drugs and Poisonings (opiates, benzodiazepines, barbiturates), Metabolic, Poliomyelitis, Myopathy, Guillian Barre Syndrome, spinal cord lesions
• Hypovolemia, Shock, Pulmonary Emboli	
• Pneumothorax, Trauma, rib injury	
• Decreased chest wall compliance	Pleural effusion, massive ascitis

Pulmonary Gas Exchange

The adequacy of gas exchange in the lungs is determined by the balance between ventilation and pulmonary capillary blood flow. This balance is commonly expressed as the ventilation-perfusion (V/Q) ratio. A perfect match between ventilation and perfusion is a V/Q ratio of 1.0. A V/Q more than 1 means excessive ventilation, and a V/Q < 1 indicates intrapulmonary shunting.

Dead Space Ventilation (Fig. 4.1)

When ventilation is in excess of capillary blood flow, the excess ventilation, known as dead space ventilation, does not participate in gas exchange

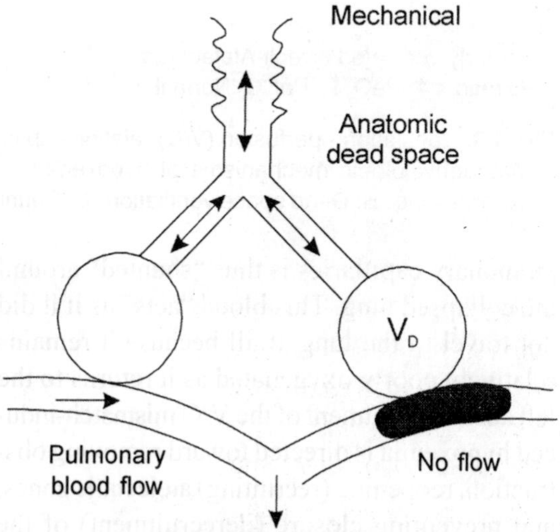

Fig. 4.1: Dead space

with the blood. *Anatomic dead space* (V_A) is the gas in the large conducting airways that does not come in contact with capillaries. Approximately 50% of the anatomic dead space is in the pharynx. *Physiological dead space* (V_D) is the alveolar gas that does not equilibrate fully with capillary blood. This represents excess alveolar ventilation relative to capillary blood flow. In normal subjects, dead space ventilation (V_D) accounts for 20% to 30% of the total ventilation (Vt.); that is, $V_D/Vt = 0.2$ to 0.3. An increase in V_D/Vt results in both hypoxemia and hypercapnia. The hypercapnia usually appears when the V_D/Vt rises above 0.5.

Dead space ventilation increases when the alveolar blood flow is reduced (e.g., heart failure, pulmonary embolism), or when alveoli are overdistended.

Intrapulmonary Shunt (Fig. 4.2)

When blood leaves the lung without participating in gas exchange, such as in patients with consolidation it is 'true shunt'. Here V/Q is zero. **Venous admixture represents** the capillary flow that does not equilibrate completely with alveolar gas (V/Q above zero but less than 1.0).

The fraction of total cardiac output (Qt) that represents intrapulmonary shunt is known as the *shunt fraction (Qs)*. In normal subjects the shunt fraction (Qs/Qt) is less that 10%. The shunt fraction increases when the small airways are

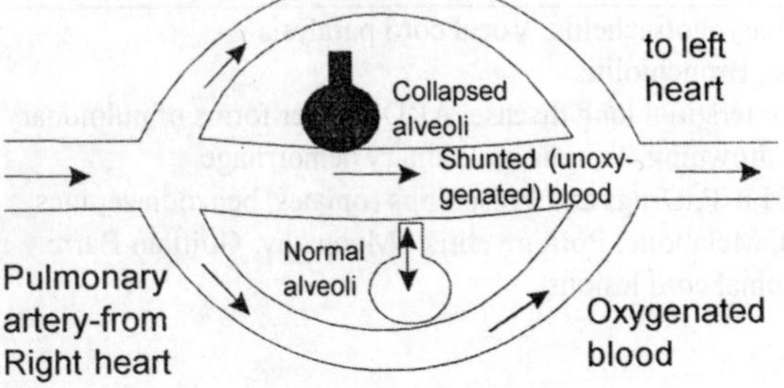

Fig. 4.2: Pulmonary shunt

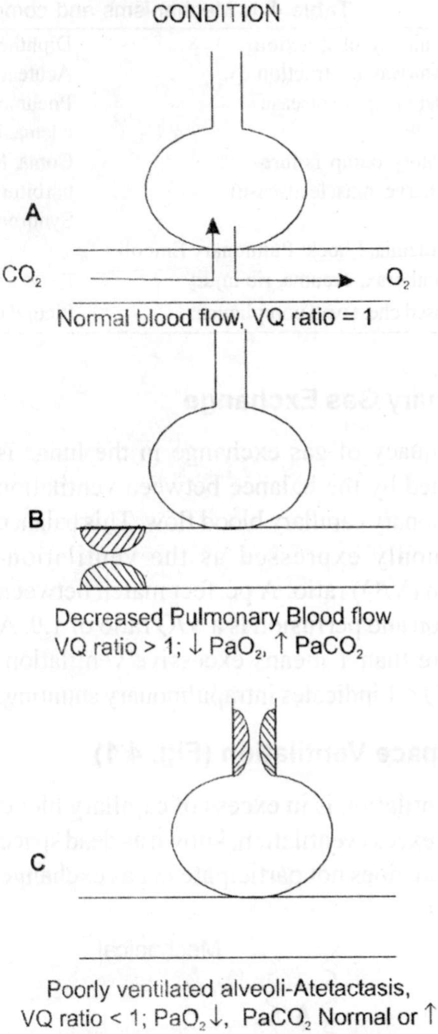

Fig. 4.3: Ventilation - perfusion (V/Q) relationship in pathophysiologic mechanisms of hypoxemia
A. Normal lung B. Dead space ventilation C. Shunt

occluded (e.g., asthma), when alveoli are filled with fluid (e.g., pulmonary edema, pneumonia) or when alveoli collapse (e.g., atelectasis).

The PaO_2 falls progressively as shunt fraction increases, but the $PaCO_2$ remains constant until the shunt fraction exceeds 50%. The $PaCO_2$ may be below normal in patients with increased intrapulmonary shunt as a result of hyperventilation due to disease process (e.g., pneumonia) or from the accompanying hypoxemia.

The shunt fraction also determines the influence of inspired oxygen on the arterial PO_2. As intrapulmonary shunt increases, the increase in fractional concentration of inspired oxygen (FiO_2) produces less of an increment in the arterial PO_2. The diminished influence of inspired oxygen on arterial PO_2 as shunt fractions rises has important implications for limiting the risk of pulmonary oxygen toxicity. In conditions associated with a high shunt fraction (e.g., acute respiratory distress syndrome), the FiO_2 can often be reduced to levels considered nontoxic (i.e., FiO_2 below 50%) without further compromising arterial oxygenation.

A. Hypoxemia

Mismatch of alveolar ventilation (V) and pulmonary perfusion (Q) (Fig. 4.3): Disease processes which cause progressive obstruction or atelectasis result in less oxygen being available in distal airways for uptake, allowing relatively more unoxygenated blood to circulate past the airways. A portion of venous blood entering the pulmonary capillaries is thus "shunted" around the collapsed lung. This blood "acts" as if it did not travel to the lung at all because it remains relatively poorly oxygenated as it returns to the left atrium. Treatment of the V/Q mismatch-induced hypoxemia is directed toward removing obstruction, reopening (recruiting) atelectatic zones, and preventing closure (derecruitment) of the affected lung units.

Other less common causes of hypoxemia include:

- Decreased diffusion of oxygen across the alveolocapillary membrane complex due to interstitial edema, inflammation, etc.
- Alveolar hypoventilation.
- High altitude and decreased ambient oxygen of other etiologies.

Alveolo-arterial PO_2 Difference [P (A-a) O_2 Gradient]

The gradient between the partial pressure of oxygen in the alveolus (PAO_2) and in the arterial blood (PaO_2) is P (A-a) O_2 gradient. The PaO_2 is obtained from an arterial blood gas while the patient breaths room air. The PAO_2 is estimated from the modified alveolar air equation:

$$PAO_2 = FiO_2\,(PB\text{-}47) - 1.25\ PaCO_2$$

PB is barometric pressure (PB=760 mmHg), and 47 is parteiral pressure of water vapor. $PaCO_2$ is obtained from the same arterial blood gas measurement.

In normal young children, the P(A-a) O_2 gradient should be <10 torr. A normal gradient suggests the hypoxemia is likely due to the hypoventilation, whereas an increased gradient suggests parenchymal changes (V/Q mismatching, intrapulmonary shunting, etc.) are causing the hypoxemia. The usefulness of this assessment is limited as most measurements would be done while the patient receives oxygen.

One of the causes of hypoxemia is an imbalance between oxygen delivery (DO_2) and oxygen uptake (VO_2) in the systemic circulation (DO_2/VO_2 imbalance). In this situation, the peripheral O_2 extraction is increased due to a low O_2 delivery or an increased O_2 uptake and thus mixed venous PO_2 gets reduced.

B. Hypercapnia

The carbon dioxide level in arterial blood ($PaCO_2$) is directly proportional to the rate of CO_2 production by oxidative metabolism ($V\ CO_2$) and inversely proportional to the rate of CO_2 elimination by alveolar ventilation.

Rate of CO_2 elimination is determined by alveolar minute ventilation, which is expressed as:

$$MV = (V_T - V_D)\ f$$

Where MV is minute alveolar ventilation, V_T is tidal volume, V_D is dead space, and f is respiratory frequency. Hypercapnia is caused by abnormality of one or more factors in the equation.

Hypercapnia may result from hypoventilation i.e. decreased V_T or f as occurs with CNS depression, neurologic injury, fatigue etc. An elevated $PaCO_2$ normally increase ventilatory drive. Therefore, hypercapnic respiratory failure may also imply that the patient is:

- Unable sense the elevated $PaCO_2$ due to drugs e.g., benzodiazepine poisoning, opiates
- Unable neurologically to stimulate effector mechanisms of ventilation eg. meningitis, encephalitis, Guillain - Barre Syndrome, critical care neuropathy
- Unable to effect a response from the muscles of respiration due to fatigue, malnutrition, shock, critical illness myopathy, myasthenia gravis, Mg++ depletion.

Increased physiologic dead space (V_D) may also produce hypercapnia and represents the other type of V/Q mismatch. When gas flow to and from airways remains adequate but blood flow is absolutely or relatively diminished, CO_2 does not have the opportunity to diffuse from the pulmonary artery blood and CO_2-rich blood is returned to the left atrium. Increased dead space ventilation may occur in hypovolemia, pulmonary embolus, poor cardiac output, or when the regional airway pressure is relatively higher than the regional perfusion pressure produced by the regional pulmonary blood flow.

Because of high solubility of CO_2, a diffusion barrier for CO_2 only occurs in terminal lung failure such as advanced acute respiratory distress syndrome (ARDS). *Rarely, increased CO_2 production may contribute to hypercapnia* if excessive nutritional calories are given or in extreme hypercatabolic conditions (e.g. burns).

C. Combination

Commonly, patients demonstrate characteristics of both pathophysiologic categories of ARF during the course of illness. Several related disease process often combine and act in concert or synergistically to compound respiratory failure.

CLINICAL MANIFESTATIONS

A. **Evidence of increased work of breathing** i.e. tachypnea, hyperpnea, nasal flaring, use of accessory respiratory muscles, intercostals/ suprasternal/supraclavicular retraction, or a paradoxical or dysynchronous breathing pattern.

B. **Signs and symptoms of hypercapnia, hypoxemia or both.** These include:
- Altered mental status ranging from agitation to somnolence.
- Cyanosis of mucosal membranes (tongue) or nail beds.
- Diaphoresis, tachycardia, hypertension and other signs of "stress" catecholamine release.

It is extremely important to recognize tachypnea, nasal flaring, grunting and retractions as early signs of respiratory failure. Cyanosis, lethargy and bradycardia are late signs.

Various laboratory measures are important in assuring adequate tissue oxygenation.

Clinical Assessment of Respiratory Failure

- **Is the airway patent?** Seems like an easy question to answer, but this assessment is often skipped in favour of assessing adequacy of breathing. Partial airway obstruction resulting in retractions and increased work of breathing may mistakenly be judged to have pulmonary pathology if the adequacy of the airway is not assessed.
- **Is the child breathing and is it adequate**? Often a more important assessment, and certainly a more difficult assessment than simply establishing whether or not a child is breathing. Children frequently require intervention even if breathing is present, due to inadequacy of breathing or fatigue with a risk of respiratory failure.
  Breathing can be thought of as providing two separate functions, oxygenation and ventilation. Both can be judged as to their adequacy in an ill child.
- **Oxygenation:** Clinical findings may be used to judge adequacy of oxygenation:
  - **Color:** Check nailbeds, lips, and tongue for evidence of cyanosis.
  - **Oxygen saturation (SpO_2) measurement:** Much less invasive than an arterial blood gas, but will only give information about oxygenation, not about adequacy of ventilation.
  - **Level of consciousness:** Normal level of consciousness is reassuring in that adequate levels of oxygen are reaching the brain.
- **Ventilation:** Adequacy of ventilation may be more difficult to assess than oxygenation. An arterial blood gas will give objective information about CO_2 levels, but represents only a single moment in time. Since minute ventilation=tidal volume × respiratory rate, these are used to clinically judge adequacy of ventilation.
  - *Air entry:* is essentially a clinical estimate of tidal volume. Fairly straightforward assessment is if air entry (depth of inspiration) is very good or very poor but quite subjective if air entry is somewhere in between.
  - ***Beware of respiratory rates that are too low:*** Avoid being lulled into a false sense

of security if the breathing rate falls quickly or the child presents with a low respiratory rate and a depressed level of consciousness. It is likely that this represents inadequate ventilation.

- **Work of breathing:** Even if oxygenation and ventilation are judged to be adequate, increased work of breathing may eventually lead to fatigue and respiratory failure in a child. Clinical indicators of increased work of breathing include the following:
  —*Respiratory rate:* abnormally high rate.
  —*Retractions:* includes retractions of intercostal muscles, suprasternal and substernal areas.
  —Use of accessory muscles.
  —"Abdominal paradox".

DIAGNOSTIC EVALUATION

Hypoxemia

Use of three variables A-a PO_2 gradient, PvO_2 and inspiratory pressure (Pimax) may pinpoint the source of hypoxemia (Fig. 4.4).

Normal A-a PO_2: Indicates a hypoventilation state rather than a cardiopulmonary disorder. In this situation, the most likely problems are drug-induced respiratory depression and neuromuscular weakness.

Increased A-a PO_2: Indicates a V/Q abnormality (cardiopulmonary disorder) and/or a systemic DO_2/VO_2 imbalance. When the A-a PO_2 gradient is increased, a mixed venous PO_2 (or central venous PO_2) is needed to identify a systemic DO_2/VO_2 imbalance.

Normal Venous PO_2 indicates that the problem is solely a V/Q abnormality in the lungs. If the venous PO_2 is 40 mm Hg or higher, then the lungs may be the source of the hypoxemia. Low venous PO_2 indicates a systemic DO_2/VO_2 imbalance. A mixed venous PO_2 below 40 mm Hg indicates either a decreased rate of oxygen delivery (anemia, low cardiac output) or an increased rate of oxygen consumption.

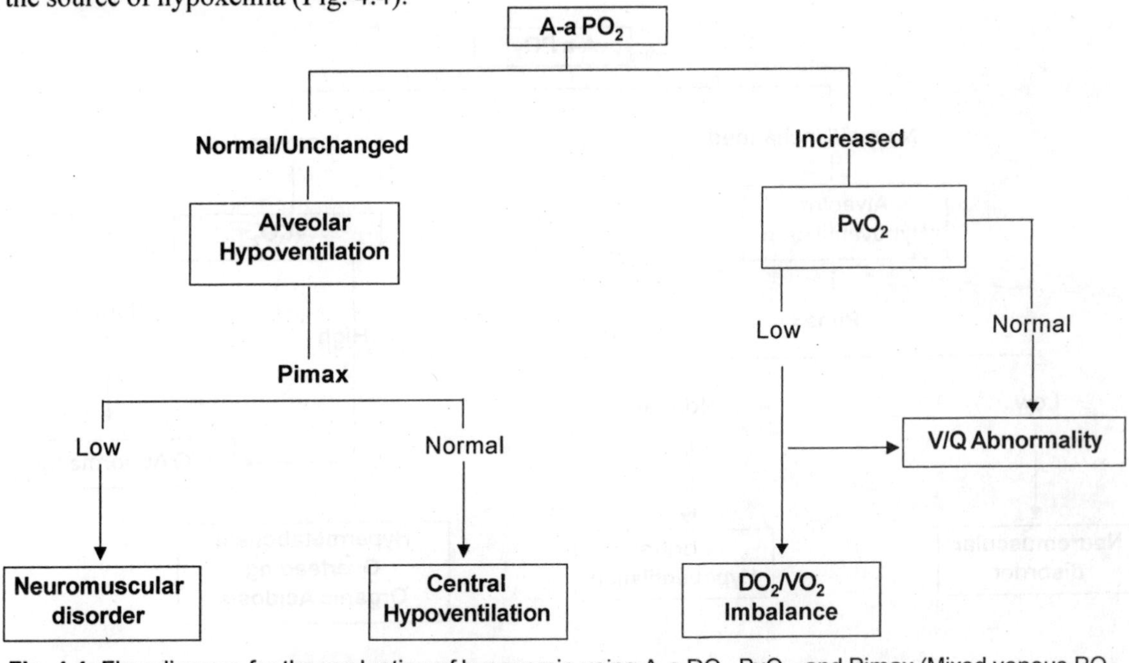

Fig. 4.4: Flow diagram for the evaluation of hypoxemia using A-a PO_2, PvO_2 and Pimax (Mixed venous PO_2, PvO_2, approximately equals central venous PO_2, PvO_2)

Hypercapnia

Before beginning the evaluation of hypercapnia ($PaCO_2$ >45 mm Hg), check as to whether the increase in arterial $PaCO_2$ is not be a compensatory response to metabolic alkalosis. If this is not so, the evaluation may proceed as shown in figure 4.5. The evaluation begins with the A-a PO_2 gradient. An increased A-a gradient indicates an increase in dead space ventilation (i.e., a pulmonary disorder), possibly complicated by an increase in CO_2 production. A normal or unchanged A-a PO_2 gradient indicates that the problem is alveolar hypoventilation.

MANAGEMENT

A. Oxygen Supplementation

Oxygen plays a vital role in the prevention of incipient respiratory failure and management of established failure. The movement of oxygen across the alveolar-capillary membrane complex is driven by the oxygen partial-pressure gradient between the PAO_2 and the PO_2 of the pulmonary capillary blood. In most cases of respiratory failure, the PAO_2 can be substantially increased by use of supplemental oxygen, increasing the gradient across the membrane and improving the PaO_2. Addition of oxygen to inspired air improves hemoglobin saturation and increases concentration of oxygen dissolved in plasma. This provides an appreciable additional source of oxygen for the tissues, when considered in relation to the total amount of oxygen uptake by the tissues from the blood.

Most of the conditions characterized by hypoxemia and increased work of breathing respond well to increased ambient oxygen. It should be administered to any child who is cyanosed or has wheezing or stridor or tachypnea with intercostal recessions. This should be considered a temporizing intervention while the primary etiology of hypoxemia is diagnosed and treated.

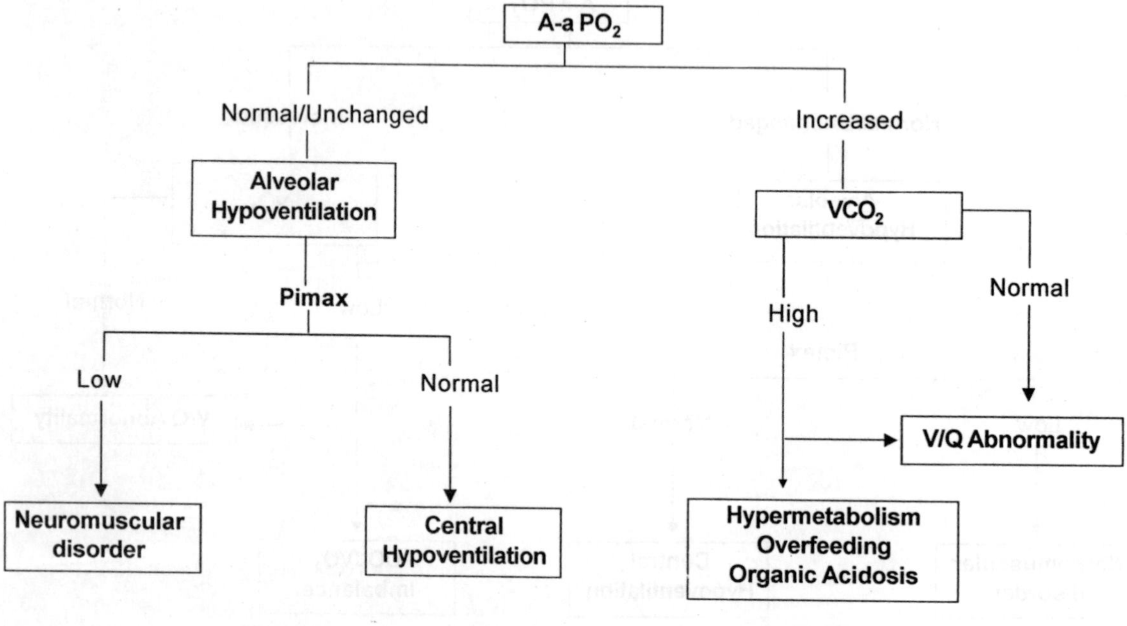

Fig. 4.5: Flow diagram for the evaluation of hypercapnia

Supplemental oxygen can be given by a variety of devices. The effectiveness of each is determined by the capacity of the device to deliver sufficient oxygen at a high enough flow rate to match the patient's spontaneous inspiratory flow rate. It may be given by an intranasal catheter at a flow rate of 1-3 L/min, a flow rate too high is wasteful. The catheter should be inserted one half of the distance between the tip of nose and the tip of ear. If the catheter is inserted, too far it may enter the esophagus and cause gastric dilatation and further respiratory embarrassment. Nasal cannula, Oxygen tent, a mask, or a head box may also be used. Nasal cannula is generally well tolerated and allow the patient feeding and at a flow rate of 2-4 L/min achieves satisfactory levels of O_2 in infants. Oxygen is best given those over 5 years by a face-mask. The masks usually provide 25 to 40 percent oxygen. Some of the masks may provide upto 50 percent oxygen concentration in inspired air at a flow rate of 8-10 L/min, while > 80% oxygen concentration can be achieved in a head box (Table 4.2). "Oxygen therapy should not be interrupted except for therapeutic reasons".

Table 4.2: Oxygen concentration (FiO_2) that can be delivered through various devices

FiO_2	*Device (Flow rate/min)*
25-50%	Nasal cannula (l-6L)
35-65%	Simple Face mask (6-l2L)
24-60%	Graded Ventury mask (graded 4-l2L)
60-80%	Oxyhood (10-15 L)
>90%	Non rebreathing masks (10-12 L)

B. Noninvasive Positive-Pressure Ventilation

NPPV may be accomplished using a tightly fitted face or nasal mask connected to a standard mechanical ventilator or to a smaller ventilator made specifically to deliver noninvasive mechanical ventilation.

NPPV is not recommended unless the patient is alert, oriented, cooperative. It is also not recommended for patients with swallowing dysfunction, difficulty in clearing secretions, hypotension, uncontrolled arrhythmias or acute gastrointestinal hemorrhages.

Initially, a pressure-support mode with 8 to 12 cm H_2O inspiratory pressure (PIP) is advised. If assist-control volume ventilation is used via a standard ventilation, initial tidal volume of 10 mL/kg should be used. Subsequently pressure, volume, and FiO_2 are titrated upward to achieve appropriate PaO_2 and $PaCO_2$ levels. Oral intake should be restricted until effectiveness in reversing acute ventilatory failure is assured.

C. Endothracheal Intubation

In child with severe respiratory distress, altered mental status, cyanosis or impending respiratory failure endotracheal intubation is the preferred treatment. It protects the airway and permits the delivery of the high concentrations of oxygen and application of CPAP and mechanical ventilation. (For details see the chapters on Recognition and Stabilization of critically ill children page 7, and Airway management page 27).

D. Continuous Positive Airway Pressure (CPAP)

In the CPAP system, the child breaths spontaneously from a continuous flow of humidified gases, and exhales against a desired pressure resistance. This positive pressure prevents air-way closure and maintains patency of alveoli at the end of expiration.

A 'T-piece' CPAP or an indigenous CPAP facility can be easily established in any emergency room. The air flow (or air+oxygen mixture) during CPAP should be 2 to 3 times that of patient's minute volume. It can be given by a face mask for a short period of time. Problem with this method is in obtaining a consistent tight fitting seal. There is also a danger of pressure necrosis of eyes and face. For a longer duration, it is therefore, preferable to give CPAP with nasal prongs or endotracheal tube.

The optimal CPAP requirements vary widely among different patients. It is generally acceptable to start CPAP at 5 cm H_2O; all children with respiratory compromise will tolerate this. This can be gradually increased in increments of 2 to 3 cm H_2O while monitoring PaO_2 and $PaCO_2$. At higher levels of CPAP (>10 cm H_2O) cardiac output should be monitored, if possible.

Mechanical Ventilation (See Chapter-7 on this subject).

E. Pharmacologic Adjuncts

Many disease causing ARF produce similar anatomic and physiologic derangements, including bronchial inflammation, mucosal edema, smooth muscle contraction, and increased mucus production and viscosity. Each of these processes may contribute to obstruction of airway gas flow, airway resistance, V/Q mismatch, and elevated VD/VT. Some pharmacologic agents are used for their direct effect to alter shunt or dead space effects.

- **β_2–Agonists:** Inhaled β_2–agonists—Salbutamol by nebulization to reverse small airway obstruction and epinephrine aerosol is an established therapy for upper airway obstruction.
- **Anticholinergic agents:** Ipratropium bromide by MDI or nebulization.
- **Corticsteroids:** In the asthmatic patient Methylprednisolone 10 mg/kg IV every 6 hrs or hydrocortisone to reverse small airway inflammation.
- **Antibiotics:** Antibiotics are used when there is clinical suspicion of bacterial infection. These should be selected to effectively treat usual pathogens.
- **Surfactant replacement in selected cases.**

Removal of Secretions

Agents to hydrate or to otherwise alter the composition, elasticity, or viscosity of mucus such as n-acetylcysteine and mucolytics.

- Nasotracheal suctioning.
- Postural drainage.

Treatment of Hypercapnia

Treatment of hypercapnia that is caused by decreased VT or respiratory rate may require reversal of sedation or other drugs, intubation and mechanical ventilation to rest fatigued muscles, nutrition, treatment of other possible primary causes.

Therapy of increased VD/VT may require reduction in peak or mean airway pressures if the patient is receiving mechanical ventilation, augmentation of intravascular volume and/or cardiac output (Table 4.3).

Table 4.3: Treatment modalities to correct and treat hypercapnia with respect to pathophysiologic mechanism

Cause of High $PaCO_2$	*Treatment to lower $PaCO_2$*
1. Hypoventilation	
– Neuromuscular	Reversal of drug effect, sedation, mechanical ventilation
– Central	
2. Airway obstruction	Maintain airway patency, treat the cause
3. Increase in dead space ventilation	– Increase expiratory minute volume RR/ V_E
a. Low cardiac output	– Increase cardiac output with inotropes
b. Pulmonary embolism	– Use heparin/ventilators
c. Vasoconstriction in pulmonary circulation	– Withdraw vasoconstrictors/give vasodilators
4. Increase in CO_2 production	
a. Body temperature increased	– Maintain normothermia
b. Muscular activity increased	– Sedation/neuromuscular block
c. Parenteral nutrition with a high carbohydrate	– Decrease carbohydrate load

Chapter five

Airway Management

A stable airway must be established in all sick children. Securing an airway in a distressed child is more difficult than in a neonate. Children in acute respiratory distress are frightened and very anxious. The upper airway of infants and children is proportioned and angled differently than adults. Teeth also come in the way. A considerable part of the airway is occupied by lymphoid tissues, adenoids and tonsils, and a relatively large tongue. Children also have more secretions than adults. All these contribute to obstruction to air flow through oropharynx, and make stabilisation of airway difficult.

OROPHARYNGEAL AIRWAY

Oral airway is used to provide a patent airway when breathing is spontaneous. The airway must be of a size appropriate to a child's mandible. The flanged end should protrude from the lips and the curved end should reach the angle of mandible. It should be placed either by direct visualisation, after flattening the tongue with a tongue blade, or inserted upside down with the convexity facing up until it reaches the throat and then twisted into position. It may be stabilised by the use of a tight fitting mask or a band around head. Proper length of the oropharyngeal airway can be estimated by holding one end at the corner of the mouth and the other to the ear. An airway that is too long pushes the epiglottis down and compresses the larynx, reducing the capacity to ventilate and, worse, increases the risk of gastric insufflation. Too short an airway pushes the tongue posteriorly, aggravating the obstruction.

ENDOTRACHEAL INTUBATION

Indications for endotracheal intubation include:

- Functional or anatomic airway obstruction.
- Inadequate central nervous system control of ventilation.
- Loss of protective airway reflexes- aspiration is a risk.
- Need for mechanical ventilatory support.
- Excessive work of breathing, which may lead to fatigue and respiratory insufficiency.
- Need for high peak inspiratory pressure or PEEP to maintain effective alveolar gas exchange.
- Potential for any of the above in a patient who needs transport.

The Endotracheal Tube

The endotracheal tube should be sterile, disposable and constructed of translucent polyvinyl chloride with a radiopaque marking. An endotracheal tube of uniform internal diameter is preferable to a tapered tube. The shouldered tracheal tube is not recommended because it may cause laryngeal injury. A standard 15-mm adapter is firmly affixed to the proximal end for attachment to a ventilating device. The distal end of the endotracheal tube may have an opening in the side wall (Murphy eye) to reduce the risk of right-upper-lobe atelactasis. The Murphy eye also reduces the likelihood of complete endotracheal tube obstruction if the end opening is occluded. The endotracheal tube should have distance markers (in centimeters) for use as reference points during placement and to facilitate detection of unintentional endotracheal tube movement. A vocal cord marker is also desirable to guide position of tube at the level of the glottic opening to ensure that the tip of the tube is in a mid-tracheal position.

A cuffed endotracheal tube should have a low-pressure, high-volume cuff and is generally indicated for children aged 8 years or more. In children younger than 8 years, the normal anatomic narrowing at the level of the cricoid cartilage provides a functional "cuff". If a cuff is present, inflation is appropriate if an audible air leak is present when ventilation to a pressure of 20 to 30 cm H_2O is provided. An appropriately selected uncuffed endotracheal tube should also allow an air leak at the cricoid ring at a peak inflation pressure of 20 to 30 cm H_2O.

The absence of an air leak may indicate that the cuff is inflated excessively, or the endotracheal tube is too large, or that laryngospasm is occurring around the endotracheal tube. These conditions may lead to excessive pressure on surrounding tissues. However, if successful intubation has been difficult, even a "tight" endotracheal tube should be left in place until the patient has been stabilized.

A 3-mm or 3.5-mm internal diameter endotracheal tube is adequate for term new born and small infants, a 4-mm endotracheal tube during the first year of life, and a 5-mm endotracheal tube in the second year of life. A simple visual estimate of appropriate endotracheal tube size can be made by choosing a tube with an outside diameter approximating the diameter of the child's little finger. Several other methods and formulas have been developed for estimating the correct endotracheal tube size. In one such formula (used for children older than 2 years) the endotracheal tube size (internal diameter in millimeters) may be approximated as follows:

$$\text{Endotracheal Tube (internal diameter—mm.)} = \frac{\text{Age in years}}{4} + 4$$

An alternative method of endotracheal tube size selection is based on the relationship between the child's length and endotracheal tube size. Length-based determination of endotracheal tube size is more accurate than age-based determination. Resuscitation tapes based on length may help identify the correct endotracheal tube size. These strategies give an approximate estimate tube size. Endotracheal tubes 0.5 mm smaller and larger than the estimated size should be readily available. Recommended endotracheal tube sizes are given in the Table 5.1.

The proper distance (depth) of insertion in centimeters (alveolar ridge to mid-trachea) for

Table 5.1: Suggested size of endotracheal and tracheostomy tubes and suction catheters for infants and children

Age	*Endotracheal tube ID (mm)**+	*Tracheostomy tube ID (mm)*	*Length (mm)*	*Suction Catheter*
Newborn Term	3.0	3.4	30-40	6
6 months	3.5	3.9	41	8
3 years	4.5	4.8	44	8
5 years	5.0	5.0	46	10
6 years	5.5	5.0	46	10
8 years	6.0	5.0	46	10
12 years	6.5	7.0	67	10

* ID = Internal diameter

\+ Length of tube (cm) = 12 + (age/2)

children older than 2 years can be approximated by adding one half the patient's age to 12.

Use of this formula will generally result in placement of the tip of the endotracheal tube above the carina. Alternatively, the distance of insertion (in centimeters) can be estimated by multiplying the internal diameter of the tube by 3. For example:

Internal diameter = 4.5 mm

Depth of insertion = $4.5 \times 3 = 13.5$ cm

The Laryngoscope

The laryngoscope consists of a handle with a battery and a blade with a light source. The blade is used to expose the glottis by moving the tongue laterally, placing the blade tip in the valecula, and lifting the base of the tongue onto the floor of the mouth. If the glottic opening is not exposed by this maneuver, the blade is advanced so that it lifts the epiglottis directly. Adult and pediatric laryngoscope handles fit all blades interchangeably and differ only in diameter and length. The laryngoscope blade may be curved or straight. Several sizes are available. A straight blade is preferred for infants and toddlers since it provides better visualization of the relatively cephalad and anterior glottis, but a curved blade is often preferred for older children since its broader base and flange facilitate displacement of the tongue and improve visualization of the glottis.

Laryngoscopy permits a visual axis through the mouth and pharynx to the larynx, through which an endotracheal tube, a suction catheter, or Magill forceps can be passed for intubation, suctioning, or extraction of foreign material, respectively.

Post-intubation Assessment

Immediately after intubation, the position of the endotracheal tube tip must be clinically assessed by:

- Observation for symmetrical chest movements
- Auscultation for equal breath sounds over each lateral chest wall high in the axillae
- Documentation of absence of breath sounds over the stomach
- Notation of the end-tidal CO_2 on capnograph level (if available).

In low cardiac output states, e.g. during cardiac arrest endtidal CO_2 levels may be minimal, especially in infants. If these clinical criteria are not met or if epigastric distention occurs during positive-pressure ventilation via the tube, esophageal intubation is suspected. The endotracheal tube should be removed and ventilation maintained with a bag-mask device.

If chest movement or breath sounds are asymmetrical, bronchial intubation is suspected. The endotracheal tube should be slowly withdrawn until equal breath sounds are heard bilaterally and chest expansion is symmetrical. Proper position of the endotracheal tube should be confirmed by chest x-ray as soon as possible.

If the endotracheal tube is properly placed but lung expansion is inadequate, or if inadequate oxygenation or ventilation is documented by pulse oximetry, end-tidal CO_2 monitoring, or arterial blood gas analysis, one of the following problems should be considered:

- *The endotracheal tube is too small, producing a large air leak:* Replacement of the tube with a large one may be necessary. In the child older than 8 years, the endotracheal tube cuff should be inflated until the air leak just disappears (at 20 to 30 cm H_2O).
- The pop-off valve on the resuscitation bag is not occluded and air is escaping into the atmosphere. This problem is most likely to occur when the child's lung compliance is poor. An increase in inflation and cuff pressures may be required to produce effective ventilation in these patients.
- A leak is present at any of the several connections in the bag-valve device. Leaks may be detected by separating the bag-valve device

from the patient and by compressing the bag against occluded outlet.

- The operator is providing inadequate tidal volume. This is easily confirmed: a large volume breath is provided while the rescuer observes movement of the chest wall and auscultates breath sounds.
- Lack of lung expansion or lung collapse is occurring for other reasons (e.g., pneumothorax, obstructed endotracheal tube etc.).

After intubation, the endotracheal tube should be secured to the patient's face with adhesive to prevent unintentional extubation. Before the endotracheal tube is taped in place, correct position should again be re-confirmed by auscultation. The distance marker at the lips should be noted in the chart to allow detection of unintentional endotracheal tube displacement.

Care of Endotracheal Tube

Attention must be paid to maintain the patency of the tube. Small plugs of mucous or debris may decrease the radius of an already small bore tube thus increasing the tube resistance. All intubated children must receive the following care:

1. ***Humidification*** of inspired air/gases, either through bubble humidifiers.
2. ***Suction and pulmonary toilet to avoid tube blockage.*** Children have more secretions than adults and this tendency may be exaggerated during disease process. Caution is necessary as suctioning may sometimes cause hypoxemia and reduction in functional residual capacity of lungs in infants.

The respiratory secretions create a blanket that covers the mucosal surface of the airways The inner layer keeps the mucosal surface moist. The outer layer composed of a meshwork of mucoprotein strands traps particles and debris in the airways,

Saline Instillation to clear the secretions, is ill-advised for two reasons. First saline cannot liquefy or reduce the viscosity of respiratory secretions The second is the risk for infection). Saline injections into tracheal tubes can dislodge these bacterial biofilms and provide a vehicle for transporting bacteria into the lower airways.

3. ***Sedation*** to prevent excessive movements of the patient in order to avoid telescoping of glottis over tracheal tube and any accidental extubation. Liberal use of sedatives must be made. Sedation may be obtained with morphine (0.1–0.2 mg/kg, IV, 4 hourly), or diazepam (0.1 mg/kg, IV, 4 hourly) or midazolam (0.2 mg/kg/dose).
4. ***Mucolytic Therapy***: Mucolytic agent like N-acetylcysteine can help to disrupt the plug and relieve the obstruction The drug can be given as an aerosol spray, or injected directly into the airways. Direct instillation of NAC into the tracheal tube is preferred, especially when there is an obstruction.

If intratracheal injection of NAC does not relieve an obstruction, bronchoscopy should be done. Following relief of the obstruction, NAC can be instilled two or three times a day for the next day or two. Daily use of NAC is not advised

Aerosol therapy: Use 10% NAC solution. Mix 2.5 mL NAC with 2.5 mL saline and place mixture (5mL) in a small volume nebulizer for aerosol delivery. This can provoke bronchospasm, and is not recommended in asthmatics.

Tracheal injection: Use 20% NAC solution. Mix 2mL NAC with 2 ML saline and inject 2 mL aliquots into the trachea. Excessive volumes can produce bronchorrhea.

5. ***Intravenous fluids*** to maintain good hydration.
6. ***Nasogastric tube insertion*** to remove swallowed air and decrease the risk of aspiration.

Extubation

Extubation should be considered when the child has protective airway reflexes, no longer has respiratory distress, has minimal tracheal secretions and maintainable airway. Before extubation clear the nose, pharynx, stomach, suction ET tube, and preoxygenate with 100% O_2. *Remove the tube while suctioning.* After extubation watch for stridor or laryngeal edema. Severe stridor or laryngeal edema may require re-intubation. Mild laryngeal edema may be treated with oral or parenteral steroids, and adrenaline nebulization.

Problems and Complications of Endotracheal Intubation

1. Endotracheal intubation may occasionally cause bradycardia, dysrrhythmia, laryngospasm, damage to larynx and dentition. Sedation and muscle relaxants given before the procedure prevent risk of such problems (See RSI Appendix-6).
2. Malpositioning of ET tube is particularly common in PICU patients and may lead to complications. Intubation of right main-stem bronchus occurs in up to 11% patients who apparently have an 'uneventful' intubation. Physical examination may be inaccurate in determining the ET tube position. X-ray chest must be obtained to confirm the position. Endtidal CO_2 measurement has been shown to be a quick and reliable way of assessing ET tube position in children.
3. Ulceration of lips, cheeks, oral mucosa, pharynx and palatal injury with prolonged orotracheal tubes.
4. Sub-glottic stenosis, tracheomalacia, tracheo-esophageal fistula have been reported even with uncuffed tubes.

Attention to proper size, shape and fixation of the tube and allowing small airleak reduces the risk of these complications. When using cuffed tubes release of pressure periodically and daily revaluation of cuff pressure may help.

Tracheostomy

It is indicated in presence of upper airway obstruction, vocal cord paralysis, facial burns or trauma, or when it is difficult to maintain patency of an endotracheal tube because of secretions, infection or bleeding. Replacement of tracheal tube with a tracheostomy is also recommended for those patients who require intubation and/or ventilatory support for prolonged period. It may provide a more secure airway for long term care, facilitate tracheo-bronchial toilet, improve patient comfort and allow the patient to communicate with family. Guideline for size of tracheostomy tube at various ages are given in Table 5.1.

Tracheostomy is technically more difficult in infants and children than in adults. It needs more attention and care. Tracheostomy may cause considerable morbidity (such as bleeding, infection, pneumothorax) except in skill hands. Percutaneous tracheostomy may decrease risk of complication; the safety and ease of the procedure has been shown in adults. Long-term complications include fusion of vocal cords, tracheal stenosis etc.

Decannulation must be done in PICU, in stages, over a period of several days, especially if the tube had been in place for longer than three weeks. A fiberoptic bronchoscopy/laryngoscopy should be done before attempting decannulation.

Chapter six

Shock: Diagnosis and Management

"Shock" is a clinical syndrome of acute, circulatory dysfunction and consequent failure to deliver sufficient oxygen and other nutrients to meet the metabolic demands of tissue beds. The critical event is poor perfusion of vital organs and other tissues and consequently altered cellular and subcellular metabolism and energy production.

Clinically the syndrome of shock is characterized by signs of hemodynamic instability, namely, tachycardia, poor capillary refill, relative or absolute hypotension and signs of poor perfusion of skin, and major organs such as diminished urine output, changes in mental status etc.

A rational approach to the patient presenting in shock not only requires a thorough understanding of the dynamic nature of shock, but also warrants early recognition, hemodynamic monitoring and use of specific agents employed to combat the shock syndrome.

PATHOPHYSIOLOGY AND CAUSES

A decrease in oxygen delivery to meet tissue oxygen requirement can be caused by any of the three basic abnormalities:

1. Hypovolemia (decreased circulating volume).
2. Cardiac function impairment (decreased myocardial contractility).
3. Inappropriate distribution of cardiac output secondary to abnormal vasodilatation and capillary leak (distributive shock).

Pathophysiology of shock based on these functional etiologies are discussed below:

Hypovolemic Shock

Hypovolemic shock is the most common form of shock in children and continues to claim millions of lives each year. In true hypovolemia there is an actual rapid loss of circulating blood volume, as a consequence of loss of fluid and electrolytes (diarrhoea, vomiting) or acute blood loss (internal or external). Relative hypovolemia occurs secondary to peripheral pooling of blood volume and 'third space' losses caused by loss of vascular tone and increased capillary permeability. It is most often seen in septic shock. It must be appreciated that because of small size, the total volume of fluid or blood loss that may cause shock is much less in a child as compared to an adult.

Important aspects of hypovolemic shock are the extent and the rapidity with which hypovolemia occurs. The loss of circulating blood volume is followed by a series of cardiac and peripheral homeostatic adjustments directed at restoration of systemic arterial blood pressure and perfusion of vital organs such as heart and brain. Whether these adjustments are adequate to maintain cardiovascular homeostasis is determined by patient's pre-existing hemodynamic status.

Cardiogenic Shock

Cardiogenic shock is best viewed as a 'pump failure'. The common event is an inadequate stroke volume mostly as a result of decreased myocardial contractility and infrequently due to mechanical obstruction to the flow of blood. Low cardiac output, decreased blood pressure and poor tissue perfusion produce a rapid downhill spiral of inadequate oxygen delivery to tissues and microcirculatory failure. Children rarely go through a compensated phase of cardiogenic shock.

Distributive Shock

In this type of shock there is maldistribution of the blood volume. Common to all the conditions causing this form of shock is massive injury to capillary endothelium resulting in loss of its integrity and leakage of fluid to interstitial space or so-called "third-space". Septic shock is a classical example of this type. Other example is anaphylactic shock.

Septic shock is often seen in emergency room and is one of the most common causes of mortality in pediatric intensive care units. The etiology of sepsis varies with the age of child, presence of septic focus such as pneumonia, peritonitis or urinary tract infection and certain predisposing conditions causing immunodepression (see chapter on Severe Infection: Diagnosis and Antibiotics).

Stages of Sepsis Response and Septic Shock

1. *Systemic inflammatory Response (SIRS)*: fever with tachycardia, tachypnoea and leukocytosis.
2. *Sepsis:* SIRS with documented infection.
3. *Severe sepsis*: Sepsis with evidence of altered organ hypoperfusion and dysfunction, such as altered mental status, oliguria or increased lactate.
4. *Septic Shock:* Severe sepsis with hypotension. Septic shock can be recognized, before hypotension occurs, by a clinical triad that includes hypothermia or hyperthermia, clinical signs of decreased perfusion such as prolonged capillary refill >2 seconds, altered mental state and peripheral vasodilatation (warm shock) or mottled cool extremities (old shock), and decreased urine output.
5. *Multiorgan failure*: Simultaneous dysfunction of two or more organs.

The clinical manifestations of sepsis and septic shock are as a result of complex interplay between microbial product and host mediator systems. Microbial factors that are important are gram negative lipopolysaccharides (LPS), peptidoglycans from gram-positive organisms, certain polysaccharides and extracellular enzymes (Streptokinase) or exotoxins (TES-1 and enterotoxins of *Staphylococci*).

A variety of host factors have been implicated in the pathogenesis of septic shock. These include components of coagulation cascade, complement and kinin systems as well as factors released from stimulated macrophages and neutrophils, like cytokines, tumor necrosis factor-α (TNF-α), and interleukin-1 (IL-1), vasoactive peptides (histamine) and products of arachidonic acid metabolism (Eicosanoids).

Interaction of host with these mediators produces a series of metabolic alterations at the cellular and subcellular levels and massive injury to capillary endothelium resulting in loss of its integrity and leakage of fluid to interstitium of so-called "third-space" and maldistribution of the blood volume. The end result of all this is multiorgan dysfunction syndrome.

CLINICAL PROGRESSION AND STAGES OF SHOCK

Shock is a progressive disorder, which if left untreated, spirals down to severe hemodynamic and metabolic deterioration. The progression may be fulminant and the patient may go into profound shock within minutes; often it evolves over hours.

This progression has been arbitrarily divided into two stages:

1. "Early", "Compensated" shock and
2. "Progressive", "decompensated" shock.

'Early', 'Compensated' shock implies that vital organ function is maintained by intrinsic compensatory mechanisms such as tachycardia and peripheral vasoconstriction. At this stage symptoms and signs of hemodynamic impairment, which are commonly observed in adults, have the potential to remain subtle in children for a longer period of time, leading to delays in recognition and underestimation of shock states. Because of this a high degree of clinical suspicion is required to identify shock in children. Blood pressure (B.P.) is usually maintained, heart rate is increased, pulse pressure is narrow and signs of peripheral vasoconstriction (decreased skin temperature and impaired capillary refill > 3 seconds) are present. Children with dehydration exhibit in addition, signs of interstitial fluid loss such as sunken anterior fontanel, sunken eyes, dry buccal mucosa, poor skin turgor. Children with "capillary leak" because of sepsis on the other hand may have none of above signs. Children may attempts to compensate for the metabolic acidosis and decreased tissue oxygen supply by increasing respiratory rate and depth of breathing. If shock is identified and vigorously treated at this stage, the syndrome may often be successfully reversed.

The progressive, decompensated stage appears with persistence of shock. There is continued fall in cardiac output and despite intense arteriolar constriction and increased heart rate, blood pressure declines. This leads to lowered perfusion pressure, progressive blood stagnation, anaerobic metabolism and release of proteolytic and vasoactive substances. Platelet aggregation and release of tissue thromboplastin produce hypercoagulability and disseminated intravascular coagulation.

Patient may demonstrate impairment of major organ perfusion which may manifest as altered mentation (impaired cerebral perfusion), oliguria (renal hypo-perfusion) and myocardial ischemia (coronary flow impairment). The external appearance of patient reflects excessive sympathetic drive with cold and clammy extremities and acrocyanosis. It is evident at this point that the patient has deteriorated. Rapid aggressive intervention is required to halt the progression of shock to irreversible stage.

Not all forms of shock progress in similar manner or go through these stages. **Neurogenic shock** is characterized by hypotension at onset due to diminished or absent sympathetic activity and loss of vascular tone. The classic example is shock following trans-section of the spinal cord in the cervico-thoracic region. Reduced peripheral vascular tone leads to pooling of blood in the extremities and inadequate venous return. Initially the patient has warm extremities, low diastolic pressure and a very wide pulse pressure. Ultimately perfusion pressure falls and acidosis develops.

Septic shock often follows a trimodal pattern of clinical presentation: "Warm" shock, "Cold" shock and "multisystem organ failure". In the early stages, there is a decrease in systemic vascular resistance and thus diastolic pressure and an increase in cardiac output ("Warm" shock). Hemodynamically it is characterised by low cardiac filling pressure, tachycardia, bounding pulses, wide pulse pressure and decreased oxygen consumption. The latter effect is due to impaired mitochondrial oxygen utilization and deficient oxygen delivery to cells despite an increase in overall cardiac output (maldistribution of cardiac output). Vital organ functions may be maintained during this period by compensatory mechanisms such as tachycardia.

Late in sequence of septic shock there is myocardial depression, decline in cardiac output and hypotension with severe acidosis, hypoxemia and hypoxia ("Cold" shock). This leads to lowered perfusion pressure, increased pre-capillary arteriolar resistance, progressive blood stagnation, anaerobic metabolism and release of proteolytic and vasoactive substances. Platelet aggregation and release of tissue thromboplastin produce hypercoagulability and disseminated intravascular coagulation.

The prolonged hypo-perfusion of brain, heart kidneys and lungs leads to ischemic cell death in these organs with progressively worsening coma, renal failure and acute respiratory distress syndrome (ARDS). A generalized endothelial damage disrupts the integrity of cell membrane with unrestrained shifts in fluids and electrolytes between cells and interstitial space, accounting for the often repeated statement, "shock not only stops the machine, but also wrecks the machinery".

RECOGNITION AND ASSESSMENT

To apply aggressive therapeutic interventions, early recognition of shock is crucial. *It requires a high index of suspicion* and knowledge of the conditions, which predispose to septic shock. Clearly, children who are febrile, have an identifiable source of infection and are hypovolemic from any cause are at a greater risk of developing shock. It may be very difficult to determine which children have crossed over from a state of being febrile to a state of fully developed shock.

It is possible to identify signs reflecting the underlying physiologic process as shown in Table 6.1. The most significant physical findings result from autonomic response to stress. In children, ***tachycardia*** occurs early and is the sole determinant of cardiac output. True tachycardia is noticed well before any notable alterations in blood pressure. The respiratory rate is usually elevated.

Decreased tissue perfusion can be identified by decreased surface temperature, impaired capillary refill (>2 seconds) and impaired function of several organs. Body surface temperature is a time-honored, simple and effective method of assessing adequate tissue perfusion. Cold extremities or increased peripheral core temperature gradients (>2°C) reflects homeostatic mechanisms compensating for hypovolemia by cutaneous vasoconstriction and indicates early shock.

Table 6.1: Signs and symptoms of shock

Signs of infection

i. Fever
ii. Focus of infection

Signs of initial autonomic response to low cardiac output

i. Tachycardia (most important early sign)
ii. Tachypnea, hyperpnoea
iii. Blood pressure normal, Bunding pulses, Flush CFT.

Signs of decreased tissue perfusion (Helpful but not absolutely reliable)

i. Color: pale, ashen-gray
ii. Prolonged capillary refilling time (>2 sec)
iii. Decreased surface temperature – cold, clammy skin
iv. Increased difference between core and peripheral temperature > 2^0C

Signs of Major organ dysfunction (late signs)

Brain	: Anxiety, confusion agitations, stupor-coma, ischemic brain injury
Kidneys	: Acute renal failure; Oliguria, anuria
GIT	: Erosive gastritis (upper GI bleed), ischemic pancreatitis, Nasogastric aspirates, decreased bowel sounds
Liver	: Ischemic hepatitis; elevation of transminases and bilirubin
Hematological	: Coagulation abnormality; elevated prothrombin time and PTTK in all forms of shock, severe DIC and thrombocytopenia

Decreased ***"Capillary refill"*** is a sensitive indictor of tissue perfusion. The rate of refill (return of pink color) after blanching of soft tissues of palm or sole or nail beds with gentle pressure is related to the site, temperature and the amount of circulation through the microvasculature. Normally a blanched area disappears extremely rapidly; in less than 2 secs. A *greater than 3 secs* delay in refill is clearly abnormal. Although capillary refill is a very non-specific indicator of tissue hypoperfusion, *serial determination at frequent intervals is an excellent indicator of response to treatment.* A gradual improvement in capillary refill occurs as the shock syndrome is successfully reversed.

"Vital organ hypo-perfusion" can be assumed to occur if *oliguria* from renal hypo-perfusion coexists, or if child develops *impairment sensorium* with disorientation, lethargy, confusion or hallucinations.

Physical examination in early septic shock usually reveals fever (though neonates may be hypothermic), chills, increased peripheral pulse rate and volume, warm overperfused extremities, widened pulse pressure and a hyperdynamic precordium and tachypnoea. At this stage presence of acidosis supports the diagnosis of early septic shock. Table 6.1 summarizes rapid initial clinical assessment of a child in shock. Based on initial screening examination a child can be placed in one of the pathophysiologic stages of shock. **"Irreversible"** shock is a term that is applied to the clinical situation in which even correction of hemodynamic derangement does not halt the downward spiral. The prolonged hypo-perfusion of brain, heart, kidneys and lungs leads to ischemic cell death in these organs with progressive worsening leading to coma, renal failure myocardial failure and myocardial failure and onset of adult respiratory distress syndrome (ARDS).

Initial Haematological/Biochemical Determinations

Initial laboratory determinations should include complete blood counts, serum electrolytes, and arterial blood gases to help in selection of immediate therapeutic interventions. Additional laboratory parameters should be obtained as warranted by the patient's condition and the most likely etiologies for shock state. Directing laboratory investigations to assess the function of various organ systems as shown in Table 6.2 is a useful practical approach as a given patient may have multiple organ dysfunctions.

Table 6.2: Laboratory tests in patients in shock

Cardiovascular System	**Gastrointestinal, liver**
ECG	Stool occult blood
Chest X-ray	Gastric pH,
Blood gases	Liver function tests
Echo-cardiogram	
Serum lactate	
Respiratory System	**Metabolic**
Blood gases	Serum Na, K, Ca
Lung function tests	Blood glucose
	Serum proteins
Renal System	**Infection Screen**
Urine –Sp. Gravity, Na,	Cultures – Blood, CSF
Sediment, protein, sugar	Urine, Stool, Pus
Urea, Creatinine	
Hematologic System	
Complete blood counts,	
Coagulation screen	
Platelet count, FDPs,	
D-diamers	

MONITORING OF SHOCK

Adequate monitoring of shock serves the following purpose:

1. Allows definition of pathophysiologic stage to plan diagnosis and treatment.
2. Permits continuous assessment of vital organ function.
3. Provides a means to assess the efficacy of therapeutic intervention.
4. Prevents complication by early recognition of correctable problems.

A competent observer must make a repeated and careful examination of the child's physiological status. The emphasis must be on frequent assessment of alteration in peripheral perfusion (capillary refill), color, presence of cyanosis, characteristics of the pulse, blood pressure, respiratory rate and pattern, and level of consciousness. In addition, the minimum monitoring of a child with shock or at risk for shock should include continuous ECG monitoring, temperature (skin and core), and blood pressure measurements, and a strict intake and urine output record.

In children with fluid refractory shock or if myocardial compromise is suspected consideration must be given to central venous pressure (CVP) and other invasive monitoring. Central venous pressure monitoring is principally a measure of right ventricular function and venous return. The CVP may not be useful as a single absolute value since the range of normal (5 to 15 cm) is large. However, a low CVP is an indicator of decreased preload or hypovolemia. CVP monitoring is useful in assessing response to fluid resuscitation. The CVP of hypovolemic patient will change little in response to an initial fluid bolus, but the CVP of a patient who is euvolemic, hypervolemic or in cardiogenic shock will have a large sustained increase to a fluid challenge. In the absence of right ventricular outflow obstruction, the CVP during volume resuscitation in children generally reflects left ventricular function.

Arterial pressure monitoring should be considered and used in children with fluid refractory shock. Use of pulmonary artery catheter to monitor pulmonary artery wedge pressure may be useful in select group of children with septic shock (see for details Chapter 12, Monitoring of a patient in PICU).

MANAGEMENT OF SHOCK

The major objectives in the management of shock are:

1. Rapid recognition of shock state and resuscitation.
2. Correction of secondary consequences of shock.
3. Maintenance of function of vital organs.
4. Identification and correction of aggravating factors.

All the objectives are approached simultaneously in an organized way so as to ensure optimal therapy.

Airway and Oxygen

The initial resuscitation involves securing patent-airway, administration of oxygen and establishment of intravenous access. Oxygen is a drug, and its use should be guided by considerations applicable to the use of other drugs in treatment of shock. In general, oxygen should be administered initially to all patients in shock, in view of impaired peripheral oxygen delivery. An attempt should be made to achieve an arterial oxygen saturation of 90 percent or higher. Continuous assessment of oxygenation can be guided by the use of pulse oximetry, but significant alterations in management must be based upon direct assessment of arterial blood gases. Lung compliance and work of breathing may change precipitously. The decision to intubate and ventilate should be taken early based on clinical assessment.

Intravenous Access

Emergency intravenous access during the first 2-3 minutes of resuscitation of a shock patient is a difficult but realistic goal. As a standard technique cannulation of peripheral vein with short catheters is preferred; however, peripheral vein catheterization may be unsuccessful in children with severe shock. In such cases use of intraosseous route could be life saving. Placement of a central catheter will be needed for vasoactive drug infusions.

Fluid Resucitation (Optimization of preload) (Figure 6.1)

Early rapid fluid resuscitation is fundamental to septic shock survival. Pre-load needs to be optimized to improve cardiac output and thus oxygen delivery. Fluid resuscitation is best initiated with rapid infusion normal saline or Ringer's lactate. Recent evidence clearly support the use of crystalloid (Normal saline) in pediatric septic shock. There may be a role of colloids (albumin,

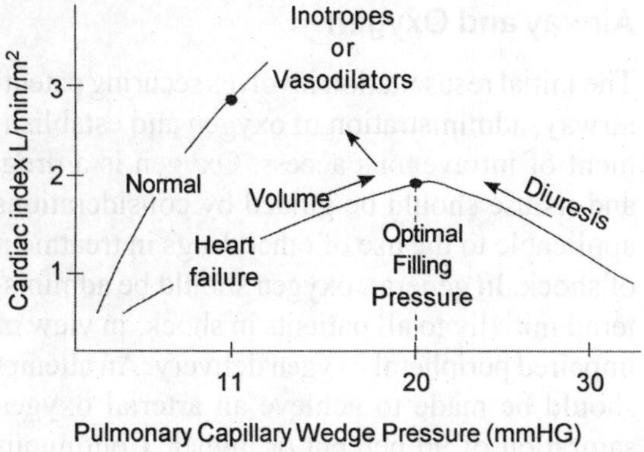

Fig. 6.1: Effect of fluid and vasopressors and cardiac output in a failing heart

dextrans, starch and gelatine in saline) in patients with a pre-existing low plasma oncotic pressure state such as protein energy malnutrition, nephrotic syndrome, acute severe burns or liver disease, in patients with malaria and dengue shock syndrome.

In hypotensive patients, fluids should be given as rapidly as possible in aliquots of 20 ml/Kg using a syringe and a 3-way stopcock and rapid pull-push or pressure bag system to achieve therapeutic goals. In patients with normal blood pressure fluids should be given in aliquots of 20 ml/Kg over 15-20 min. In a randomised trial from Chennai that compared slow and fast infusion rate, fast infusion did not result in faster resolution of shock but incidence of pulmonary edema requiring intubation doubled if fluids were given at rate of 40 ml in 15 minutes, compared to 20 ml over 15 minutes.

Children with septic shock usually require 40-60 ml/kg, sometimes up to 90-110ml/kg in the first hour of resuscitation. It may go upto 200ml in 6 hours or 240 ml in 8 hours in vasodilatory shock or shock due to gastrointestinal sepsis and staphylococcal diseases presenting with septic shock.

Initial fluid requirement should be titrated to clinical parameters e.g., combination of heart rate, systolic blood pressure, peripheral perfusion, urine output and level of consciousness. Hepatomegaly occurring with rapid fluid resuscitation in children is a reliable indicator of adequate fluid resuscitation. Patient should be monitored for clinical signs suggestive of myocardial dysfunction or pulmonary edema during fluid therapy. The incidence of cardiogenic or non-cardiogenic pulmonary edema of severe sepsis is more likely with inadequate fluid resuscitation. The tendency to develop pulmonary edema and capillary leak during administration of large volume of fluids during resuscitation may be countered by providing ventilation using self inflating or flow-inflating ventilation bags in the ED. An attempt should be made to achieve all the end-points to define shock resolution in fluid and inotrope responsive shock. Discontinuing fluid therapy based on achievement of some and not all the goals result in inadequate resuscitation.

If signs suggestive of myocardial dysfunction or pulmonary edema are noted during fluid therapy, further fluid administration is interrupted briefly for endotracheal intubation. Intubation and positive pressure ventilation to resolve pulmonary edema is necessary before further administration of fluids is possible. Since shock can worsen during or following intubation, initiation of an appropriate inotrope infusion often improves the safety profile of this procedure. Following intubation and positive pressure ventilation with bag valve mask or flow inflating ventilation bags, features of pulmonary edema and hepatomegaly usually resolve while shock persists. Further fluid aliquots of 10- 20 ml/kg over10-20 minutes are recommended until shock resolves or pulmonary edema and hepatomegaly recurs.

If there is persistence of signs of shock with signs of fluid overload, or reappearance of signs of pulmonary edema and hepatomegaly after initial fluid resuscitation (Fluid refractory shock), use central venous pressure (CVP) monitoring to guide further fluid therapy. CVP measurement may be useful in evaluating the need for further fluid therapy. CVP should be interpreted in light of serial clinical assessment, as it is likely to be influenced by rapid heart rate and increase in intrathoracic pressure. A low CVP <10 cmH_2O suggest need for further fluids. Though, further fluid resuscitation beyond a CVP of 15 cmH_2O may increase the risk of pulmonary edema, it should be remembered that large volumes of fluid for acute stabilization in children with septic shock have not been shown to increase the rate of acute respiratory distress syndrome or cerebral edema.

Clinical indicators of excessive fluid resuscitation include pulmonary rales on auscultation, palpable liver edge, increased jugular venous pressure, S_3 gallop and a decrease in SaO_2.

Cardiovascular Support

Cardiogenic shock and late stages of septic shock are characterized by impairment of myocardial function. Hence therapeutic endeavours to optimize cardiac output are the cornerstone of therapy. Therapy is directed towards increasing myocardial contractility and decreasing left ventricular afterload (Fig. 6.2). Unfortunately no single agent appears to produce the desired effects in all the patients. Proper choice of drugs requires knowledge of exact hemodynamic disturbance and pharmacology of these drugs (Tables 6.3 to 6.5).

The sympathomimetic amines are the most potent positive inotropic agents available; besides inotropy they also possess chronotropic effect and complex effects on vascular beds of various organs. In higher doses they may have undesirable vascular actions or toxic effects on myocardium. Hemodynamic effects at various doses, site of action and dosage for various sympathomimetic amine is given in Table 6.4.

Following adequate intravascular volume repletion, continued presence of hypotension and or poor perfusion (fluid refractory shock) warrants the consideration of vasoactive therapy, which should be goal directed. Begin inotrope Dopamine 10 μg/kg/min by intravenous route. Obtain central venous access. Reverse cold shock by titrating dopamine, or if resistant (normal or low blood pressure) titrate central epinephrine (0.05-0.3 μ/kg/min). Reverse warm shock with wide pulse pressure and/or low blood pressure by titrating central nor-epinephrine.

Table 6.3: Gradation of shock with respect to hemodynamic disturbance and response to therapy

Cold or warm shock: Decreased perfusion including decreased mental status or decreased urine, with capillary refill > 2 secs, diminished peripheral pulses, and mottled cool extremities (cold shock), or flash capillary refill, bounding peripheral pulses (warm shock), urine output<1ml/kg/hr.

Fluid-refractory/dopamine-resistant shock: Shock persists despite > 60 ml/kg fluid resuscitation in first hour and dopamine infusion > 10 μg/kg/min.

Catecholamine resistant shock: Shock persists despite use of catecholamines - epinephrine or norephinephrine.

Refractory shock: Shock persists despite goal – directed use of inotropic agents, vasopressors, vasodilators, and maintenance of metabolic (glucose and calcium) and hormonal (thyroid and hydrocortisone) homeostasis.

If signs of shock persist despite adequate volume replacement and perfusion of vital organs is jeopardized, vasoactive drugs may improve cardiac output and perfusion. Optimal preload is essential before vasoactive therapy is contemplated. Regardless of the vasoactive drug therapy used, increasing cardiac output and oxygen delivery to supranormal levels is not recommended; these have failed to demonstrate benefit in critically ill patients with sepsis.

The choice of vasoactive drug used would depend on patient's condition after adequate volume resuscitation. Some of pediatric patients may have adult type manifestation of high cardiac output, vasodilatation and hypotension.

Table 6.4: Properties of various sympathetic receptors, their properties and effect of cardiovascular support drugs

Receptor	*α*	*β_1*	*β_2*
Receptor	1-vasoconstrictor	Heart rate	Vasodilation
Property	2-decreased Central sympathetic Flow, vasoconstrictor	Contractility Conduction	
Drugs			
Dopamine (high)	++++	+++	++
Dobutamine	+	+++	++
Phenylepherine	++/+++	-	-
Adrenaline	++++	++++	+/++
Nor-adrenaline	++++	++++	++
Isoproternol	-	++++	++++
Dopexamine	-	-	+++

Table 6.5: Cardiotonic and vasodilator agents

Drug	*Dose (mcg/kg/min)*	*Predominant site of action*	*Comments*
Dopamine	0.5 – 5	Dopaminergic	Vasodilator to renal and cerebral beds
	5 – 10	β_1	Inotropic dose
	> 10	α_1	Pressor dose, arrhythmogenic
Dobutamine	2 – 20	β_1 and β_2, and Dopa	Inotrope, weak chronotrope, selective mid vasodilator, useful in low output high SVR shock
Isoproterenol	0.1 – 5	β	Inotrope, chronotrope, vasodilator, arrhythmogenic (tachyarrhythmia)
Nor-adrenaline	0.05 – 1	α_1, β_1	Strong inotrope and vasoconstrictor, useful and preferred for high output, low SVR state septic shock, may cause reflex bradycardia, splanchnic and peripheral ischemia
Adrenaline (epinephrine)	0.03 – 0.1	β	Inotrope
	0.1 – 0.2	$\alpha_1\beta_1$ and β_2 mixed	Inotrope and Pressor effects,
	> 0.2	α	Vasoconstriction and arrhythmogenic
Dopexamine	0.5 – 6	β_2 and Dopa	Inotrope, vasodilator, improves splanchnic blood flow
Phenylepherine vasoconstrictor	0.2-1	α_1	Inotrope, vasodilator, improves splanchnic blood flow
Amrinone	5 – 10		Inotropic, vasodilator (inodilator), Loading dose 2 – 3 mg/kg IV over 30 min
Milrinone	0.75 – 1.0		Loading dose 75 mg/kg. For every increase of infusion by 0.25 mg/min extra loading dose of 25 mg/kg
Ca-chloride	10–20 mg/kg	–	
Nitroglycerin	0.75 – 1.0	–	Venodilator, limited experience in children
Nitroprusside	10–20 mg/kg	–	Vasodilator, arterial>venous, cyanide toxicity a problem

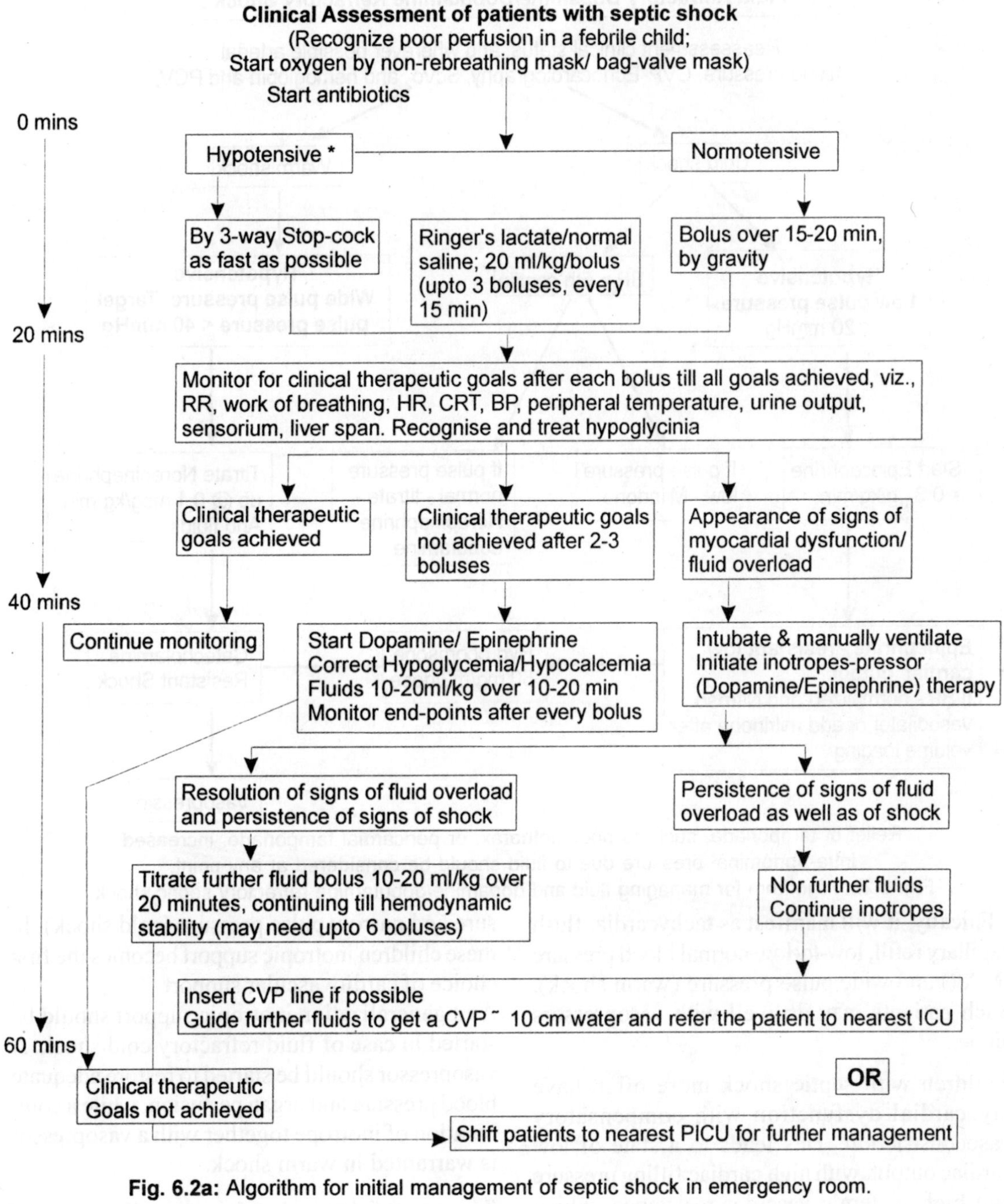

Fig. 6.2a: Algorithm for initial management of septic shock in emergency room.

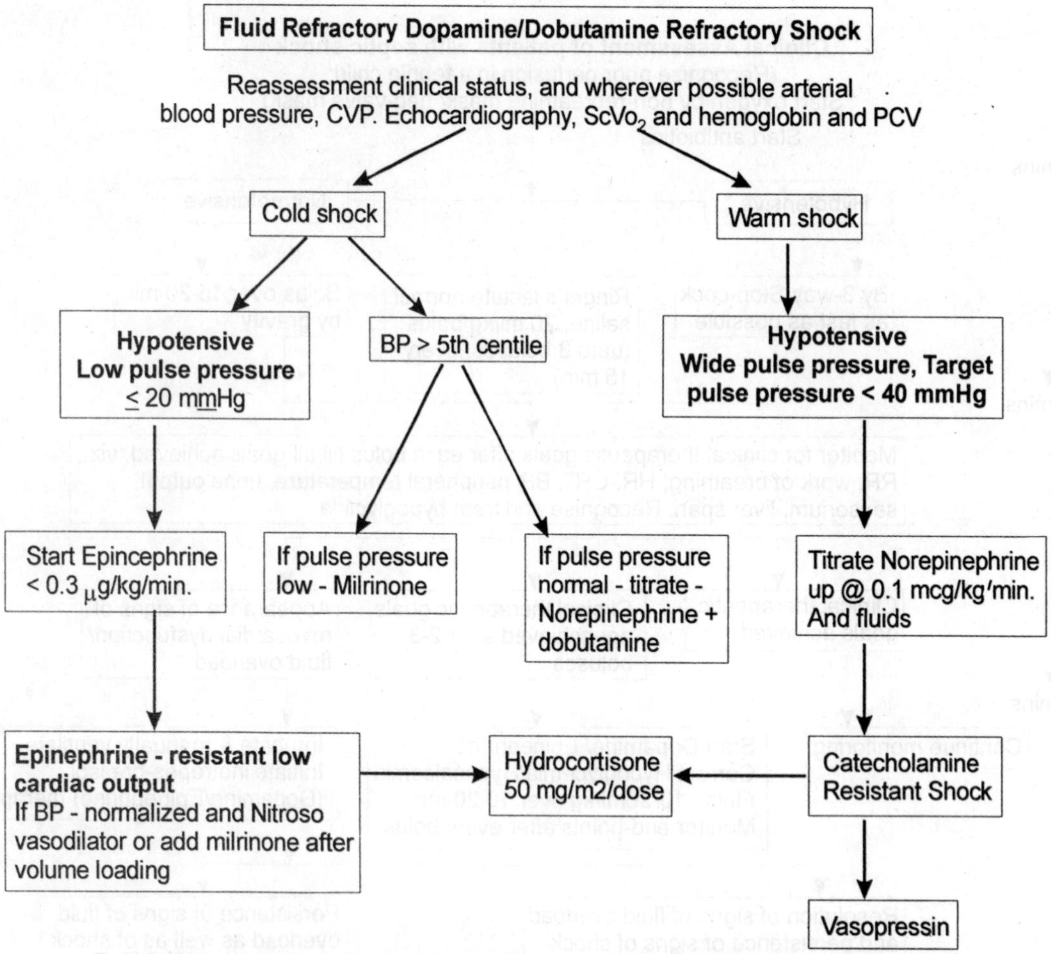

Relief of tamponade, such as pneumothorax, or pericardial tamponade, increased intra-abdominal pressure due to fluid should be considered at any point.

Fig. 6.2b: Algorithm for managing fluid and dopamine/dobutamine refractory septic shock.

Clinically, it will manifest as tachycardia, flush capillary refill, low-to-low normal blood pressure (MAP) and wide pulse pressure (warm shock). Such patients may do well with vasopressors alone.

Children with septic shock more often have myocardial dysfunction with compensatory vasoconstriction. This leads to a state of low cardiac output, with high cardiac filling pressure and high systemic vascular resistance, which clinically manifests as tachycardia, signs of hypoperfusion, prolonged capillary refill, cold extremities and low-to-low normal blood pressure and narrow pulse pressure (cold shock). In these children inotropic support becomes the first choice of cardiovascular support.

As a generalization inotropic support should be started in case of fluid refractory cold shock. A vasopressor should be started to restore adequate blood pressure and organ perfusion, while a combination of inotrope together with a vasopressor is warranted in warm shock.

The use of dopamine is generally accepted as the first line vasopressor for fluid refractory hypotensive shock in the setting of low systemic vascular resistance. Children with septic shock more often have myocardial dysfunction and low cardiac output hence it is preferable to combine inotropy with a vasopressor effect. ***Dopamine in mid or higher doses can be used as first line drugs for giving this kind of support.*** Dopamine increases MAP through an increase in cardiac output and peripheral resistance (primarily by increasing cardiac index). However in children the age specific insensitivity to dopamine has to be kept in mind before starting dopamine particularly in infants < 6 months.

Patients with low cardiac output (myocardial failure) despite adequate fluid resuscitation will require inotropy. Dobutamine (5 μg to 20 μg/kg/min) is the agent of choice for inotropic effect. However, dobutamine alone may be inadequate in a hypotensive patient. In absence of cardiac output measurement, hypotensive patients with sepsis may have low, normal or increased cardiac output. Therefore dobutamine (inotrope) is usually combined with a vasopressor such as dopamine or norepinephrine to increase the peripheral vascular resistance.

The low cardiac output state, characterized by persistent narrow pulse pressure and/or prolong capillary refill, even after use of dopamine, may be improved with addition of dobutamine (up to 20μg/Kg/min) or low dose epinephrine (<0.3 μg/Kg/Min)

When a child in septic shock doesn't improve and the goals of treatment are not achieved even after dopamine and or dobutamine infusion the shock is labeled as ***fluid refractory, dopamine/dobutamine resistant shock***. Dopamine resistant shock may reverse with epinephrine or norepinephrine infusion. (figure 16.2 B). Epinephrine is usually not considered first line therapy for septic shock due to its negative effects on gastric blood flow and lactate. Its use should be limited and should be reserved for cases of extreme hemodynamic collapse like a post arrest state. The dose should be titrated to minimum required for the desired effect; higher doses cause severe vasoconstriction, splanchnic ischemia and lactic acidosis.

At this stage Children in shock may be classified into 2 broad categories: warm shock and cold shock.

Children in cold shock may be further categorized in two sub-groups. First are children with low blood pressure. In these children the dose of epinephrine should be titrated to achieve normal mean arterial pressure for age. Once this is achieved but the other goals of therapy are not yet achieved one should consider adding a vasodilator such as nitroprusside and nitroglycerine, which are pure vasodilators with very short half life, or milrinone having both vasodilator as well as inotropic effects. Nitrosovasodilators are used as firstline therapy for children with epinephrine- resistant low cardiac output and elevated systemic vascular resistance. Use of phosphodiestrase inhibitor milrinone (50-75 ug/kg/min) should be strongly considered if low cardiac and high vascular resistance state persists inspite of epinephrine and nitrosovasodilators. Starting milrinone may require additional fluid bolus, and titrating up the dose of epinephrine to check the vasodilatation and maintain BP.

Second category is that of children with normal blood pressure. In these children, further action would depend on the pulse pressure. If the pulse pressure is low phosphodiestrase inhibitor such as milrinone would be the drug of choice. However, if the pulse pressure is normal or high norepinephrine and doubtamine should be titrated up. Children with 'warm shock' are likely to have a wide pulse pressure. A vasopressor norepinephrine is the drug of choice in such patients. Norepinephrine causes a clinically significant increase in mean arterial pressure due to its vasoconstrictor effects, with little changes in heart rate or cardiac output. It should be used only to restore adequate values of mean arterial pressure that is sufficient to restore urine output. The usual dose is 0.05-1.00 μg/kg/min.

Vasopressin in shock: There is a limited experience with vasopressin in children as a rescue therapy in catecholamine resistant shock. Vasopressin therapy may be considered as a last resort if patient has warm shock with low blood pressure unresponsive to norepinephrine. In pediatric patients, suggested dose is 0.3 to 2 milliunits/kg/min (equivalent to 0.0003 to 0.002 units/kg/min or 0.01 to 0.12 units/kg/hr). The infusion should be titrated to optimize blood pressure and perfusion. Vasopressin may have deleterious effects on renal functions and platelet counts.

Vasoactive drugs- Practice points: Accurate dose delivery is an important component of vasoactive drug therapy. This can only be achieved with infusion pumps. When infusion pumps are not available the infusions may be given using micro-infusion sets whose drop size has been standardized (and confirmed by the user). When several infusions are being administered through the same intravenous access close monitoring of actual delivery of each infusion should be ensured. Even a small change in rates of infusion of vasoactive drugs can have a profound effect on the circulatory status; constant monitoring of the drops rate in such situations is required. One should avoid administering boluses of fluid through single lumen catheters used for vasoactive drug infusion to avoid inadvertant infusion of high doses of the vasoactive drugs.

Mixing of more than one vasoactive drug in the same infusion set or infusion syringes is not recommended even when limited numbers of intravenous access ports are available. These drugs can be infused through the intraosseous route till the time that an intravenous access becomes available.

A meticulous search for the causes of persistent catecholamine resistant shock should be made if therapeutic goals are not achieved in spite of adequate volume loading and high doses of appropriate vasoactive agents. One must rule out mechanical causes of catecholamine resistant shock such as tamponade due to pericardial effusion, pneumothorax or increased intrabdominal pressure.

End Points

Reversal of hypoperfusion, hypotension and endorgan dysfunction (normal urine output and mental status) are early priorities; optimising cardiac output is next priority.

Early goal directed therapy aimed at achieving a CVP. 8-12 mmHg, BP > 5th centile, normal urine output and a central (superior vena cava) or mixed venous oxygen saturation $\geq$ 70% has made a significant impact on survival from septic shock in adults and children.

Antiarrhythmic Therapy

Cardiac output in young children is highly dependent on heart rate. The wide variation in heart rates associated with metabolic derangements may significantly impair cardiac performance. In each case therapy should be directed towards the derangement present.

Treatment of arrhythmias includes correction of acidosis, hypoxia, hypocalcemia and hypokalemia or hyperkalemia. Specific cardioactive drugs that may be used are atropine and isoproterenol for bradyarrhythmias, adenosine or digoxin for supraventricular tachyarrhythmias and lidocaine for ventricular ectopy (See chapter on arrhythmia).

Intraortic Counter Pulsation: Ballon Pumping

It improves coronary blood flow, reduces ventricular afterload, and increases cardiac output. It is best used when the ventricular performance is expected to improve and the cause of shock is reversible.

Antibiotics

Therapy with appropriate antibiotics in appropriate dose should be initiated in all cases suspected of septic shock as soon as specimens for cultures are obtained (Table 6.6). Obtain at least two blood cultures and cultures from other

Table 6.6: Doses of various antibiotics in pediatric septic shock

Ampicillin	50 mg/kg/dose	6 hourly	IV,IM
Ampicillin + Sulbactam	50 mg/kg/dose of ampicillin	6 hourly	IV or IM
Amikacin	> 10 years: 20 mg/kg on Day 1, then 15 mg/kg, 1 week-10 years: 25 mg/kg on Day 1, then 18 mg/kg Neonates: < 30 weeks: 15 mg/kg on day 1, then 7.5 mg/kg > 30 weeks—Term: 10 mg/kg, term 15 mg/kg	OD	IV or IM
Amoxycillin	50 mg/kg/dose	8 hourly, 12 hourly (for babies < 1 wk), 6 hourly (2-4 weeks)	IV, IM
Amoxycillin + Clavulanic acid	Dose same as Amoxicillin 4:1	8 hourly	IV, IM
Amphotericin B	0.5-1.5 mg/kg/day Total dose 30-35 mg/kg	Infusion with D5W over 4-8 weeks	IV
Amphotericin B-lipid/ Liposomal	2-3 mg/kg/day over 1 hour Total dose 20-60 mg/kg	Infusion with D5W over 2-4 weeks	IV
Fluconazole	12 mg/kg stat, 6-12 mg/kg/dose	OD	IV
Itraconazole	5 mg/kg/dose	12-24 hourly	IV, Oral
Voriconazole	6 mg/kg/dose stat over 2 hours, Repeat after 12 hours, then 4 mg/kg/dose	12 hourly	IV IV, Oral
Ceftriaxone	50 mg/kg/dose	12 hourly	IV or IM
Cefepime	50 mg/kg/dose	8 hourly	IM or IV
Cefotaxime	50 mg/kg/dose	4-6 hourly 12 hourly for neonates	IV
Ceftazidime	50 mg/kg/dose	6-8 hourly	IV, IM
Gentamicin	> 10 yrs: 7 mg/kg on day 1, then 5 mg/kg/dose, 1 wk-10 years: 8 mg/kg on day 1, then 6 mg/kg, Neonates: 5 mg/kg	OD	IV, IM
Cloxacillin	50-100 mg/kg/dose	4-6 hourly	IV
Vancomycin	10 mg/kg/dose Neonates: 10 mg/kg/dose	6 hourly 8 hourly	IV over 1 hour
Piperacillin + Tazobactam	Piperacillin: 75-100 mg/kg/dose	6 hourly	IV
Ticarcillin + Clavulanic acid	50-75 mg/kg/dose	6 hourly	IV
Meropenem	40 mg/kg/dose	8 hourly	IV
Imipenem + Cilastin	25 mg/kg/dose	6 hourly	IV

IV—Intravenous, IM—Intramuscular, D5W—5% dextrose solution in water.

sites such as CSF, urine, wound and other body fluids. It is preferable to provide empirical broad-spectrum antibiotic coverage taking into consideration, primary site of infection, local bacterial sensitivity pattern and immunocompetence of the host. In addition, pus anywhere in the body should be drained surgically (for more details See Chapter-18, Severe infections and antibiotics).

Metabolic Correction

Acidosis

A significant secondary complication of shock is the development of metabolic acidosis. Severe acidosis impairs metabolic processes, impedes normal neurovascular interactions, and may prevent effective pharmacologic actions of various vaspopressor and inotropic agents administered to the patient. Correction is indicated when marked metabolic acidosis exists (arterial blood pH < 7.15). Sodium bicarbonate is given in an initial dose of 1 to 2 mEq/kg. Subsequent doses are based on body weight and base deficit (mEq = body weight in kilograms × base deficit × 0.3). Bicarbonate should be used only to partially correct the pH to levels which do not pose a serious immediate threat to life. Care must be taken to avoid over correction as this may impair cardiac function and cause paradoxical acidosis.

Glucose

Pediatric septic patients frequently have hypoglycemia and hypocalcemia as their unique response to sepsis/septic shock. At the time of resuscitation, hypoglycemia is of major concern for its negative inotropic effect and associated severe neurological damage and should be identified rapidly and corrected immediately. It may be treated with 5 ml/Kg of 10% dexrose solution or 2 ml/Kg of 25% dextrose solution. A regular monitoring protocol should then follow to maintain normal blood sugar; *Hyperglycemia should be avoided*. Treatment of hyperglycemia is probably not a significant management issue during initial resuscitation. Hyperglycemia should be taken care of at an appropriately later stage after essential initial resuscitation is over, especially if it is associated with polyuria. *Intensive insulin therapyhowever, is not recommended at this time to achieve strict glycemic control in sepsis.*

Serum Sodium

Disorders of serum sodium concentration may cause cerebral injury. The levels should be monitored and maintained within normal range.

Calcium and hypocalcaemia

Before cardiac output and perfusion pressure are restored with vasoactive drugs, ionized hypocalcemia that might impair cardiac performances should be corrected. Ionized hypocalcemia is common in neonates and children with sepsis admitted to PICU and may be reversible contributor to cardiac dysfunction and hypotension. Administration of calcium in septic patients with ionized hypocalcemia (<4.2 mg/dl) may improve blood pressure for period lasting for. However, there is no evidence to suggest a survival benefit. In absence of facility to identify ionized hypocalcemia, a bolus dose of calcium (1-2 ml/kg of 10 % calcium gluconate solution by infusion) may be given empirically before labelling septic shock as dopamine-resistant shock.

Phosphorus

Phosphorus is essential to muscle, nervous system and functioning of blood cells and is also important in the entire process of generating and storing energy. Consequences of severe hypophosphatemia include acute respiratory failure, altered myocardial performance, platelet dysfunction, hemolytic anemia, hepatocellular damage and neurologic abnormalities. To correct hypophosphatemia, 5 to 10 mg/kg of potassium phosphate is given intravenously over six hours. Complications of phosphate therapy include hypocalcemia and hypotension.

Respiratory/Ventilatory Support

The lung is the most sensitive organ in shock, respiratory failure can develop rapidly and is frequently the cause of death. The work of breathing is substantially increased so as to result in respiratory muscle fatigue. Therefore, patients in shock should be given oxygen supplements, intubated early and treated with positive pressure ventilation. Pulmonary edema caused by fluid extravasations from lung capillaries is not uncommon; it may be worsened by excessive fluid resuscitation. Attention should be paid to avoid pulmonary edema.

Indication for mechanical ventilation in the management of a patient in shock are:

1. Apnea or ventilatory failure (acute respiratory acidosis).
2. Failure to adequately oxygenate with high flow systems i.e. ventury masks or nasal prongs.
3. Respiratory fatigue – for relief of metabolic stress of the work of breathing.
4. Adjunctive therapy for other interventions (post operative state).

In a patient requiring positive pressure ventilation, an attempt should be made to achieve desirable arterial oxygen concentration with a FiO_2 of 0.6 or less. This may be facilitated by judicious use of positive end expiratory pressure (PEEP). Close observations of chest movements, ventilator pressures and flow and arterial blood gases are essential to ensure adequate oxygenation and ventilation. Changes in compliance or obstruction of the endotracheal tube can lead to inadequate alveolar ventilation and must be constantly watched for. High pressure and high tidal volume should be avoided.

Lung injury and air leaks and its sequelae are quite common in children on positive pressure ventilation. Frequent posture changes and vigorous physiotherapy to promote drainage of secretions and avoid atelectasis are essential.

Cerebral Protection

Early correction of hypoxia, hypoglycemia and cerebral edema should be given full attention. CNS infection should be actively excluded if necessary by CSF exam and CT scan. Hyponatremia should be looked for and if present should be corrected cautiously. Good cardiac output should be maintained as cerebral blood flow is correlated with cardiac index in septic shock.

Renal Salvage/Replacement

The hypotension and hypoperfusion associated with shock state affects renal perfusion pressure and may often lead to renal failure. Aggressive fluid replacement is necessary to support urine output. Nevertheless, should hyperkalemia, refractory acidosis, hypervolemia and altered mental status occur, dialysis should be seriously considered. Administration of nephrotoxic drugs should be avoided. Continuous veno-venous hemofiltration (CVVH) offers easier management in hemodynamically unstable patients. (See chapter on Acute Renal Failure).

Gastrointestinal Support

Gastrointestinal disturbances after shock include stress bleeding and ileus. Ileus may result from hypokalemia and may lead to abdominal distension with respiratory compromise. Stress ulcer and gastrointestinal blood loss can be prevented by using antacids, sucralfate and/or H_2-receptor blockers (See chapter 18 for details). Attempts should also be paid to maintain the patient normothermic in order to optimize tissue oxygen utilization. Splanchnic circulation may be unfavorably affected. At present there is no specific agent that can correct it, though dopexamine has given encouraging result. Initiation of enteral feeding should be delayed during resuscitation phase of septic shock treatment.

Hematological Support

Activated protein C (APC): Recombinant human APC is recommended in adult patients at high risk of death such as those in septic shock, sepsis with multi organ failure and sepsis induced ARDS. Current data does not support its use in pediatric septic shock.

Hematocrit should be maintained in the range of 30% (Hb 9-10 g/dl) with the use of packed red cells transfusions. Critical Care Society recommends that during first 6 hours of resuscitation of septic shock, if central venous oxygen saturation or mixed venous oxygen saturation (SVO_2, or $SCVO_2$) of 70% is not achieved with fluids and inotropes and a CVP of 8-12 mmHg, then the patient should receive packed red blood cells to achieve a hematocrit of $\geq$ 30%.

DIC frequently complicates shock. The use of fresh frozen plasma and platelet transfusion to correct laboratory clotting abnormalities is not recommended. These should be used if there is bleeding or invasive procedure is planned.

Platelets transfusion is recommended when counts are < 5000/ mm^3 regardless of bleeding or if there is bleeding and counts are less than 40,000/ mm^3.

Nutritional Support

Nutritional support is a frequently overlooked but extremely important aspect of the care of the shock patient. Excessive catabolism with destruction of lean body mass is the most common nutritional abnormality in shock states. Nutritional support of shock patient should be started as soon as possible. Patients on ventilator, nasogastric tube is placed for initial gastric decompression and then is converted to gastric feeding tube. Transpyloric route may be used. Enteral nutrition is more physiological and preferred. Close monitoring of daily caloric intake and determination of serum albumin, electrolytes and liver function tests should be done. Continuing assessment of vitamin and essential trace metal level is important in long-term care of these patients.

Corticosteroids Therapy

Although adrenal insufficiency (absolute/ relative) is common in children with severe sepsis and septic shock, corticosteroids are not recommended routinely in the treatment of septic shock, except in those cases where stress dose corticosteroid (hydrocortisone 1-2 mg/Kg or 50mg/ m^2 followed by 50 mg/m^2/day in 4 divided doses intravenously for 5 to 7 days) is required. This group includes patients with proven adrenal insufficiency or at high risk of adrenal insufficiency. Children at risk for adrenal insufficiency include those who have or are suspected to have pituitary or adrenal abnormalities, who have received corticosteroids for chronic illness or those who present with septic shock and purpura. Corticosteroids are also recommended for catecholamine-resistant septic shock in children. The recommended dose varies between hydrocortisone 1-5mg/kg/day.

The enthusiasm associated with use of low dose (physiological stress doses) corticosteroids for a longer duration because of beneficial results in terms of mortality reduction and reversal of shock in adult patients has come down. At present, there is insufficient evidence to determine role of low dose hydrocortisone in children with septic shock. In an exploratory study from Chandigarh, there was a trend towards earlier reversal of shock and lower inotropes requirement in the hydrocortisone treated patients as compared to controls; however, the difference was not statistically significant. There is no large randomized study in children to support the use of corticosteroids in septic shock. There is also a concern about higher mortality and adverse effects associated with use of corticosteroids in children with critically ill children.

Intravenous Immunoglobulins (IVIG)

IVIG *may* be considered in children with severe sepsis if cost is not an issue. It is known that endogenous and exogenously administered IVIG can neutralize endotoxins (IgM is more potent than IgG) and can attenuate the overshooting inflammation in patients of sepsis. There is evidence that it has some benefit in children, and may possibly have some benefit in neonates. A recent RCT of polyclonal IVIG in Pediatric sepsis showed a significant reduction in mortality and fewer complications. However, large clinical trials and recent consensus guidelinesdo not recommend widespread use of IVIG in patients with severe sepsis or septic shock. Cost being an additional consideration in resource limited settings use of *IVIG is not routinely recommended* in patients of severe sepsis and septic shock.

Anti-inflammatory and Immunotherapy

Convincing evidence that septic shock and its morbid consequences are a direct result of endogenous protein and phospholipid mediators secreted by the host has prompted the use of many anti-inflammatory and experimental immunomodulatory therapies with outcome of septic shock. These were directed toward blocking the inflammatory response to sepsis, and counteract deleterious effects of endotoxins. However, these efforts have not met with clinical success so far. The interventions considered include ibuprofen, pentoxyphylline, immunoglobulins, endotoxin antibodies, TNF antibodies, interleukin–1ra, PAF –antagonists, bradykinin antagonists etc.

Extracorporeal Membrane Oxygenation

Full cardiopulmonary bypass via percutaneous femoral arterial and venous approaches, utilizing a portable cardiopulmonary bypass machine with membrane oxygenator may be used if other therapies has not worked. Limited success has been reported with this technique in patients with refractory shock or cardiac arrest.

Indications for referral to an ICU

1. Need for intubation and ventilation.
2. Failure to respond to fluid infusion and need for vasoactive drug therapy.
3. Need for major surgery.
4. Renal or any other organ failure.

It is always advisable that the patient is stabilized before transfer.

Minimum Facilities Needed in an Unit Treating Shock

Defined area, trained nurses, facilities to monitor vital signs, urine output, BP, CVP, body temperature, ECG, oxygen-saturation, invasive BP (optional), electrolytes, urea, hemoglobin, support services, X-ray, microbiology.

Titrated oxygen therapy, mechanical ventilation, controlled drug infusion systems, availability of IV fluids, antibiotics, vasoactive drugs, access to renal support, nutrition.

PROGNOSIS AND ASSESSING OUTCOME

Aggressive and early management of shock is associated with intact survival of a child. The mortality depends upon the underlying etiology, and may be as high as 30-40% with septic shock. Therapeutic goals for management of shock are now defined. In recent times a remarkable improvement in survival has been noted with early focussed aggressive fluid and vasoactive therapy in children with meningococcal and dengue shock, and adults with septic shock. Outcome is improved in patients with early normalization of heart rate (<24 hours), increased cardiac output, elevated oxygen consumption and elevated oxygen extraction and without significant pulmonary disease. On the other hand low body temperature (<37°C) pulmonary disease, low cardiac index (<3.3 lit/min/m^2) and decreased oxygen utilization are all poor prognostic indicators in shock.

Chapter seven

Mechanical Ventilation

Optimal use of mechanical ventilation requires a thorough knowledge of physiology and applied mechanics of lungs, and recognition of diverse mechanisms of respiratory failure. A good understanding of the available ventilators, various modes of ventilation and ventilatory adjustment is also essential. Recognition and understanding of each patient's pathophysiology combined with appropriate use of the available ventilatory options are the most vital elements in minimising morbidity and mortality caused by our supportive efforts.

Components of respiration may be divided into ventilation and oxygenation. **Ventilation** deals with the movement of air in and out of the lungs. **Oxygenation** deals with the process of gas exchange within the lungs at alveolar level (external) or at the tissue level (internal).

Ventilation requires the development of a pressure gradient between the mouth and the alveoli (transpulmonary pressure). During spontaneous breathing, this gradient is achieved by contraction of the respiratory muscles that enlarges the pleural cavity and lower pleural and intra-alveolar pressure to sub-atmospheric. This pressure gradient causes air to move into the lungs. Expiration is usually passive; the natural elastic recoil of the lung tissue causes an increase in intra-alveolar pressure to reverse the pressure gradient to allow air to flow out of the lungs.

Mechanical Ventilation

Mechanical ventilation helps with 'ventilation' and does not necessarily influence the 'gas exchange'. It involves an external device connected directly to the patient, which provides the movement of air in and out of the lung. Mechanical ventilation may deliver a volume of gas to the patient's lungs in one of two ways.

a. *Positive Pressure Ventilation*: Positive pressure is applied directly to the airways, which forces air down the airways, and into the lungs.
b. *Negative Pressure Ventilation:* Negative pressure is applied externally to the chest cage which will change the pressure dynamics so that gas flows from the relatively positive atmosphere to the relatively negative air spaces. Although negative pressure ventilation is more physiological, the apparatus is cumbersome and access to the patient is limited.

Applied Pulmonary Mechanics

The predominant factors, which influence distribution of inspired gases, are compliance of lungs and thoracic wall and airway-resistance.

Compliance (C) is a measure of the 'stiffness' of the chest and is determined by elastic forces of the lung, chest wall, and surface tension generated within the alveoli. It is defined as the change in volume per unit change in pressure and is expressed in litres/cm of H_2O as $C= \Delta V/\Delta P$. Normal lungs are highly compliant (less stiff). Diseased lungs may have reduced compliance (increased stiffness) requiring higher pressures to produce lung expansion e.g. Acute Respiratory Distress Syndrome (ARDS), pneumonia, pulmonary edema.

Airway resistance (R): Airway resistance is the pressure difference between the mouth and alveoli and is expressed in cm H_2O/litre/second.

The resistance is determined by various factors, the most important of which is the radius of the airways. Even minor degrees of narrowing from bronchospasm, edema or mucus accumulation can cause significant increase in airway resistance.

Functional residual capacity (FRC) is the volume of gas that is present in the lung at the end of expiration. FRC results from the balance between forces that favor alveolar collapse and those that maintain alveolar inflation. The normal FRC is about 30 ml/kg. Residual volume is the volume of gas present in the lung at the end of maximal expiratory effort that cannot be expelled from the lung.

Closing capacity (CC) refers to the volume of gas, present in the lung at which small conducting airways begin to collapse. When FRC exceeds CC, as is the case normally, the small airways and the alveoli remain open because the lung volume remain above CC. When CC exceeds FRC, on the other hand, the small airways and alveoli tend to collapse. In children older than 6 years FRC exceeds CC. However in infants and in children less than 6 years, CC exceeds FRC. This explains the tendency for atelectasis in infants and young children.

Time constants: The time constant is the product of airway resistance and compliance (RxC) and is measured in seconds. It is a measure of how quickly the lungs can inhale or exhale or how long it takes for pressures delivered in the proximal airways to reach the alveoli. One time constant fills in 63% of an alveolus and three fill in 95%. Three to five time constants are required for complete filling or emptying of an alveolar unit. In a normal infant, one-time constant equals 0.15 seconds and three time constants equal 0.45 seconds. Thus, the minimum inspiratory or expiratory time should be about 0.5 seconds. If sufficient time is not allowed in expiration air trapping will occur.

Various diseases can alter the time constant. An understanding of this concept aids greatly in selecting the safest and most effective ventilator setting for an individual patient. In normal lungs the difference between the inspiratory and expiratory time constant is minimal. In some situations, the inspiratory and expiratory time constants may be different, as the airway calibre and lung compliance vary with different stages of the respiratory cycle. The difference may be accentuated in various diseases. In diseases that cause increased airway resistance such as asthma, the time constants of alveolar units will increase, causing slower filling and emptying of alveoli (slow alveoli). In diseases that result in decreased compliance or 'stiff' lung the time constant will decrease, causing faster filling and emptying of the alveolar units (fast alveoli).

BASIC TERMINOLOGY

Tidal Volume (Vt)

This is the volume of gas that flows in and out of the chest during quiet breathing. In adults, the normal tidal volume is 500 ml. In children the tidal volume is 6 ml/kg.

Frequency/ Ventilatory Rate (f)

The rate of mechanical breaths per minute set on the ventilator. The preset rate depends on the indication for ventilation and the physiologic norm for the patient's age.

Minute Ventilation (MV)

This is the product of the tidal volume and the ventilatory rate and reflects the volume of the gas moved in and out of lungs in a minute. It is expressed in litres/minute.

Inspiratory Time and I:E Ratios

The I:E ratio refers to the relationship between inspiratory time (I) and expiratory time (E). The normal I:E ratio is usually 1:2 to 1:3. Adjustment of the inspiratory time is the primary method by which the I:E ratio is altered. Normal settings for inspiratory time range from 0.4 to 1.5 seconds depending on the ventilatory rate and underlying lung disease. Expiratory time should not be decreased to <0.5 seconds except in conditions associated with reduced compliance and shortened time constants.

Peak Inspiratory Pressure/Pressure Limit (PIP)

This is the highest pressure during the inspiratory period. It depends upon Vt, inspiratory time, rate of gas flow, compliance of chest and lungs. The PIP level is usually kept as low as possible since it has been implicated as cause of barotrauma.

Positive End Expiratory Pressure (PEEP)

PEEP is the base-line (minimum) positive pressure in the airway during expiration. It is designed to keep alveoli from collapsing at the end of expiration. The technique is very useful when lungs are diffusely non-compliant and have tendency to atelectasis. A normal level of PEEP (Physiological PEEP) is 2-3 cm H_2O.

FiO_2 stands for fractional inspired oxygen concentration where 100% oxygen is represented as 1.0, oxygen in room air (21%) as 0.21 and so on.

Mean Airway Pressure (MAP)

MAP is a measure of average positive pressure generated in the lung throughout the respiratory cycle. It is not a ventilator setting but a result of ventilator settings. It is determined by several factors including PIP, PEEP, inspiratory time and flow rate. MAP is a critical factor in determining both the oxygenation and the potential for barotrauma. Many ventilators have the ability to continuously monitor and display MAP allowing the clinician to see the effects of ventilatory adjustments on this value.

Sensitivity/Trigger

This refers to the ease with which a ventilator can sense the patient's demand for a breath. It is usually expressed as the amount of negative pressure (pressure trigger) or change in flow (flow trigger) that a patient must create through spontaneous breathing efforts to 'switch ON' the ventilator to deliver a mechanical breath. Setting the sensitivity too high may increase the work of breathing as the patient must create a higher intra-thoracic negative pressure in order to get assistance from the ventilator. Setting the sensitivity too low may lead to over-triggering and the patient being over ventilated (See Table 7.1 for other ventilator related definitions).

Table 7.1: Some ventilator related definitions

- Initiation of Ventilation—MODE
  By Ventilator—controlled ventilation
  By Patient—assisted or spontaneous ventilation
- Completion of Inspiration—LIMIT
  By Preset pressure, volume, flow, or TIME
- Beginning of Expiration—CYCLING
  By preset time, pressure or flow

MODES OF VENTILATION (Fig. 7.1)

This may be broadly classified as below:

- *Spontaneous mode:* Patient is breathing on his own. This includes Continuous Positive Airway Pressure (CPAP) and Pressure Support Ventilation (PSV).
- *Assist mode:* Patient's effort is assisted by the ventilator.
- *Controlled mechanical ventilation (CMV):* In this mode, all breaths are initiated and delivered by the ventilator, the patient does not take an active role.

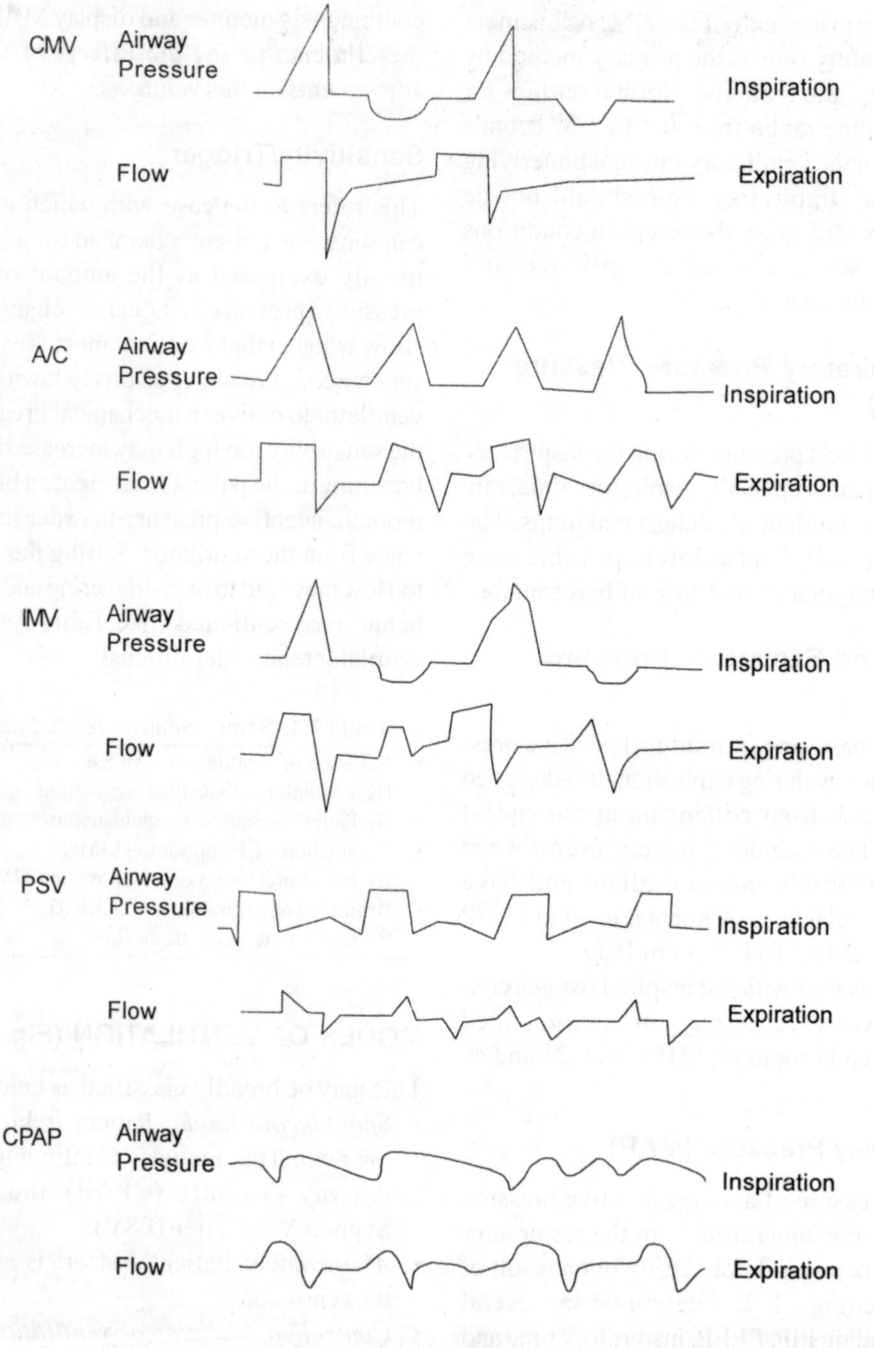

Fig. 7.1: Schematic airway pressures and flow tracings for different modes of mechanical ventilation. (CMV—Controlled Mechanical Ventilation; A/C—Assist-Control; IMV—Intermittent Mandatory Ventilation; PSV—Pressure Support Ventilation; CPAP—Continuous Positive Airway Pressure)

Continuous Positive Airway Pressure (CPAP)

CPAP is usually defined as positive pressure maintained in the airways throughout the respiratory cycle during spontaneous respiration. CPAP should not be confused with PEEP, which refers to the elevation of baseline pressure during mechanical ventilation.

Technical Considerations

Many devices have been developed to deliver CPAP. All work on the same principle, using a continuous gas flow, a reservoir bag, a valve to maintain positive pressure above atmospheric and a humidification device. CPAP is most commonly applied to the patients' airways via an endotracheal tube. Other modes of application include face mask or nasal prongs.

Physiologic Effects of CPAP

CPAP improves arterial oxygenation by opening up collapsed alveoli (recruitment) and decreasing intra pulmonary shunting. This allows the clinician to decrease the FiO_2 to non-toxic levels in many cases while maintaining acceptable arterial oxygen levels.

Side Effects of CPAP

1. Barotrauma secondary to alveolar over distension.
2. *Cardiovascular*: An increase in thoracic pressure because of CPAP may decrease venous return to the heart and consequently decrease cardiac output.
3. *CNS*: Aggravation of intracranial hypertension, cerebral ischemia or both.
4. *Renal effects:* Stimulation of reflex secretion of antidiuretic hormone (ADH) leading to decreased urine output and significant water retention.

Indications and Applications of CPAP

The primary indication is in acute lung injury e.g. ARDS and HMD. Other conditions in which CPAP is useful include apnea, tracheobronchomalacia and weaning from mechanical ventilation.

Controlled Mechanical Ventilation

When ventilator controls all the ventilation while patient has minimal or no respiratory effort it is called Controlled Mechanical Ventilation (CMV). It delivers a pre-selected ventilatory rate, tidal volume and inspiratory flow rate, which are independent of spontaneous effort of patient. Indications for CMV include apnea, depression of central nervous system (drug overdose) neuromuscular paralysis or significant fatigue of the ventilatory muscles. Although paralyzing critically ill patients is done infrequently, the use of CMV with muscle paralysis may prove effective in patients with severe status asthmaticus or with severe multi-organ failure. It is the mode often used at initiation of mechanical ventilation.

Continuous positive pressure ventilation (CPPV), like CMV delivers a positive pressure breath followed by a fall in airway pressure to a previously selected positive pressure plateau. The airway pressure never returns to zero. This prevents alveolar collapse during the ventilator's expiratory phase, and thereby improves and maintain overall alveolar ventilation-to-perfusion (VA/Q) relationships.

Assisted Mechanical Ventilation

It is "patient-triggered" positive-pressure ventilation. If the patient initiate a spontaneous breathing effort, the ventilator will deliver a mechanical breath. Assisted mechanical ventilation is often used to promote spontaneous breathing during weaning of patients from CMV. Usually a decrease in breathing circuit pressure generated by spontaneous effort is used as trigger. The greatest operational difficulty with assisted mechanical ventilation is that many of the assist mechanisms, which trigger the inhalation phase, are unreliable. The patient's condition change rendering 'trigger-sensitivity' too low resulting in repetitive cycles or too high, so that the ventilator fails to cycle.

Assist-Control Ventilation

The technique combines assisted mechanical ventilation and CMV. The ventilator may be triggered by the patient's spontaneous inspiratory efforts or by a timing device, whichever comes first. If the patient attempt to breath, the negative pressure so generated triggers the ventilator, which releases a pre-set volume of air-oxygen mixture to the patient. If the patient fails to initiate the breathing within a prescribed time, ventilator triggers the breathing and provides a controlled breath. The patient may trigger the ventilator "ON" at any time, but the timer determines a minimal pre-selected rate. Hence, in this mode CMV acts as a backup should the patient become apneic or attempt to breathe at a lower rate.

Further refinement in assisted modes of ventilation are the outcome of sensitive microprocessor technology, which allows very rapid interaction between patient and ventilator. The breath by breath on line monitoring of flow, pressure, volume and respiratory mechanics available in more advanced ventilators have been used to improve one or more aspects of mechanical ventilation. The benefits that the newer modes offer are—an improvement in ventilation perfusion balance, minimization of positive pressure related cardiovascular compromise, decrease in work of breathing or facilitation of weaning.

Intermittent Mandatory Ventilation (IMV)

IMV delivers a preset number of controlled breaths at preset intervals. In between these breaths patient is allowed to breath spontaneously. The mechanical ventilatory rate, like CMV, cannot be influenced by the patient. Between sequential mechanical breaths, an unrestricted flow rate of gas equal to or greater than the patient's peak spontaneous inspiratory flow rate demand is provided.

The IMV rate should be titrated to deliver the support, which in conjunction with spontaneous breathing maintains normal alveolar ventilation and $PaCO_2$. IMV is extremely useful in regulating $PaCO_2$ and pH compared with CMV.

Synchronized Intermittent Mandatory Ventilation

Synchronized intermittent mandatory ventilation (SIMV) like IMV, allows the patient to breathe spontaneously between mechanical breaths. The ventilator delivered "mandatory" breath is synchronized to begin with patient's own breathing efforts analogues to assisted mechanical ventilation. This technique was introduced because of concern that a mechanical breath might be superimposed on a spontaneous breath, which might predispose to increase in peak inflation, mean airway, and mean intrapleural pressures. However, no difference between IMV and SIMV modes were noted with respect to cardiac output, stroke volume, intrapleural pressure and intrapulmonary shunting.

Peak inflation and mean airway pressures do increase significantly with IMV, and breath stacking may also occur but there are no demonstrable adverse effects. SIMV does not seem to offer any physiological advantage compared with IMV.

Mandatory Minute Volume Ventilation

Mandatory minute volume (MMV) ventilation guarantees a pre-selected minute volume, either through spontaneous ventilation or as positive-pressure breaths from the ventilator. If the preset minute volume is not met by patient's spontaneous effort, the ventilator delivers the remaining volume automatically. Because it ensures a minimal level of support, mandatory minute volume has been advocated for weaning patients from mechanical ventilation.

Minimal Minute Ventilation (MiMV)

Like MMV, MiMV ensures delivery of a preset minute volume. In MiMV the patient has to generate spontaneous breath for assistance. The respiratory drive therefore should be intact.

Airway Pressure Release Ventilation (APRV) and Inverse Ratio Ventilation (IRV)

Both these modes are specifically aimed at patients with Acute Respiratory Distress Syndrome (ARDS). IRV with inspiratory: expiratory ratio of 2 : 1 upto 4 : l achieves better oxygenation by an increase in airway pressure (Paw) and progressive stabilization and recruitment of collapsed alveoli. However, an increased Paw may cause air-trapping and clinical deterioration. In APRV, there is intermittent release from positive airway pressure to an ambient pressure. The pressure wave form of APRV closely resembles that of IRV, but in APRV the patient is allowed to breathe spontaneously, which facilitates CO_2 elimination and reduces Paw.

Pressure Support Ventilation (PSV)

In PSV mode all of the patient's ventilatory efforts are supported ('boosted') by the ventilator to various degrees determined by the operator. The patient triggers breathing and ventilator delivers air and gas mixture at a preset positive pressure in the ventilator circuit (Fig. 7.3). The pressure is actively sustained until the end of inspiration. Patient determines own inspiratory time, and tidal volume. This mode provides additional inspiratory flow through a demand valve in response to a spontaneous breathing effort. The additional gas flow rapidly produces a positive inspiratory airway pressure and enables a full tidal volume breathing, thus reducing the patient's work of breathing and diaphragmatic fatigue. The airway pressure, flow and lung volume changes during pressure support ventilation are more akin to assisted mechanical ventilation.

This mode may be used by itself so that all breaths are initiated by the patient and pressure supported by the ventilator or it may be combined with SIMV (SIMV + PSV mode). In the combined mode the patient receives some mechanical breaths and some pressure supported spontaneous breaths. It is popular as a weaning mode. With this mode categorically induced respiratory alkalosis and 'fighting' against the ventilator is uncommon because it is the patient who controls the respiratory frequency and duration of inspiration.

Air flow pattern and pressure changes with various modes of ventilation are shown in Figures 7.1 to 7.3. Advantages and disadvantages of various modes are summarized in Table 7.2.

Proportional-assisted Ventilation (PAV)

In this mode the positive ventilation pressure sums itself to the pressure that the respiratory muscles generate. As a result, the ventilation pressure increases the effect of spontaneous breathing to the expansion of the lungs and reduces work of spontaneous breathing. The patient himself determines the timing and the depth of each breath.

The increase in assisted pressure is proportionally to tidal air volume. The intensification (the degree of assistance of spontaneous breathing) is set at a pressure per unit or respiratory volume in cmH_2O/ml elastic unloading. The elastance of breathing work is therefore reduced. Pressure increases proportionally to respiratory gas flow. The intensification is set as pressure per respiratory gas flow in $cmH_2O/i/sec$ resistive unloading. The resistive breathing work is reduced.

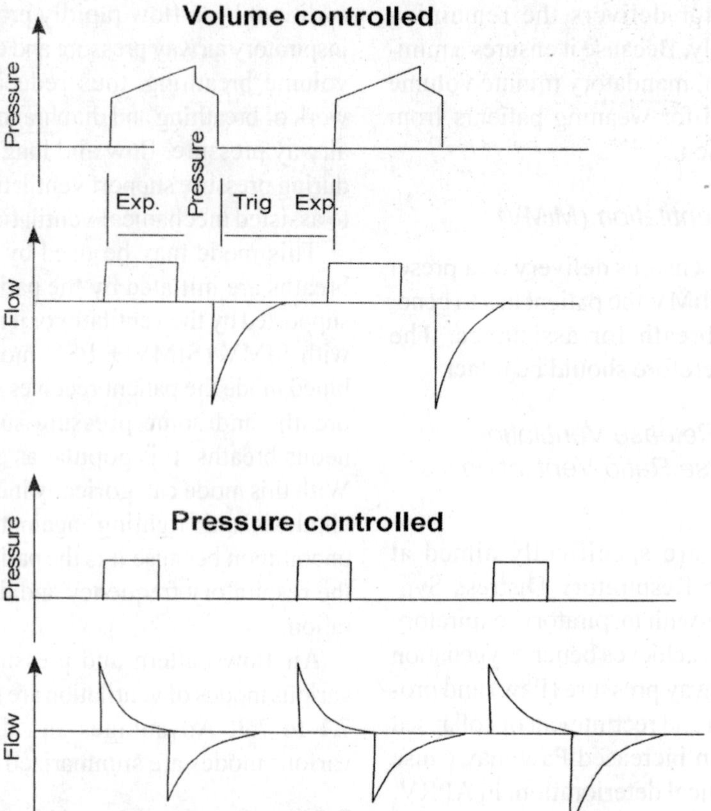

Fig. 7.2: Pattern of airflow and pressure generated during volume controlled and pressure controlled ventilation

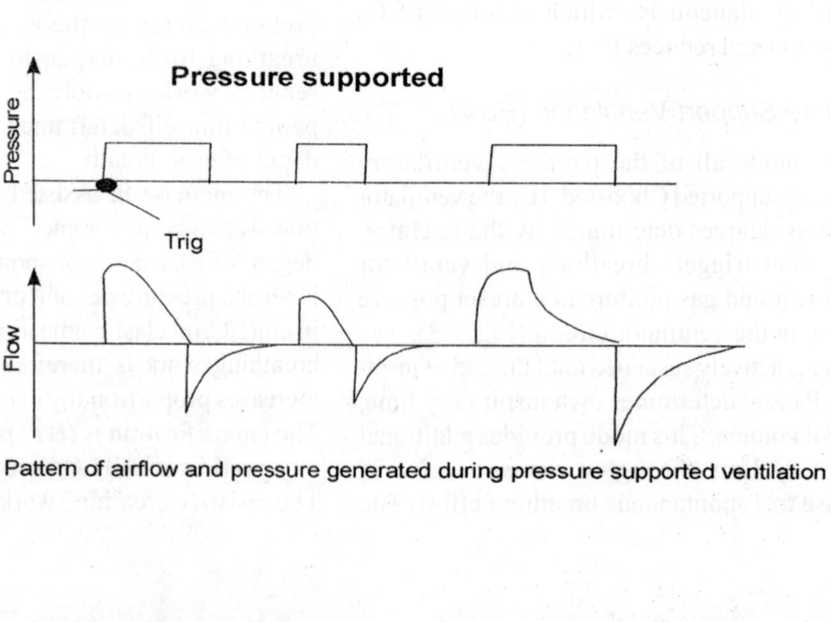

Fig. 7.3: Pattern of airflow and pressure generated during pressure supported ventilation

Table 7.2: Advantages and disadvantages of various modes

- Controlled mechanical ventilation (CMV)
  - Rests muscles of respiration
  - No patient-ventilator interaction; requires use of sedation/neuromuscular blockade; potential adverse hemodynamic effects
- Pressure-controlled ventilation (PCV)
  - Allows limitation of peak inspiratory pressures, control of inspiratory/expiratory ratio
  - Potential hyper-or hypoventilation with lung resistance/compliance change
- Assistant control ventilation (AC)
  - Patient determines amount of ventilatory support; reduces work of breathing
  - Potential adverse hemodynamic effects; may lead to inappropriate hyperventilation
- Synchronized intermittent mandatory ventilation (SIMV)
  - Improved patient-ventilator interaction; less interference with normal cardiovascular function
  - Increased work of breathing compared to AC
- Pressure-support ventilation (PSV)
  - Patient comfort; improved patient-ventilator interaction; decreased work of breathing
  - Apnea alarm is only back-up
  - Variable effect on patient tolerance

Table 7.3: Parameters used for ventilation "cycling"

Time
Divided into inspiratory (Ti) and expiratory (Te) periods and is expressed in seconds or by the relation to inspiratory time to expiratory time expressed as an i:e ratio

Pressure
A measure of the Vt delivered by the ventilator to the patient's airways and lungs generated as a result of airway resistance and lung-thorax compliance expressed in cm H_2O mm hg

Flow rate
A measure of the rate at which the gas volume is delivered to the patient, is expressed as L/sec or L/min

Benefits

- Lower transpulmonary pressure.
- Better synchronization of spontaneous breathing and ventilation pressure patterns.
- Training of the respiratory regulation and respiratory muscles.

The main indications for PAV are respiratory failure as a result to obstructive and restrictive changes and weakening or respiratory muscles. It is contraindicated in patients with paralysis of the respiratory muscular system and diaphragmatic hernia.

High Frequency Ventilation (HFV)

HFV is a generic term, which refers to all systems of ventilation at high rates. There are three subcategories of HFV based primarily on frequency range, tidal volumes and operational characteristics. These are:

- High Frequency Positive Pressure Ventilation (HFPPV)
- High Frequency Jet Ventilation (HFJV)
- High Frequency Oscillation (HFO). In this mode, using special high frequency ventilators very high respiratory rates—upto 900/min, with very small tidal volume are delivered. HFPPV and HFJV are no longer used due to their poor results.

Cycling Mechanisms

The changeover to the exhalation phase, i.e. the process used to "switch off" the inspiratory phase is called "cycling". A preset time, volume, pressure and flow rate, which are interrelated variables, are used for cycling. The cycling mechanism of a ventilator is used to describe spontaneous and mechanical positive pressure ventilation.

Time-Cycled Mechanical Inhalation

Time cycling gives a physician freedom to set desired inspiratory and expiratory time and adjust it to patient's need. Mechanical inhalation is terminated after a pre-selected inspiratory time elapses. Duration of the inhalation phase is controlled by the operator. The Vt delivered is the product of inspiratory time (sec) and inspiratory flow (ml/sec), thorax compliance and directly proportional to airway resistance.

Pressure-Limited, Time-Cycled Mechanical Ventilation

A pressure limit is applied by presetting a limit to PIP to a selected value. Once the pressure limit is reached, airway pressure is held at that the level until the ventilator time cycles "OFF". Limited peak inflation pressure can reduce the risk of barotrauma. The delivered tidal volume (Vt) depends upon inspiratory time (Ti) and flow rate of gases (Vi):

$$Vt = Ti \times Vi$$

and the peak inflation pressure generated is inversely proportional to compliance (C):

$$PIP = \frac{Vt}{C} = \frac{Ti \times Vi}{C}$$

Volume-Cycled/limited Mechanical Inhalation

Volume-cycled mechanical inhalation is terminated after a pre-selected Vt has been delivered to patient irrespective of the peak inflation pressure, inspiratory time, and inspiratory flow rate. The peak inflation pressure generated is directly proportional to inspiratory time, and inspiratory flow rate and inversely proportional to compliance (C).

A common misconception is that Vt delivered to the patient is always constant despite increases in peak inflation pressure (either because of decreases in compliance and/or increase in airway resistance). No ventilator currently available delivers constant Vt. It should be understood clearly that the ejected Vt is distributed in the ventilator breathing circuit tubing and the patient's lungs. The greater the peak inflation pressure, the greater is the fraction of Vt compressed and "left behind" in the breathing circuit, and the less volume delivered to the patient. When high peak inflation pressures are required, noncompliant and nondistensible tubing should be used and the humidifier should be full. Exhaled Vt should be measured to ascertain the actual, delivered Vt that the patient receives.

Volume limited ventilators continue to deliver a preset tidal volume, irrespective of the pressure required for the delivery. In conditions where lung compliance is decreased, this may be high enough to cause alveolar rupture, pulmonary air-leaks, and barotrauma.

Pressure-Cycled/Limited Mechanical Inhalation

Pressure-cycled mechanical inhalation is terminated when a pre-selected peak inflation pressure is achieved within the ventilator breathing circuit, irrespective of the Vt, inspiratory time, or inspiratory flow rate. When the pre-selected peak inflation pressure is reached, inspiratory flow rate and the exhalation valve opens to allow passive exhalation. Delivered Vt and inspiratory time are related directly to lung-thorax compliance. A decrease in lung-thorax compliance and/or increase in airway resistance predispose to a decrease in inspiratory time, and Vt.

$$Vt = PIP \times C$$

Because pressure cycled ventilators deliver air till a set pressure limit is reached this is desirable in small infants. However, in conditions associated with low lung compliance, pressure cycled ventilators are less desirable. In these conditions, the pressure limit is reached quickly and adequate tidal volume may not be delivered resulting in inadequate alveolar ventilation. Careful monitoring will indicate the change in pressure or compliance and these can be taken care of.

Flow-Cycled Mechanical Inhalation

Flow-cycled mechanical inhalation is terminated when the inspiratory flow rate delivered by the ventilator decreases to a critical value. Flow cycling is employed by microprocessor-controlled mechanical ventilators operating in the pressure support ventilation mode. In the pressure support ventilation mode, when the ventilator is triggered 'ON' by patient's effort an abrupt increase in airway pressure and a high peak inspiratory flow rate is delivered immediately to the patient. The inhalation phase continues until the inspiratory flow rate decays to a predetermined percentage of the initial peak value; at this critical value, flow rate ceases (i.e., the ventilator flow cycles "OFF" and the exhalation valve opens, allowing passive exhalation).

Constant and Nonconstant Flow Generators

During mechanical inhalation several patterns of gas flow may be generated by different ventilation. It may be constant, sinusoidal, decelerating, or accelerating inspiratory flow waveform. Constant flow generators require a high driving pressure to maintain a large pressure gradient. A constant or square inspiratory flow waveform is delivered with the type of ventilator.

Whether a particular type of inspiratory flow waveform can improve the distribution of ventilation, VA/Q matching, and gas exchange is controversial.

INDICATIONS FOR VENTILATION

Indications for ventilation may be grouped as follows:

1. *Depressed ventilatory drive*—apnea, irregular breathing, shallow breathing, drug induced.
2. *Neuromuscular inability*—respiratory paralysis/weakness, exhaustion.
3. *Unable to sustain increased work of breathing*—Severe respiratory distress caused by acute pulmonary or airway problem, injury to previously normal lungs: ARDS, pneumonia, bronchiolitis, asthma, pulmonary edema, chronic lung disease.
4. *Shock and myocardial failure*—Heart disease, septic shock.

Serious respiratory depression or paralysis causing apnea or hypoventilation is the most obvious indication for mechanical ventilation (Table 7.4).

Table 7.4: Common indications for mech ventilation

1. Respiratory failure
   Apnea, respiratory arrest, irregular breathing.
   Inadequate oxygenation: $PaO_2 \leq 60$ mmHg
   - Refractory hypoxemia
   - Need for PEEP
   - Excessive work of breathing

   CO_2 retention (Ventilation Abnormalities): $PaCO_2$ 50 mmHg or more
   - Respiratory muscle dysfunction-Fatigue
   - Hypoventilation
   - Increased airway resistance and/or obstruction
2. Cardiovascular dysfunction: Myocardial failure
3. Neurological disorders: Decreased ventilatory drive, raised ICP
4. Respiratory paralysis: Neuromuscular disease, LGB syndrome, snake-bite, poisonings.

When ventilatory drive or the neuromuscular ability to breathe is partial, decision to institute ventilatory support requires critical timing. Drug-induced ventilatory depression should be assessed only when the patient is not stimulated in any manner. In these patients tests that reflect neuromuscular ability such as vital capacity or maximum inspiratory pressure can be fatally misleading.

Mechanical ventilation should be started in any severely distressed, cyanosed patient, whose hypoxemia persists in spite of maximal oxygen therapy and signs of exhaustion appear, and who has a reversible disease such as pneumonia, aspiration syndromes, laryngotracheitis, pulmonary oedema, bronchiolitis , asthma etc.

Patient's inability to meet the demands of increased work of breathing is a common indication for ventilation. The increased resistive breathing work is generally due to increased resistance to the flow of gas which may precipitate ventilatory failure either by acute CO_2 retention or by ventilatory muscle fatigue. Ventilatory failure due to increased elastic work of breathing is probably due to ventilatory muscle fatigue. Intervention aimed at the primary pathologic process may prevent progress to overt ventilatory failure. Close observation of these patients may allow intubation and ventilatory support more safely before the patient is moribund.

Failure of organ systems, other than the central nervous system, neuromuscular system, and lungs, may precipitate ventilatory failure. Patients with severe hemorrhagic, cardiogenic, or septic shock states and those with extensive burns or head injury should receive elective mechanical ventilation before sudden, severe, respiratory failure occurs.

The decision to ventilate a patient deserves critical assessment and mature clinical judgment. The benefit of ventilation must be carefully weighed against the potential complications of positive airway pressure, complications due to intubation, pulmonary toilet, sedation, and the sophisticated equipment.

SETTING VENTILATOR PARAMETERS

Goals of mechanical ventilation are to: (a) Improve arterial blood oxygenation [by applying high levels of inspired oxygen or by methods of recruiting non-ventilated alveoli] (b) decrease or eliminate energy consumption of the respiratory muscles by having the ventilator provide some or all of the power required to breathe and (c) control the rate of alveolar ventilation of a patient who is unable to meet the ventilatory demand, or has excessive or inadequate central respiratory drive.

To accomplish these goals of mechanical ventilation, the physician must be certain that the ventilator parameters of FiO_2, tidal volume (Vt), respiratory rate, and mode of ventilation are so set that the ventilator delivers an appropriate FiO_2 and minute ventilation.

An understanding of the pathophysiology that precipitated respiratory failure (identifying the adequacy of chest mechanics, derangements of resistance and compliance, the nature of parenchymal injury, the presence of air-trapping, the influence of nonpulmonary organ failure on lung function, and principles of airway management) may help the clinician implement mechanical ventilation and choose appropriate ventilatory mode, rate, tidal volume, inspiratory: expiratory ratio, PEEP/CPAP level, and other ventilatory variables.

Selection of Ventilation Mode

It is not possible to say which is the best overall ventilatory mode; such a panacea does not exist. Even though various modes are recommended highly by some authors, few prospective well-controlled studies comparing ventilatory options are available because of inhomogeneity of the population in need of respiratory support and to the large interpatient difference in measurable respiratory variables. The appropriate mode to choose depends on the patient's circumstances. *When the patient is first intubated, or during periods of instability, CMV or A/CMV ventilation is customarily utilized because it provide maximal ventilatory assistance and guarantees a lower limit of delivered ventilation.* When the patient is being evaluated for removal of machine support, pressure support ventilation, SIMV, CPAP modes, or combinations of these modes are employed.

During the initial stabilization phase, contribution of the patient to ventilation is kept at a minimum and the focus is on optimum delivery of positive pressure by ventilator preferably using controlled ventilation (CMV). When the patient's ventilatory drive is inadequate or if the patient has neuromuscular paralysis CMV is appropriate. When the patient begins to make ventilatory efforts, assist/control, intermittent mandatory ventilation (IMV) and SIMV modes are useful as long as the minimum number of mechanical breaths/minutes (backup rate) ensures adequate minute ventilation. Pressure support ventilation should not be used alone for those with depressed ventilatory drive because it only augments spontaneous ventilatory efforts. When ventilatory failure is due to reduced functional residual capacity (FRC) and increased extravascular lung water minute ventilation usually is elevated and does not need further augmentation. When such patients retain airway reflexes and are awake and cooperative, the hypoxemia and increased elastic work of breathing can be corrected with a CPAP mask. CPAP also can be the sole supportive mode in tracheally intubated patients whose spontaneous minute ventilation is adequate or whose lung mechanics have improved greatly after CPAP, for patients with cardiogenic pulmonary edema and acute intravascular volume overload. Patients, who suffer from an imbalance between the required work of breathing and their ability to perform such work e.g. patients with severe asthma, ARDS, severe lung infection or injury, and multiple organ failure, may be given partial ventilatory support (Assist-control, IMV, SIMV). It allows patients to perform whatever part of their work of breathing they are capable, with the ventilator performing the remainder of the work.

Fractional inspired Oxygen (FiO_2)

The goal of oxygen therapy is to increase oxygen delivery (DO_2) to the tissues so that oxidative phosphorylation and other oxygen-dependent metabolic processes may continue. Severely hypoxemic patients supplement ATP formation via anaerobic metabolism, but this pathway generates lactic acid with the subsequent problem of metabolic acidosis.

$$DO_2 = CO \times \text{Arterial oxygen content}$$

$$\text{Arterial } O_2 \text{ Content} = \text{Hemoglobin Concentration (g/dl)} \times O_2 \text{ Saturation} \times 1.3)$$

Increasing the FiO_2 alters only one of the above primary determinants i.e., hemoglobin O_2 saturation. Once the arterial oxygen tension (PaO_2) is increased to the level that fully saturates hemoglobin, only small additional amounts of O_2 are dissolved in the plasma with additional increases in PaO_2.

There are several risks associated with administering high FiO_2 levels. First, potent cellular toxins, most notably free oxygen radicals, are created at high partial pressures of oxygen. If the concentrations of free oxygen radicals overwhelm the lung's antioxidant defenses, cellular injury will occur. It is therefore prudent to maintain the FiO_2 below 60% in patients who need high FiO_2 for extended periods. The second risk of breathing very high concentrations of inspired oxygen is that poorly ventilated alveoli may collapse as oxygen is rapidly absorbed from the alveolus into capillary blood. At very high FiO_2, nitrogen is washed out and oxygen becomes the predominant gas in the lung, unless adequate alveolar ventilation is provided rapid absorption of alveolar gas will lead to instability of the alveoli and "absorption atelectasis". It can develop in less than an hour at an FiO_2 of 100% and can significantly increase hypoxemia. Placing patients with obstructive airway disease and chronic hypercapnia on a high FiO_2 can result in pulmonary vasodilation, and diversion of blood flow through nonaerated alveoli (intrapulmonary shunting). Thus oxygen therapy may increase dead-space ventilation and contribute to the increased hypercapnia by reducing the efficiency of CO_2 excretion. The shunt fraction varies with FiO_2 and is minimum at FiO_2 of 0.4-0.6.

What is appropriate FiO_2? The appropriate level of FiO_2 for a given patient depends on the etiology of the hypoxemia. Patients who are hypoxemic secondary to hypoventilation or VA/Q mismatch usually respond impressively to relatively small increments of FiO_2 above 21%. In contrast, patients who are hypoxemic from intrapulmonary or intracardiac shunting such as pulmonary edema, lobar pneumonia, and atelectasis are refractory to oxygen and require a high FiO_2. If the shunt fraction exceeds 40%, it is not possible to obtain an adequate PaO_2, even on an FiO_2 of 100%. In this situation, nonventilated alveoli must be recruited with help of PEEP to reduce the shunt fraction. Often, the disease responsible for the patient's hypoxemia is not well defined nor is the oxygenation status known. In these situations, the patient can be placed on an FiO_2 of 100% for a short period until measurement of PaO_2 is collected. The FiO_2 then can be adjusted to the lowest level necessary to achieve a hemoglobin oxygen saturation of $\geq$ 92%; ideally at 0.4 or less.

Tidal Volume and Ventilatory Rate

The minute ventilation is the product of Vt and ventilatory rate (MV = Vt × f). The desired Vt is chosen not only to satisfy minute ventilation requirements, but also to arrest the progressive atelectasis that can occur in supine patients when they are ventilated monotonously with only a physiologic Vt of 5 ml/kg. A practical approach to determine an adequate tidal volume is to evaluate the desired degree of chest expansion through manual ventilation and to reproduce that when patient is connected to a ventilator. A desirable expiratory Vt in most patients is 8 ml/kg. Thus, in most patients, the Vt is set at 10-12 ml/kg, is to allow for the volume compressed and lost in the ventilator circuit. Lower tidal volume may be selected in patients with severe airway obstruction where there is a concern about air-trapping, in patients with only one lung, or in patients in whom the pressure required to deliver a Vt of 10-12 ml/kg is very high (>30 cmH_2O) and injure the lung. Also if one chooses to increase the FRC to more normal level with PEEP of 4-8 cmH_2O, smaller tidal volumes should be used.

In pressure-controlled ventilation the rate of air flow decreases as the alveolar pressure rises with increasing alveolar volume and ceases entirely when alveolar pressure equals the applied airway pressure. The airway resistance and the compliance of the lung and chest wall determine the rate at which the equilibrium occurs. The patient is not guaranteed a constant Vt or specific flow pattern when a set level of pressure is applied to the airway. Instead, the delivered Vt is a function of the mechanical properties of the chest, the time allotted for inspiration, and the alveolar pressure at the beginning of inspiration. As compliance decreases, less volume enters the lung for any applied airway pressure. When airway resistance increases, inspiratory air flow decreases to the point that alveolar and airway pressures do not equilibrate at the end of inspiratory time and the alveoli do not reach their full equilibrium volume. If there is positive pressure in the alveoli at the beginning of inspiration because of air-trapping or applied PEEP, then higher applied pressure is required to maintain Vt. During pressure-controlled ventilation, Vt can rise or fall if compliance or airway resistance change.

In volume-controlled ventilation, the flow rate is predictable and predetermined. Inspiratory flow ends when a preset Vt or a preset inspiratory time has been achieved. The ventilator applies to the airway whatever pressure necessary to maintain the flow pattern against opposing resistive and elastic forces during the inspiratory phase of the respiratory cycle. For a similar Vt and mean flow rate, the peak airway pressures usually will exceed than those seen during pressure-controlled ventilation. These excessive peak pressures may contribute to lung injury.

The choice of Vt and respiratory rate are straightforward in a paralyzed patient or in a patient otherwise unable to ventilate spontaneously: the respiratory rate and Vt are set to provide the appropriate minute ventilation. The situation is more complex when the patient is able to initiate a breath. Under these conditions response can be characterized by whether the ventilator ignores patient efforts (controlled mechanical ventilation—CMV); whether it allows patients to breathe passively through the ventilator circuit continuously (CPAP) or alternating with machine assistance (IMV or SIMV) or whether the ventilator delivers increased pressure to the airway in response to the patient's inspiratory efforts (assist/control ventilation—A/CMV and pressure support ventilation). Several adjustments in ventilator settings may be needed to maintain minute volume in such patients. The large tidal volume ventilation is accompanied by high PIP, increased surfactant turnover, increased surface tension and decreased lung compliance. Increased surface tension predisposes to alveolar collapse, which is more pronounced in normal lung units. This results in decreased interstitial fluid pressure leading to transudation of fluid from extra-alveolar vessels and development of pulmonary edema. Application of PEEP (up to 10 cm H_2O) may improve the balance between surfactant generation and loss in such situations.

Respiratory Rate

During full ventilatory support with tidal volumes of 10-12 ml/kg a mechanical ventilatory rate appropriate for age (for infants 20-25 breaths/minute, for older children 15-20/min) will usually provide adequate minute volume sufficient to meet ventilatory requirement and normocarbia. Higher rates allow less time for expiration; increase mean airway pressure and cause air trapping, especially in the presence of increased airway resistance. However, in conditions where low tidal volume is used higher rates may be needed. The rates may be adjusted with guidance of $PaCO_2$ and oxygen saturation.

Inspiratory Flow Rate and the Inspiratory: Expiratory (I/E) Ratio

Time in seconds required by the ventilator to complete one inhalation (inspiration) and exhalation (expiration) is called the cycle time. Both occur within the same cycle and their ratio is called the inspiratory: expiratory (I/E) ratio. The time required to complete inspiration is a function of the average flow rate and Vt.

Ti = Vt/ Flow rate.

A larger Vt will take longer time and same Vt will take longer to deliver if flow rate is less. The inspiratory flow pattern has an impact on inspiratory time and the I/E ratio. During constant flow, the average flow rate is about equal to the peak inspiratory flow rate set on the ventilator. During decelerating or sinusoidal flow pattern the inspiratory flow rate is again equal to the peak inspiratory flow rate, but the average flow rate is lower and the inspiratory time is, therefore, longer for the same settings of peak flow and Vt.

There are several considerations guiding flow rate selection. First, higher flows require greater airway pressures to deliver the same Vt. Second, at higher flow rates rapid changes in the volume increase shear forces, risking airway and parenchymal damage. Third, in certain patients, there is a higher inspiratory flow demand because the respiratory center signals that gas be delivered to the lung at a faster rate, particularly if the minute ventilation requirements are high. If the machine flow rate is set lower than the patient's inspiratory flow demand, then the patient will pull or fight against the ventilator, increasing energy consumption. Fourth, a low inspiratory flow rate causes increase in inspiratory time and consequently shorten the available expiratory time. In patients with airflow obstruction, it may cause dangerous air trapping if the flow rate is set too low.

Several guidelines can be used while selecting a flow rate. Patients with high ventilatory requirements usually require a flow rate of at least four times the minute ventilation. In patients who initiate breaths spontaneously, the flow rate should be adjusted at the bedside to match inspiratory effort. Relatively higher flow rates should be used for patients with airflow obstruction. During pressure-controlled ventilation, the inspiratory flow rate is a function of the driving pressure, the airway resistance, and the compliance of the respiratory system. The flow rate cannot be adjusted independently from these variables.

Inspiratory time must be selected to allow sufficient time for all lung segments to be inflated. In heterogenous lung disease with varying regional time constants, a short inspiratory time may not be sufficient to inflate all lung segments and may contribute to underventilation and underinflation. Similarly, sufficient expiratory time must be provided for all lung segments to empty. If inspiration starts before the lung has completely emptied, this will result in airtrapping and inadvertent positive end-expiratory pressure.

The inspiratory time is selected to provide an I/E ratio of 1:2 to 1:3. It can be set either as percentage of total respiratory cycle or as a fixed time in seconds depending on the ventilator. In most circumstances, the I/E ratio is set at about 33% i.e. 1:2 and more typically 1:3. Lower I/E ratios provide longer expiratory times. However, under conditions of high airway resistance, a short inspiratory time will result in a lower Vt, since the alveoli do not achieve their full equilibrium volume. In such a situation higher I:E ratio may be needed. Increasing the I/E ratio (greater than 50% or 1:1), however will increase mean airway pressure and may cause air trapping. I/E ratio greater than 1:1 is generally avoided except under special circumstances. Increasing inspiratory time will distribute gas more evenly to abnormal areas and improve oxygenation, but normal alveoli may suffer barotrauma because of extended exposure to high pressure. In diseases with airway obstruction such as bronchial asthma longer expiratory time is required. A typical I:E ratio in such patients is l:4, PEEP should be avoided.

Inspiratory Pause

Lung inflation at full inspiration can be sustained by setting an inspiratory pause or plateau. The inspiratory pause control occludes the expiratory port for a set time following the delivery of the Vt. It allows variation in the I:E ratio during volume-cycled ventilation independently of the flow rate. An inspiratory pause shortens the expiratory phase of the respiratory cycle, increasing the I/E ratio. The inspiratory pause may be used for estimating alveolar pressure at end-inflation. With flow in the airway stopped, alveolar pressure equilibrates with that measured at the proximal airway by the ventilator's manometer. If end-expiratory alveolar pressure is known (PEEP or auto-PEEP), static compliance of the respiratory system can then be estimated (Compliance = Vt -[Palv-PEEP]).

PEEP (Positive-end-expiratory pressure)

PEEP has received considerable attention as a means to improve oxygenation. It is provided by a valve in exhalation limb of ventilatory circuit and is set by the physician. Physiologic PEEP/CPAP of 2-3 mmHg is an acceptable method of preventing microatelectasis during mechanical ventilation, especially when lower tidal volumes are used. In conditions associated with air trapping, reduced lung compliance, noncardiogenic pulmonary edema, and a tendency to atelactasis, use of PEEP may be needed to prevent airway closure and enhance gas exchange. Extubation of the trachea from these low PEEP levels rather than from ambient pressure may improve post-extubation pulmonary function. Goals of using PEEP are shown in Table 7.5.

Early aggressive use of PEEP in those with early evidence of lung injury may decrease duration of ventilator therapy. PEEP does not reduce extra-vascular lung water and may cause it to increase. Nevertheless, in patients with pulmonary edema, PEEP effectively increases FRC by opening (recruiting) closed airways and alveoli

Table 7.5: Goals of PEEP

- Reduction of FiO_2 to nontoxic level – 0.4 to 0.6
- Maintain PaO_2 > 60 mmHg (SpO_2 > 90%)
- Increase FRC above closing volume
- Reduce work of breathing

and prevent their collapse during expiration. It also flattens the edema fluid on the wall of respiratory tree, improves compliance, and reduce work of breathing. PEEP thus reduces V/Q mismatching and improves oxygenation.

Application of PEEP result in a higher mean airway pressure, and mean lung volumes. The optimum PEEP is the level at which there is an acceptable balance between the desired goals and undesired adverse effects. The desired goals are achieving adequate PaO_2 using "nontoxic levels" oxygen concentration while improving lung compliance.

Level of PEEP depends on clinical circumstances. Customarily PEEP is started at a low level of 3-5 mmHg and gradually increased to achieve PaO_2 between 60-90 mmHg. Currently the standard of care is to achieve SpO_2 >92% with the lowest level of PEEP that allows FiO_2 to be reduced to nontoxic levels i.e.<0.6. (See flow chart for adjusting PEEP in Procedure section). Not all hypoxemic patients are responsive to PEEP. High PEEP should therefore be used only if it allows reduction of FiO_2 to non-toxic levels or by demonstrably improving lung compliance. When using the PEEP one must be familiar with the system's mechanical characteristics.

Arbitrary limits cannot be placed on the level of PEEP or mean airway pressure that will be required to maintain adequate gas exchange. When the PEEP is high, peak inspiratory pressure may be limited to prevent it from reaching dangerous levels that contribute to airleaks and barotraumas. In children with tracheomalacia or bronchomalacia, PEEP decreases the airway resistance by distending the airways and preventing dynamic compression during expiration.

If the expiratory time is too short to allow full exhalation, the next lung inflation is superimposed upon the increased residual gas in the lung causing "breath stacking". This process may result in hyperinflation of the lung and the occurrence of PEEP not preset on the ventilator. This is called auto-PEEP or intrinsic, inadvertent, or occult PEEP. Auto-PEEP can be quantified using manual methods or through electronic programs within some ventilators. The potentially harmful physiologic effects of auto-PEEP on airway pressures and upon lung injury or cardiovascular function are the same as preset PEEP.

Reduction in undesirable auto-PEEP is usually accomplished by extending the expiratory time to allow full exhalation of tidal volume. The expiratory time can also be lengthened by prolonging the cycle time if the preset respiratory rate is reduced.

Peak Inflation Pressure (PIP)

The PIP is the amount of pressure needed to inflate the lungs. The peak inspiratory pressure that moves the chest wall is usually adequate to achieve alveolar ventilation. Diseased lungs require high PIP.

The peak inflation pressure (PIP) generated is influenced by at least five variables; the lung-thorax compliance (C) and airway resistance (Raw) of the patient, and delivered tidal volume (Vt), inspiratory flow rate (Vi) and baseline pressure (i.e., level of continuous positive airway pressure) from the mechanical ventilator. PIP varies inversely with compliance and directly with Vt, Raw and Vi. These factors may be represented mathematically by the following equation:

$$PIP = (Vt/C) + (Raw \times Vi) + \text{Baseline Pressure}$$

If the patient's compliance suddenly decreased and all other variables were essentially unchanged, then the PIP would increase. Similarly, a marked increased in Raw or in the delivered Vt and Vi from the mechanical ventilator would result in proportional increases in PIP.

High PIP and PEEP, both increase intrathoracic pressure, which may lead to reduction in venous return, cardiac output and pulmonary blood flow and reduced oxygen delivery. In addition, myocardial function may be compromised because of increased right heart after-load with right ventricular distension. This may shift intraventricular septum and affect left ventricular mechanics. To minimize these effects, high PIP should be applied only for a short time (less than 50% of a respiratory cycle), and the end expiratory pressure should be kept to minimum, so that the mean increase in intrathoracic pressure is minimal.

Alarms

Alarms on ventilators warn about potentially dangerous problems: disconnection of the patient from the ventilator: apenic episodes; and dangerously high airway pressures. The low exhaled volume and low pressure alarms detect inadequate volume or pressure delivery to the airway and alert personnel in the ICU to the possibility of machine failure, circuit disruption, ventilator disconnection, or even large bronchopleural fistulae.

Airway Pressure

The difference between the peak and plateau (end-inspiratory) airway pressure is used diagnostically. A large difference signifies abnormally increased resistance due to a narrow tracheal tube, bronchospasm, and excessively high inspiratory flows causing turbulence. Setting the low-pressure alarm at approximately 5 cm H_2O below peak inspiratory pressure will detect not only ventilator disconnection, but also the development of a leak or improved resistance. Setting the high-pressure alarm 5-10 cm H_2O above peak airway pressure will give early warning of increased resistance, decreased compliance, or the patient coughing or 'fighting' the ventilator.

The peak airway pressure alarm should be set at a level that will alert the physician to the potential for barotrauma - >40 cm H_2O. The high-pressure alarm prevents the ventilator from delivering excessive pressure to the airway during ventilation. If the airway pressure exceeds the high-pressure limit, then the ventilator depressurizes the airway, shunting the remaining volume into the expiratory port. This alarm system reduces delivered Vt. Often, the high pressure limit is reached during coughing efforts or during the dysynchronous effort of an agitated patient. Repeated alarming of the high pressure limit should prompt a careful reassessment of the patient, searching for endotracheal tube kinking, mucus plugging, bronchospasm, intubation of the right main bronchus, or a tension pneumothorax.

Potential adverse effects from high inspiratory pressure include barotrauma and reduced cardiac output. High peak inspiratory pressure usually correlates with an important indicator of alveolar distension, the inspiratory plateau pressure (IPP).The inspiratory plateau pressure is the airway pressure immediately after cessation of gas flow into the lungs during a mechanical inhalation. It can be measured at the bedside using an inspiratory hold/ pause method and best correlates with ventilator-related lung injury. The IPP should be maintained below 30 cm H_2O as far as possible. Elevated peak or plateau airway pressure may be reduced by:

- Decreasing PEEP, this may secondarily decrease oxygenation.
- Decreasing VT; this may secondarily reduce alveolar minute ventilation and lead to hypercapnia. When high pressures need to be controlled, hypercapnia may be accepted. "Permissive hypercapnia" should not be used in patients at risk for elevated intracranial pressure (ICP).
- Increasing inspiratory time; this will shorten the expiratory time and may lead to auto-PEEP.

Minute Ventilation–CO_2 Elimination

The primary determinant of CO_2 elimination during mechanical ventilation is alveolar minute ventilation, calculated as $MV = (V_T - V_D) \times rate$. Where V_T is tidal volume and V_D is dead space ventilation. CO_2 removal can be enhanced by increasing the tidal volume or rate. The physiologic V_D represents, in general, lung units that are relatively well ventilated but underperfused. The patho-physiologic effect of high amounts of V_D is hypercapnia. V_D may result from the pathological process in the lung, over distension of alveoli because of high airway pressures, low intravascular volume or low cardiac output. If hypercapnia persists during mechanical ventilation despite use of the preset V_T and appropriate rates, consultation should be sought. It may be necessary to use a low V_T to avoid high airway pressure and/or a low respiratory rate to avoid auto-PEEP, thus permitting hypoventilation and hypercapnia. This "permissive hypercapnia" technique should be initiated only with careful consideration and expert advice.

Oxygenation

On the pressure wave form of a ventilator administered breath MAP (Mean Airway Pressure) is the area under the curve it directly affects oxygenation. It is affected by PIP, PEEP, IT and flow rate. Increasing any of the above parameters will increase the MAP and hence improve oxygenation (Fig. 7.4). Most ventilators digitally display MAP. If there is a need to improve the oxygenation then either FiO_2 or the MAP may be increased.

It is difficult to give actual settings of controls of ventilators for all circumstances. If the need for assistance is because of central respiratory failure or muscular paralysis with reasonably healthy lungs, low pressure IPPR (PIP up to 25 cm H_2O) and physiologic PEEP is adequate. In diseased lungs, high pressures upto 30-40 cmH_2O may be required. The initial settings may be as follows:

Provision of Adequate Alveolar Ventilation (CO_2 removal)

- *Select rate:* Physiologic norm for age, 20-25 for children under 2 years and 15-20 for older children.
- *Select tidal volume:* 10-15 ml/kg (Volume controlled) OR Select PIP—15-25 cmH_2O (Pressure controlled). Tidal volume (10-15 ml/kg) should be adjusted to achieve visible chest excursion simulating normal breathing and audible air entry, while maintaining an oxygen saturation (SaO_2) of >90%.

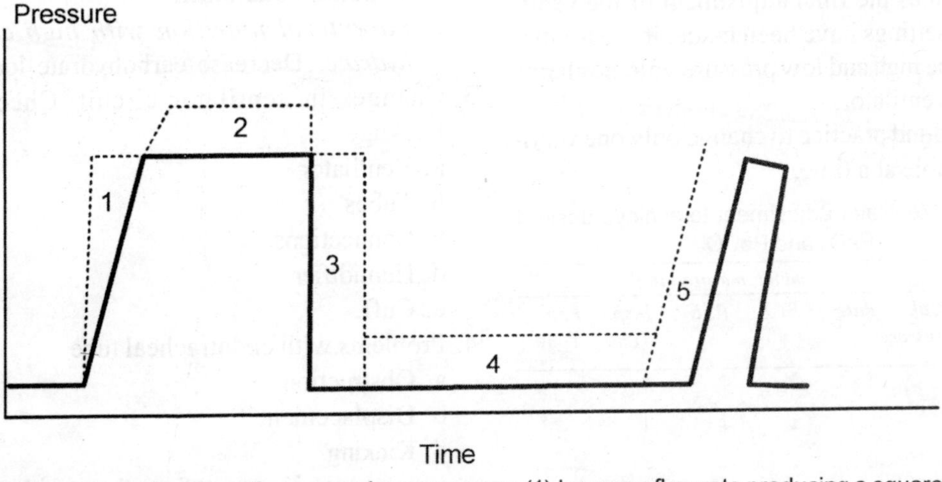

Fig. 7.4: Five ways to increase the mean airway pressure (1) Increase flow rate producing a square waveform (2) Increase PIP (3) Reverse the I : E ratio or prolong the IT (4) Increase PEEP (5) Increase ventilator rate by reducing Expiratory Time without changing IT

- *Select inspiratory time*: 0.5 second (0.35 – 0.75 second), resulting in I:E ratio 1:2 -(In obstructive lung disease set at 1:3 or 1:4- to provide prolonged expiratory time and slow rates).

Maintenance of Adequate Oxygenation

- Set FiO_2 at 0.6- 0.9, FiO_2 should be decreased to <0.5 as soon as possible to prevent oxygen toxicity and absorption atelectasis.
- PEEP—3 mmHg or higher as needed. After setting PEEP immediately assess for signs of adequate oxygenation (colour, pulse oximetery) and signs of perfusion, and measure oxygen saturation, PaO_2 and FiO_2. While maintaining PaO_2 >60 mmHg or oxygen saturation >90% in lung disease with decreased compliance, set PEEP as needed to achieve PaO_2> 60 mmHg with FiO_2 0.5- 0.6.
- Once the preliminary settings are made, the patient is connected to the ventilator. The optimum PIP and tidal volume are then assessed by listening to the air entry and exit, observing chest excursion and performing an arterial blood gas analysis. Ventilator parameters that can be changed to achieve desired PaO_2 and $PaCO_2$ are shown in Table 7.6.
- As soon as the final adjustment of the ventilatory settings have been made, it is essential to set the high and low pressure/volume alarms on the ventilator.

It is a sound practice to change only one ventilator variable at a time.

Table 7.6: Ventilator adjustment to achieve desired PaO_2 and $PaCO_2$

Desired change	*Parameter manipulated*					
	Peak pressure	*Rate*	*FiO_2*	*PEEP*	*Insp. Time*	*Exp. Time*
↑ PO_2	↑	↑	↑	↑	↑	-
↓ PaO_2	↓	-	↓	↓	↓	-
↑ $PaCO_2$	↓	↓	-	-	-	↓
↓ $PaCO_2$	↑	↑	-	↓	-	↑

Methods that Decrease O_2 Demand

1. Ventilatory.
2. Sedation/neuro-muscular block.
3. Body temperature. Maintain normothermia.
4. Adequate Cardiac output. In many patients with severe acute respiratory failure cardiac output should be kept higher than normal.

High or rising $PaCO_2$: Methods to lower $PaCO_2$ based on the cause

1. If increase in dead space ventilation:
   a. *Increase expiratory minute volume RR/ V_E*
   b. *If low cardiac output:* Increase cardiac output with inotropes
   c. *If effective PEEP too high:* Reduce PEEP
   d. *Pulmonary embolism:* Use heparin/ ventilators
   e. *Vasoconstriction in pulmonary circulation:* withdraw vasoconstrictors/give vasodilators.
2. If increase in CO_2 production
   a. *Body temperature increased:* Maintain nomothermia
   b. *Muscular activity increased:* Sedation/ neuromuscular block
   c. *Parenteral nutrition with high carbohydrate:* Decrease carbohydrate load.
3. Changes in ventilator circuit: Check for Leakage
   a. Ventilator
   b. Tubes
   c. Connections
   d. Humidifier
   e. Cuff.
4. Problems with endotracheal tube
   a. Obstruction
   b. Displacement
   d. Kinking.

In most patients, apart from those with a brain injury, a high–normal $PaCO_2$ seems preferable.

VENTILATION STRATEGIES IN COMMON CONDITIONS

To achieve ventilation, i.e. inflation of lung, one needs to negotiate airway resistance and overcome the elastic recoil of lung and chest wall. The ventilation strategies and settings therefore, mainly depend on compliance and airway resistance in a given patient. Conditions that cause decreased compliance are shown in Table 7.7.

In infants who weigh < 10 kg, time-cycled pressure –limited ventilation is the most common form of mechanical ventilation. Peak inspiratory pressure (PIP) is generally started at low levels (18-20 cm H_2O) until a pressure is reached that provides adequate chest movement. PIP can also be adjusted by monitoring tidal volume to achieve a VT in the range of 10 to 15 mL/kg. Since tidal volumes measured at the ventilator also incorporate breathing circuit expansion and gas compression volumes, the inhaled VT values may need to be ≃ 10-12 mL/ kg in infants and small

Table 7.7: Factors associated with decreased total respiratory compliance

Decreased lung compliance

1. Sufactant deficiency or dysfunction: Respiratory distress of the newborn; Acute respiratory distress syndrome
2. Interstitial inflammation : Diffuse pneumonitis, fibrosis
3. Pulmonary edema, alveolar edema, interstitial edema
4. Hyperinflation: Airway obstruction – both upper and lower, excessive CPAP/PEEP or auto-PEEP.
5. Atelectasis.

Decreased chest compliance

1. Restrictive pleural disease: Pleural collection of air or fluid, fibrosis
2. Increased intercostal muscle tone: upper motor neuron disease, drugs
3. Restrictive chest diseases: Deformation – kyphosis, scoliosis, ankylosis, restrictive bandages.

Diaphragmatic restriction

1. Abdominal distention
2. Abdominal binding
3. Increased abdominal pressure – peritoneal dialysis, post laparotomy, and so on.

children. In older children volume ventilation is the most commonly chosen mode for the initiation of mechanical ventilation. Suggested initial ventilator settings for children: VT 10 mL/kg, an inspiratory time of 0.6 to 0.7 secs for babies, 0.8 secs for toddlers, and 0.9 to 1.0 secs for school-age children and teenagers. Rates > 20 breaths/ min are usually not necessary in patients with normal lungs.

A low physiologic level of PEEP, 2 to 4 CmH_2O, is used to prevent alveolar collapse on exhalation in normal lungs, but may be increased if alveolar recruitment is a desired goal.

In conditions where the lung condition is normal ventilation depends on the specific cause: In conditions where there is pump failure i.e. respiratory muscle paralysis we need to provide synchronized mandatory ventilation (SIMV) if the patient has some muscle power and a normal ventilatory drive to continue his own respirations. If there is total muscular paralysis then controlled mechanical ventilation should be used. Volume controlled mode is preferred over pressure-controlled mode. Normal tidal volume 10 ml/kg and normal respiratory ratio ranging between 15-25 breaths/min should be set with an I:E ratio of 1:3 or 1:2 and FiO_2 0.21-0.40. Once the patient begins to regain his muscular power, the controlled mode can be gradually weaned off to SIMV/ Pressure support ventilation and then off the ventilatory support.

In a patient with raised intracranial pressure, controlled ventilation may be required to achieve necessary level of ventilation. In this case the patient is paralyzed and ventilated by volume controlled mode tidal volume (V_T) 12 ml/kg, RR = 30/min, I:E—1:3, FiO_2 - 0.21-0.4, VR is to be so adjusted that $PaCO_2$ will range between 30-35 mm of Hg. Hyperventilation may be given for a short period of time if there is an acute rise of intracranial pressure.

Pneumonia

It is better to ventilate such patients with a pressure controlled mode of ventilation as chances of air leak syndromes are maximum in these cases when too high peak inspiratory pressures are used for obtaining optimal oxygenation. While ventilating such patients the pathogenesis of desaturation should be kept in mind. Volume controlled modes may be used with low tidal volumes, I:E ratio 1:2-1:1, and high VR to maintain a good minute volume. High tidal volumes in this situation are not much useful because it increases the risk of volutrauma or barotrauma. Most atelactatic and consolidated areas give rise to significant shunting as well as ventilation perfusion mismatch. Therefore, use of very high FiO_2 (> 0.6) is not beneficial in achieving the desired SpO_2.

If $PaCO_2$ is high initially higher ventilatory rates 30 per minute and I:E ratio 1:3 may be used but after the CO_2 normalizes the rate should be accordingly readjusted. While weaning the patient synchronized intermittent mandatory ventilation may be used.

Obstructive Airway Disease

Mechanical ventilation for patients with asthma is designed to support oxygenation and assist ventilation until airway obstruction has improved. Mechanical ventilation of patients with obstructive airway disease may produce hyperinflation, auto-PEEP, and secondary hypotension. Therefore, careful attention is needed to balance cycle, inspiratory, and expiratory times.

The initial V_T should be 8 to 10 mL/kg, and the minute ventilation adjusted to a normal pH. The flow rate should be set to an optimal expiratory time (I:E) so as to allow complete exhalation. Such management reduces breath stacking and the potential for auto-PEEP. If flow rates are too high, however, inspiratory pressure may increase, potentially increasing the risk of barotraumas and lung injury.

While the patient is supported with mechanical ventilation, airway obstruction should be aggressively treated. As airflow obstruction improves, the patient will tolerate higher V_T levels and longer inspiratory times.

Acute Respiratory Distress Syndrome (ARDS)

The primary goal of any form of respiratory assistance is to treat arterial hypoxemia and prevent tissue hypoxia. Because AV shunt is the major cause of hypoxemia in ARDS, increased FiO_2 does not markedly improve PaO_2. On the contrary, inspired O_2 more than 60% can convert areas of low ventilation—perfusion ratio (Va/Q) to areas of pure shunt. Therefore, FiO_2 must be kept below 0.6 as far as possible.

In ARDS, functional residual capacity of the lung is decreased and lung compliance reduced because of interstitial as well as alveolar edema. High PEEP to recruit more alveoli and achieve a Qs/Qp less than 15% is needed. Very high PEEP (15-25 cmH_2O) can be tolerated by children with ARDS without hemodynamic compromise.

The work of breathing is immensely increased because of increased airway pressure and tachypnea. This may consume 25-50% of the O_2 consumption of the body. Therefore, one of the chief benefits of mechanical ventilation in this condition is it decreases the patient's work of breathing so that blood flow can be redirected to the other vital organs.

In ARDS there is an imbalance between the synthesis, release and consumption of surfactant leading to its serious deficiency. The rate of loss of surfactant is proportional to the phasic volume and pressure changes of the alveolus. Hence, while ventilating such patient's pressure fluctuations (ΔP) should be kept to a minimum.

Lung-Protective Ventilation

The hyperinflation of normal lung regions during mechanical ventilation can produce stress fractures in the walls of alveoli and adjacent pulmonary capillaries. The alveolar damage can lead to alveolar rupture, with accumulation of alveolar gas in the pulmonary parenchyma (pulmonary interstitial emphysema), mediastinum (pneumomediastinum), or pleural cavity (pneumothorax). The damage to the pulmonary capillaries can result in the leaky-capillary type of pulmonary edema. These complications may be the result of excessive alveolar pressure (barotrauma) or excessive alveolar volume (volutrauma).

Because of the risk of lung injury with large inflation volumes, an alternative approach has evolved in recent years where reduced inflation volumes (5-7 mL/kg) are advocated. This strategy uses positive end-expiratory pressure (PEEP) to prevent collapse of alveoli and small airways. The goal is an end-inspiratory plateau pressure that is less than 35 cm H_2O. Inflation volumes of 8 ml/kg or lower can result in CO_2 retention, which is allowed if no evidence of harm exists. This latter strategy is contrary to traditional ventilatory strategy that is aimed at avoidance of hypercarbia and respiratory acidosis. This controlled hypoventilation with hypercapnia ($PaCO_2$>50 to 70 mmHg and pH >7.2) is known as ***permissive hypercapnia***, and is being practised as part of lung protective strategy.

Key elements to be followed during ventilating a patient with ARDS are:

1. Recruit maximum functional lung units using optional PEEP.
2. Maintain the patency of airway and keep alveoli open throughout respiratory cycle.
3. Avoid alveolar over distension by keeping PIP and VT low.

Optimal Ventilatory Mode

A controversy exists between the volume cycled versus pressure limited ventilation. Intermittent mandatory ventilation is preferred by some over and above the assist control mode because of the decreased risk of barotrauma.

Ventilatory Settings

Tidal volume (V_T) 6-8 ml/kg; high tidal volume at high PIP/plateau pressure should be avoided. Large VT cause alveolar over distension and injury whereas low V_T increase the atelectatic segments due to alveolar collapse. Reduction of tidal volume over 1-2 hours to a low tidal volume (6 ml/kg) while maintaining plateau pressure <30 cmH_2O is recommended.

PEEP

PEEP is initially set at 5-6 cm H_2O and then increased in steps of 2-3 cm H_2O till SaO_2 >90% is achieved with an acceptable mean airway pressure and FiO_2< 0.6. PEEP as high as 15-20 cm H_2O, have been used. PEEP helps in recruitment of nonventilated lung units and maintenance of patency of recruited lung.

PIP

PIP should be < 35 cm H_2O as far as possible because rising PIP is proportional to amount of surfactant depletion and barotrauma.

I:E ratio

I:E ratio: 1:2 or even I:E ratio 1:1 with inspiratory hold if needed. In certain situations inverse ratio ventilation is preferred for optimal oxygenation as long as a minimum expiratory time of 0.5 seconds is maintained. Ventilator manipulations to achieve a desired change in PaO_2 and/or $PaCO_2$ are summarized in Table 7.8.

Hypoxemia is treated by increasing Paw without increasing PIP, low flow rate and inspiratory pause may accomplish the goals.

Asymmetric Lung Disease

Asymmetric lung disease or injury such as that associated with aspiration, contusion, or a localize pneumonia may cause abnormal distribution of ventilation and gas exchange during mechanical

Table 7.8: Suggested ventilator adjustments to improve oxygenation and carbon dioxide elimination

Improving Oxygenation

1. Increase FiO_2 – should be always a temporizing measure, should be kept <0.6
2. Increase Mean Airway Pressure (12-14 cmH_2O) Increase PIP (max. 35 cmH_2O)
3. Prolonged inspiratory time (Allows expansion of underventilated alveoli), add pause with usual I-E ratio; always keep a minimum expiratory time, 0.5 secs
4. High PEEP: Prevent collapse, recruit more alveoli
5. Increase rate: increase minute volume

$PaCO_2$ too high !

1. Check ventilation : tube patency, placement
2. Rule out pneumothorax
3. Ventilator function: check for too high PEEP, reduce it

Still high

4. Increase minute volume by increasing tidal volume
5. Increase ventilatory rate, 5 min at a time
6. Urgent CxR to rule out air leaks/chest disease

$PaCO_2$ too low (< 35 mmHg)!

1. Reduce minute volume by reducing rate: in step of 5/min till ventilator rate 10/min
2. Reduce tidal volume, if PaO_2 falls step up PEEP/FiO_2

ventilation. Because the conditioned gas from the ventilator follows the path of least resistance along the bronchi, the V_T is distributed primarily to the less affected (more compliant) lung and may overexpand it. Overdistension of the less affected lung and poor expansion of the diseased/ injured lung worsens ventilation-perfusion relationships in both lungs, and hypoxemia and hypercapnia may occur, persist, or worsen. Standard setting and principles of ventilatory support should be initiated.

A summary of ventilation adjustments in common conditions is given in Table 7.8 and achieve desired oxygenation and CO_2 in Table 7.9

CARE OF A PATIENT ON VENTILATOR

The following care is needed:

1. If cuffed endotracheal tube is used, cuffs must be released every 4 hourly for 5 minutes. During this period, deep pulmonary inflation is performed using a bag and O_2.
2. Repositioning of patient 2-4 hourly.
3. Change of ventilator tubings periodically.
4. Filling up of humidifier with sterile water daily.
5. Checking the humidifier traps, condensation and temperature.
6. Wash compressor filter daily.
7. Culture of respiratory endotracheal secretions daily to monitor the microbial flora.
8. Provision of adequate calories—Oral feeds of the ventilated child with an endotracheal tube is not possible, since the tube interfere with normal swallowing. However, the majority of ventilated children may be fed enterally via a nasogastric tube. The few patients in whom enteral feeding is not possible because of ileus or abdominal pathology should receive parenteral nutrition. Whichever the route is chosen, an attempt to meet caloric and protein requirements must be made.

Table 7.9: Suggested ventilator adjustments in common conditions

PARENCHYMAL DISEASES

1. Peak pressure—high, up to 30-35 mmHg, to achieve VT 6-8 ml/kg
2. More inspiratory time, IE ratio 1:2, 1:1, give inspiratory pause
3. PEEP—high up to 12-15 mmHg specially in ARDS, set at optimal level till it improves oxygenation
4. Rate—above physiologic range, up to 30-35/min
5. Decrease work of breathing by neuromuscular blockage

AIRWAY OBSTRUCTION

Lungs hyperinflated with atelactasis, Resistance -increased, Shunting and V/Q mismatching

1. Do not keep high pressure/ Avoid 'Pressure Control'
2. Tidal volume 8-10 ml/kg
3. More expiratory time, IE ratio at least 1:3, better 1:4
4. Low level of PEEP- 2-3 mmHg

RAISED ICP

1. Adequate minute ventilation to keep $PaCO_2$ to 30-35 mmHg
2. Avoid high PEEP, PEEP impedes venous return hence increases CVP
3. Neuromuscular blockage

9. Sedation and muscle relaxants: particular attention is needed in following situations:
   - Requirement for high airway pressure (e.g. asthma, ARDS)
   - Critically inadequate oxygenation (e.g. ARDS)
   - Ventilator intolerance in anxious patients
   - Need for controlled hyperventilation.

   Before switching to muscle relaxants (Pancuronium, vecuronium) adequate sedation and analgesia should be achieved with help of diazepam (0.2 mg/kg IV) and morphine (0.1 - 0.2 mg/kg IV).

Ongoing Clinical Appraisal to Answer

- Is the endotracheal tube patent and in place, or is it becoming occluded or misplaced?
- Are the lungs hyperinflated?
- Is there a pneumothorax?
- Is there pulmonary oedema?
- Is the systemic circulation becoming compromised?
- Is there a large leak around an endotracheal tube that is too narrow?
- Does the child require a muscle relaxant?
- Is the child ready for weaning to IMV or CPAP?

Following variables should be measured and recorded continuously or periodically to assess proper functioning of ventilator and oxygen delivery or demand:

1. FiO_2.
2. I : E ratio.
3. Tidal volume (both inspiratory and expiratory), flow rate, ventilator rate and minute ventilation.
4. Peak inspiratory pressure and mean airway pressure.
5. Confirmation of all preset alarms for gas supply, airway pressures, apnea, inspired O_2 concentration etc.
   No change in ventilator setting should be done without recording the reason and the change.
6. Temperature of inspired gas.
7. Oxygen saturation of hemoglobin (SpO_2) and end-tidal CO_2.
8. Heart rate, rhythm (continuous ECG), oscilloscopic BP–(intermittent check with sphygmomanometer).
9. Temperature (core and peripheral).

The following variables must be monitored at variable intervals depending on the clinical condition of the patient and change in ventilator settings:

1. Arterial blood gases (ABGs) and DO_2 calculation within 20-30 mins of initiating ventilation and after a change in ventilator setting and every 6 hourly unless there is a marked change in patient's condition, which requires more frequent assessment.
2. Measurement of vital capacity, negative inspiratory force, and dynamic compliance.
3. Chest X-ray—to look for position of endotracheal tube, overall lung volume—collapse or hyperinflation, air leaks, and heart size. Once daily or in two days, or if any acute deterioration occurs.

Other variables that should be monitored are:

1. Intake and output measurement and their calculation every 8 hourly.
2. Blood biochemistry—electrolytes and urea, coagulation parameters.
3. Nutritional support—Enteral and parenteral.
4. Nutritional status and weight.

COMPLICATIONS OF VENTILATION

Numerous complications may occur during mechanical ventilation which contribute to patient morbidity and mortality. These may be classified as follows:

1. Related to increased airway pressures and lung volume
   A. Barotrauma/ Volutrauma: Pulmonary interstitial pneumonia, pneumothorax, pneumopericardium, pneumo-peritonium, subcutaneous emphysema (Discussed below)

B. Decreased Cardiac filling and poor perfusion
C. Other organ dysfunction; Renal, hepatic, CNS
D. Pulmonary parenchymal damage
E. Acid base disturbances – if minute volume is incorrectly set

2. Related to Endotracheal / Tracheostomy tube
   - Tracheal, laryngeal and pharyngeal mucosal damage especially with intubations > 3 weeks
   - Sinusitis/Middle ear infection (nasal ET tubes)
   - Laryngeal edema, subglottic stenosis
3. Nosocomial Infections
   - Ventilator associated pneumonia
   - Sepsis
4. Mechanical Operational Problems
   - Mechanical failure
   - Alarm failure
   - Inadequate humidification
5. Complications of prolonged sedation and muscle relaxants use
   - Myocardial depression and hypotension
   - Critical care myopathy and neuropathy.

Some of these complications may be sudden and other gradual. A practical guide to causes of deterioration during ventilation is given in Table 7.10.

Table 7.10: Causes of deterioration during ventilation

ACUTE

Sudden fall in SpO_2, cyanosis, pallor, fall in BP, poor capillary refill, bradycardia

- Tube blockage/displacement
- Pneumothorax, pulmonary hemorrhage interstitial emphysema
- Massive bleed
- Septic shock
- Ventilator malfunction

GRADUAL

- Persistence/development of retractions
- Increasing ventilatory requirement
- Inspissated secretions in tube
- Diffuse segmental/sub-segmental atelactasis
- Pneumonia, pulmonary interstitial emphysema.

Barotrauma

The airway pressure and the tidal volumes required to maintain adequate gas exchange might contribute to lung injury. Some of these are apparent such as pneumothorax (air leaks). Other are more subtle and gradual. These are leakage of fluid, proteins and blood into tissues and air spaces or leakage of air into tissue spaces. This process is followed by an inflammatory response and possibly a reduced defense against infection. Hypoxic vasoconstriction of edema filled segment can produce a potentially insurmountable problem.

Lung impaired by disease processes face a potentially insurmountable problem. The mechanical ventilation in such a clinical setting generally presupposes the existence of some remaining, reasonably healthy pulmonary parenchyma that participates in gas exchange. These healthy regions are well ventilated and well perfused, while the remaining regions of the lungs are ventilated and perfused at abnormal VA/Q ratios. Mechanical ventilation preferentially directs the bulk of gas flow to the most compliant regions of the lung, subjecting those parts of the lungs to the bulk of airway pressure, volume and flow, and leads to overexpansion well beyond the normal. When healthy lung volume is reduced by 50%, or even 75%, to sustain adequate alveolar ventilation and hence $PaCO_2$, the ventilation of the remaining small lung will have to be increased by nearly 100% and 300%, respectively, with substantial increase in Vt and/or increase in respiratory rate. Thus the total fraction of pulmonary parenchyma taking part in gas exchange is reduced to varying degrees by the underlying disease and ventilation per unit volume is greatly increased. The higher metabolic load in sick patients may place an additional burden to increase alveolar ventilation. This combination invariably leads to a rise in peak inflation pressure and high mean airway pressure, alterations in pulmonary cellular functions and finally to barotrauma. It affects mostly the healthiest hence, the most complaint region of the lungs, and is further aggravated by structural immaturity of lungs in infants and children.

The primary offending factor causing barotraumas is high peak inflation pressure with high incidence at pressure above 40 cm H_2O. The apparent site of disruption is the common border of the alveolar base and the vascular sheath. An early indicator of barotrauma is pulmonary interstitial emphysema, which may manifest as linear air streaking toward the hilum. Its presence complicates patient management and greatly increase the risk of morbidity and mortality.

The onset of air leaks alone is a marker of underlying cellular dysfunction, indicative of type II alveolar cellular dysfunction. Those lungs become atelectatic because of surfactant depletion and require high airway pressures and positive-end-expiratory pressure (PEEP) to maintain lung volume. A brief period of mechanical ventilation could evoke significant injury to alveolar cellular function. Importantly, these changes may not be apparent immediately while on mechanical ventilation, but appear late.

Prevention

Preventing regional or global overdistension of lung parenchyma can minimize the barotrauma. Cardinal step to prevent mechanical ventilation-induced lung injury lies in lowering the peak inflation pressure. This can be accomplished by keeping tidal volumes down, construction of a compliance curve, by change in the inspiratory/expiratory ratio, by reduction in peak flow, by using higher respiratory rates, by judicious use of paralysis and sedation, by using only necessary PEEP levels, by change in body position, by control of body temperature, by tolerating mildly elevated $PaCO_2$, by limiting FiO_2 or by possible use of pulmonary surfactant, to switch from one mode of ventilation to another mode of ventilation.

Airway pressure release mode of ventilation also minimizes peak inspiratory pressure while supplying a continuous positive airway pressure. Extra pulmonary oxygenation using ECMO can facilitate lung recovery by permitting use of lower ventilatory pressures, volumes and rates.

Mechanical ventilation is well tolerated by normal lung save for the discomfort. Adverse effects from mechanical ventilation occur primarily becuase of over ambitious ventilation of greatly reduced healthy lung volume, and lung volume still recruitable, at pressures, volumes, PEEP settings, inspiratory/ expiratory ratio, types of oxygen/air flows and frequencies. Efforts to achieve ideal alveolar ventilation and adequate arterial blood gases, and to correct, in part, the VA/Q imbalance; beyond a certain point lead to primary functional and parenchymal impairment from effects of mechanical ventilation. Those adverse changes manifest in worsening in lung compliance, barotrauma, adverse changes in VA/Q ratio, changes in microvascular permeability and in rise in extravascular lung water content, in addition to alterations in the biochemical function of the lung and the resulting systemic effects.

CARDIOVASCULAR EFFECT OF MECHANICAL VENTILATION

Positive intrathoracic pressure may influence cardiac function beneficially or detrimentally, depending on the state of the patient's myocardium. The normal preload dependent heart will decrease its output. When intrathoracic pressure is raised with positive pressure ventilation and/or high PEEP the right arterial and central venous pressure increases and the gradient for blood flow to heart decreases. As a result, venous return falls lowering right ventricular pre load and stroke volume and left ventricular stroke volume. The blood pressure may decrease. These changes are more pronounced in hypovolemic patients. Improved arterial oxygenation must therefore, be carefully evaluated after institution of positive pressure maneuvers to ensure that PaO_2 has not been improved at the expense of cardiac output, and decreasing O_2 delivery. Patients with abnormally increased preload (the failing heart) improve cardiac function as raised airway pressure decreases cardiac afterload and preload.

When hypovolemia is present or suspected, appropriate intravenous fluid must be administered and a ventilatory mode that offers low mean airway pressure is preferable until euvolemia is achieved. These patients typically fair better with as much spontaneous ventilation as possible to preserve the thoracic venous pump, a slow rate of mechanical ventilation, and ambient expiratory airway pressure. Almost all ventilatory parameters alter mean airway pressure. Whether the patient's cardiovascular system, intracranial pressure, and renal and hepatic perfusion can tolerate such change must be carefully evaluated before making the changes in ventilatory settings.

Other Cause of Hypotension Associated with Initiation of Mechanical Ventilation

Tension Pneumothorax

When hypotension occurs immediately after initiation of mechanical ventilation, tension pneumothorax is most likely. It is diagnosed by decreased or absent breath sounds and hyper-resonant percussion on the side of the pneumothorax. Tracheal deviation away from the side of the pneumothorax may be observed, although is uncommon after placement of an endotracheal tube. Treatment includes emergent decompression by inserting a large-bore catheter or needle into the second or third intercostals space in the midclavicular line. Treatment should not be delayed for chest radiographic documentation. This procedure is both diagnostic and therapeutic, improving blood pressure and reversing physical examination findings. The insertion of the catheter or needle must be followed by chest tube placement.

Auto-PEEP

Auto-PEEP occurs when the combination of ventilator setting and patient physiology result in an inadequate expiratory time. Excessive end-expiratory pressure may increase intrathoracic pressure and cause hypotension due to decreased venous return to the heart and/or barotrauma. Putting the less involved lung in the gravitationally dependent (decubitus) position may be helpful in directing pulmonary blood flow to lung units receiving better ventilation. Other techniques such as differential lung ventilation may be required.

Although auto-PEEP may occur in any patient, patients with obstructive airway disease are particularly predisposed to this condition. Assessment and treatment of auto-PEEP are described on page 62.

WEANING FROM VENTILATOR

Ventilator weaning is the process of gradual decrease in ventilatory support after recovery from the disease. It should be started when there is demonstrable improvement or resolution of the problem necessitating ventilation and patient has normal central ventilatory drive.

Patients who have been ventilated for brief periods of time (e.g., overnight ventilation following major surgery) may be liberated from mechanical ventilation rapidly after termination of sedation. In contrast patients who have been critically ill for long periods of time (days), the process of withdrawal of ventilatory support is often protracted. Day-to-day changes in the patient's condition during this period of respiratory convalescence often necessitate the temporary reintroduction of more substantial mechanical ventilatory support.

Several criteria for weaning have been laid down (Table 7.11), but these may be unnecessary or difficult to measure in infants. Serial measurements of vital capacity are most useful. In infants

Table 7.11: Criteria for weaning

Clinical	
1.	Stable pulmonary status without evidence of pneumonia, severe infection or bronchospasm
2.	Satisfactory muscle power
3.	Cardiovascular stability: no need for vasoactive drugs
4.	Afebrile
Ventilation and oxygenation parameters	
1.	Tidal vol > 5 ml/kg
2.	Vital capacity > 10 ml/kg
3.	PaO_2 > 60 mmHg at FiO_2 < 0.4, normal $PaCO_2$
4.	Maximum voluntary ventilation > 2 x minute volume
5.	Maximum inspiratory pressure < -20 cm H_2O
6.	PaO_2 to FiO_2 ratio > 200.
7.	Alveolar to arterial O_2 gradient $(A\text{-}a)DO_2$ <350mmHg at 100% oxygen
8.	Shunt fraction <15%
9.	V_D/V_T ratio <0.6
10.	FRC > 50% predicted
11.	Minute ventilation <180 ml/kg/min for $PaCO_2$ of 40 mmHg.

respiratory rate and blood gas remain the major determinants for weanability. A good guide is a stable cardiovascular system, absence of metabolic abnormalities such as hypoglycemia, intact chest wall and diaphragm (capable of generating negative pressure), and stable arterial blood gases at inspired oxygen content of less than 40% (i.e.FiO_2 < 0.4).

It should be done in a timely manner supported by objective observation of pulmonary mechanics and functions. Patients who have been ventilated for a period of less than 2-3 days and who were in good health prior to their acute respiratory problem may usually be taken off straight from the ventilator and allowed to breathe spontaneously. Gradual weaning is needed in patients with severe respiratory failure or for those demonstrating ongoing ventilatory muscle fatigue at lower mechanical ventilatory. The rate of weaning should be determined mainly by the patient's clinical appearance. Factors that may delay weaning are shown in Table 7.12. Weaning may be difficult in certain patients (Table 7.13).

Table 7.12: Factors which may cause delay in weaning

1. Diminished respiratory muscle strength
   - Diaphragmatic fatigue
   - Dyselectrolytemia (K, Ca, Mg)
   - Malnutrition
   - Prolonged use of muscle relaxants
2. Respiratory muscle paralysis—Central/ Peripheral
3. Increased work of breathing
   - Laryngeal edema—airway obstruction
   - Pneumonia
   - Collapse
   - Chronic lung disease
4. Increased ventilatory requirements
   - i. Increased dead space—collapse
   - ii. Increased CO_2 production

Table 7.13: Clinical conditions associated with weaning difficulties

1. Persistence of the primary pathology
2. Untreated cardiovascular or renal failure
3. Malnutrition
4. Sepsis or pyrexia (increased metabolic demands)
5. Fluid overload
6. Residual sedation
7. Delirium/coma
8. Electrolyte imbalance (particularly Ca++, K+, PO_4^{3})
9. Anemia
10. Pain
11. Abdominal distension

Above factors must be addressed before initiating the process. Certain pre-requisite tests should also be obtained (Table 7.14). Respiratory depressant drugs should be avoided before initiating periods of spontaneous ventilation and additional humidified oxygen should be given via tube during these periods.

Table 7.14: Prerequisite tests before weaning

1. Chest X-ray – Improvement/normal/No fresh area of consolidation
2. Blood gases – pH 7.35 – 7.45, PO_2 60-80 torr. PCO_2 – 40-50 torr
3. PCV –0 35- 45%
4. Serum Na^+, K^+, Ca^+, Mg^{++} - within normal limit.

Principles of Ventilator Changes During Weaning

It is important to recognize the indication for ventilation; most patients are able to breath spontaneously. Once the reason for which the patient required ventilation is gone; ventilatory support may be discontinued. This may sound rather elementary, but the plan for discontinuation of ventilatory support should begin when the support is instituted. Daily trials of spontaneous breathing on CPAP (5 cmH_2O) or T-piece, after discontinuation of sedation and muscle relaxants can effectively identify patients ready for weaning. Prior to trials of spontaneous breathing patient should be arousable, hemodynamically stable with vasopressors, having low ventilatory and PEEP requirement, and FiO_2 need <0.4.

Gradual discontinuation of ventilatory support is done by reducing the parameters most closely associated with barotraumas viz. FiO_2 (to 0.4), PEEP (to minimum-physiological level), PIP, tidal volume and VR. The changes are made in one parameter at a time. First of all FiO_2 is brought down to 0.4 and then PEEP and PIP are brought down step by step.

Weaning from pressure-controlled ventilation is achieved by gradual reduction of PIP in steps of 2-3 cmH_2O alternating with ventilator rate (3-5 at a time). Once PIP of 20 cm of H_2O is reached further reduction should be made in ventilator rate only. On volume controlled ventilation tidal volume and rate are reduced step by step. Once minimal settings are achieved one may opt for any of the weaning modes described below.

Methods of Weaning

The most commonly used methods are IMV or SIMV, followed by T-tube or CPAP trials, and pressure support ventilation. A more recent mode is mandatory minute ventilation (MMV). No matter which method is used, majority of children can be successfully weaned from the ventilator.

IMV or SIMV is successful in most of the patients. In this mode, work of breathing performed by the ventilator is gradually decreased by slowly decreasing the IMV rate while the patient increases the number of spontaneous breaths. The work performed by the patient gradually increases. CPAP trials are used when ventilatory rate is about 15 breaths/min. The patient is kept in a CPAP circuit for a specified period of time (to start with, 5 min 4 times a day). This is followed by full ventilatory support. The time period of CPAP is gradually increased until ventilatory support is discontinued.

Intermittent Mandatory Ventilation

A rule of thumb for choosing an appropriate mechanical ventilatory rate during IMV or SIMV is to reduce the mandatory rate as long as the arterial pH exceeds 7.35 in patients with adequate ventilatory drive and no clinical signs of ventilatory muscle fatigue, particularly no increase in respiratory rate is seen. If one uses a trigger, care must be exercised to ensure that the trigger is sensitive enough and has low enough inertia so as not to increase the work of breathing. The negative airway pressure swings at the outset of spontaneous inspiration should not be more negative than 2 cmH_2O below expiratory pressure.

When using a continuous flow IMV system with an inspiratory reservoir bag, the continuous flow of air must be controlled attentively. When flow is too low, inspiratory effort will increase. When the flow is too high, it may increase the mechanically delivered tidal volume due to late closure of the valve.

Pressure Support Ventilation

In the pressure support ventilation, once the patient's inspiratory effort has triggered the ventilation, a positive pressure in the circuit enables full tidal volume breathings. The pressure initially is generally set at the same level as PIP that is about 20 cmH_2O, and the brought down in steps of 2-3 cmH_2O to 5-10 cmH_2O. At this level support is withdrawn. This method has the advantage of minimizing the work of breathing on breath-by-breath basis while making the patient initiate the breath. It also allows better coordination with the ventilator, larger tidal volume and efficient breathing. However, in very small infants this method may not be desirable.

Non-augmented, spontaneous tidal volume should be measured and followed during pressure support ventilation. PSV should be used only in hemodynamically stable patients with reliable respiratory drive.

Children who have been ventilated for a longer period need to be weaned gradually. In this phase the emphasis is on the ways of enhancing the return of full diaphragmatic function and discontinuation of mechanical ventilation. It is now well recognized that diaphragmatic fatigue is the main cause of failure of weaning. Therefore, in this phase the focus is on training the ventilatory muscles. It is done by allowing increasing period of spontaneous ventilation for several days. Initially this is done during daytime, starting with 10 minutes/hour, and increasing gradually to several hours at a time.

Throughout weaning, a close watch on the pulse and respiratory rate must be kept and blood gases must be checked at the end of each weaning period off the ventilator (Table 7.15). Never hurry. Bronchodilators such as aminophylline and sympathomimetics act as adjuncts to improve diaphragmatic functions, and may be useful during weaning.

Table 7.15: Monitoring during weaning

1. Clinical
   a. Resp. rate, pattern, depth, retraction chest expansion, air entry
   b. Signs of anxiety – diaphoresis, restlessness
   c. Cardiovascular–Heart rate, BP, Capillary refill, pallor
2. ECG—Continuous
3. Oxygen saturation, $EtCO_2$
4. Chest X-ray (after 6-12 hours)
5. Blood gases

If the patient is able to breath spontaneously, without signs of distress and anxiety, and maintain SpO_2 and $EtCO_2$, during the weaning, it is time to consider extubation.

Common Sources of Difficulty in Weaning

1. **Rapid breathing** is the most common problem in weaning. It may be because of anxiety or true weaning failure such as muscle fatigue and cardio pulmonary disease. An increase in tidal volume suggests anxiety, whereas a decrease in tidal volume suggests true weaning failure. When the tidal volume is unchanged or increased, arterial blood gases can help. A decrease in arterial PCO_2 suggest anxiety (hyperventilation) and is managed with sedation, whereas an unchanged or rising arterial PCO_2 indicates true weaning failure and resumption of ventilatory support.
2. **Abdominal paradox** during weaning is a possible sign of a diaphragmatic weakness. When the diaphragm is weak, the negative intra-thoracic pressure created by the accessory muscles of respiration pulls the diaphragm upward into the thorax. This decreases the intra-abdominal pressure and causes a paradoxical inward displacement of the abdomen during inspiration, known as abdominal paradox. It is also a sign of labored breathing, and should prompt immediate return to full ventilatory support.
3. **Hypoxemia:** One potential cause of hypoxemia that deserves mention in the setting is a decrease in cardiac output. The hypoxemia in this case is caused by a decrease in mixed venous oxygen saturation (SvO_2). SvO_2 can be an important measurement in the evaluation of hypoxemia during weaning.
4. **Hypercapnia** is an ominous sign during weaning, and should prompt immediate return to full ventilatory support. The gradient between end-tidal CO_2 and arterial PCO_2 can help identify

the problem. An increase in the $PaCO_2$ –CO_2 gradient indicates an increase in dead space ventilation from a decrease in cardiac output or hyperinflation with intrinsic PEEP whereas an unchanged gradient suggests respiratory muscle fatigue or enhanced CO_2 production.

5. **Low Cardiac Output:** The transition from positive-pressure ventilation to negative-pressure spontaneous breathing can result in a decrease in cardiac output, which is (caused by an increase in left-ventricular afterload. This can add to the difficulty of spontaneous breathing by promoting pulmonary congestion and also by impairing diaphragm function. A drop in cardiac output can decrease the strength of diaphragmatic contractions. Low cardiac output can also promote hypoxemia through a decrease in mixed venous O_2 saturation. These deleterious effects of a low cardiac output should be considered in patients with cardiac dysfunction who do not tolerate spontaneous breathing.

Detecting a Low Cardiac Output: A decrease in cardiac output will increase O_2 extraction in the systemic capillaries, and this will be reflected in an increase in the (SaO_2 –SvO) difference. The SaO_2 is easily monitored with a pulse oximeter, and the SvO_2 can be measured with a central venous catheter in the superior vena cava. The (SaO_2- SaO_2) is normally about 25%, and it will increase to 50% in low output states.

A simpler method is to calculate the difference between the arterial and end-tidal PCO_2; both are equal in healthy subjects. A decrease in cardiac output will decrease end – tidal PCO_2 relative to arterial PCO_2 and this will be reflected in an increase in the $PaCO_2$ – $PETCO_2$) difference. An increase in dead-space ventilation from lung disease will also increase the ($PaCO_2$ – $PETCO_2$) gradient. In patients who show evidence of a reduced cardiac output during breathing, CPAP can help by eliminating the increased after load caused by negative intrathoracic pressures. In patients who show a favorable response, CPAP can be continued after extubation (by face mask) if necessary.

Overfeeding

An increase in the daily intake of calories is associated with an increase in metabolic CO_2 production. If the daily intake of calories exceeds the daily caloric requirements the excess, CO_2 that is produced nust be removed by the lungs. This requires an increase in minute ventilation, and this can add to the difficulty of sustaining spontaneous breathing.

Tracheostomy during Weaning

Tracheostomy may aid weaning, particularly in patients who have been ill for some time. Advantages of tracheostomy include:

1. *Reduced sedation requirements*—most patients require little or no sedation in order to tolerate a tracheostomy, in contrast to endotracheal tubes, which are very irritating.
2. *Improved nutrition*—largely a result of reduced sedation.
3. *Improved oropharyngeal toilet*—may reduce incidence of nosocomial pneumonia.
4. Reduced airway resistance.
5. Easier access to lower respiratory tract secretions.
6. Flexibility with changes in respiratory support.

Tracheal Extubation

When the patient no longer requires ventilator support, the next step is to remove the endotracheal tube, if possible. Successful weaning from mechanical ventilation is not synonymous with tracheal decannulation. The patient should be evaluated for extubation. If there is a good cough, no evidence of excessive swelling around the endotracheal tube (e.g., passing a cuff deflation test), and the patient is neurologically intact and able to protect the airway, extubation should be performed. When a patient has successfully weaned but is not fully awake, or is unable to clear respiratory secretions, the tracheal tube should be left in place.

Tracheal extubation is usually accompanied by an increased work of breathing, presumably as a result of laryngeal edema produced by endotracheal tubes. Tracheal extubation should therefore never be performed to simply reduce the work of breathing. The signs of upper airway obstruction following extubation are labored breathing and stridor. Because the obstruction is extra-thoracic, the stridor occurs during inspiration (when the negative pressure of inspiration leads to narrowing in the extra-thoracic portion of the upper airways). Inspiratory stridor is a sign of severe obstruction (more than 80%), and should prompt immediate reintubation.

The management of severe upper airway obstruction after extubation includes reintubation followed by tracheostomy. Role of corticosteroids in reducing the severity of postextubation laryngeal edema is doubtful. Aerosolized epinephrine (2.5 mL of 1% epinephrine or 2.25% racemic epinephrine) is effective in reducing postextubation laryngeal edema in children. However, epinephrine treatments should never delay reintubation.

Removal of Tracheostomy Tubes

An evaluation for upper airway obstruction is important before removal of tracheostomy tubes. If there is no evidence of upper airway obstruction after 24 hours of breathing with the tracheostomy tube plugged, then the tube can be removed.

Tracheal stenosis following tracheostomy usually occurs at the site of the tracheal incision. This complication usually becomes evident after the tracheal stoma closes, and is thus a late complication of tracheostomy (usually appearing after the patient leaves the ICU).

WEANING PROTOCOL

1. If the criteria for weaning are satisfied obtain Chest X-ray, ABG, PCV and electrolytes (all must be normal).
2. Stop ventilatory support and allow spontaneous breathing for 5 minutes through T-tube.
3. Trial of spontaneous breathing is given for 2 hours if any two of following 3 criteria are fulfilled during this 5 minutes period.
   a. Maximum inspiratory pressure below – 20 cm of H_2O
   b. Tidal volume above 5 ml/kg
   c. Respiratory rate < 40/minute in children 1-5 years, <50 in infants.

   Monitor Respiratory rate and pattern, heart rate, chest expansion, air entry, heart rate, ECG, BP, SaO_2, ABG and chest X-ray.

   Trial of spontaneous breathing is discontinued if any of following sign develop:
   a. Respiratory rate > 40/min in children 1-5 years, > 50 / min in infants.
   b. Heart rate > 180/min or sustained increase or decrease by 20% in heart rate
   c. O_2 Saturation < 90%
   d. Anxiety diaphoresis
   e. Hypotension or Hypertension.
4. Another trial of spontaneous breathing for two hours can be given after 24 hours.

   If no respiratory distress during trial: Plan extubation immediately, except where tube is needed to prevent aspiration in patients with underlying CNS diseases.

Chapter eight

Acute Heart Failure

Heart failure occurs when the heart fails to maintain a cardiac output (CO) sufficient for the metabolic needs of the body, or when it can only do so at the expense of abnormally elevated end-diastolic pressures. Heart failure is not a diagnosis *per se,* but a clinical syndrome; the underlying disease must always be sought and treated. Heart failure is not a single entity but can be classified according to the side the heart that is involved (right-sided vs. left-sided failure) or the portion of the cardiac cycle that is affected (diastolic vs. systolic failure).

Left ventricular failure: The hemodynamic consequences of progressive left-sided heart failure are as follows: The earliest sign of ventricular dysfunction is an increase in cardiac filling pressures. The stroke volume is maintained, but at an elevated filling pressure. The next stage is a decrease in stroke volume and an increase in heart rate. The tachycardia offsets the reduction in stroke volume; CO may be maintained. The final stage is characterized by a decrease in cardiac output. Thus, increased end-diastolic volumes and pressures in left ventricle characterize left ventricular failure. These in turn result in increased pulmonary hydrostatic pressure and pulmonary edema.

Right ventricular failure involves similar processes on the right side of heart to leading to raised filling pressures systemic venous hypertension, peripheral edema, hepatomegaly, etc. Contractile failure of the right ventricle results in an increase in end-diastolic volume and only when the increase in volume of the right heart is impeded by the pericardium does the end-diastolic pressure (CVP) rise. The hemodynamic changes in right heart failure can appear like the hemodynamic changes in pericardial tamponade

Biventricular failure occurs either as a result of involvement of both ventricles in the disease process or secondary to left ventricular failure progressively embarrassing right ventricular performance. The latter occurs as a result of raised left arterial pressures and hence pulmonary hypertension, which increases the resistance against which the right ventricle has to work and left ventricular dilatation impinging on right ventricular filling.

Diastolic heart failure is a combination of impaired ventricular relaxation and a decrease in passive ventricular distensibility. In this type of heart failure, the decrease in cardiac output is due to inadequate ventricular filling, not impaired systolic contraction. Common causes of diastolic heart failure include ventricular hypertrophy, and positive-pressure mechanical ventilation. The end-diastolic pressure is increased in both types of heart failure, but an increased end-diastolic volume distinguishes diastolic from systolic heart failure.

High-output heart failure: Certain clinical circumstances (such as arteriovenous malformation, severe anemia, or-thyrotoxicosis) require an increased cardiac output to maintain tissue perfusion. The capacity of the heart to increase

CO is limited, and if requirements exceed this capacity then heart failure can develop.

Causes of cardiac failure

Impaired ventricular function: Diffuse myocardial disease, myocarditis, cardiomyopathy, arrhythmias, metabolic alterations such as hypoglycemia etc.

Ventricular inflow obstruction: Mitral or triscupid valve stenosis, constrictive pericarditis, endocardial fibrosis, left ventricular hypertrophy, pulmonary embolus,

Ventricular volume overload: Increased metabolic demand, e.g., sepsis, hyperthyroidism, intracardiac shunting, etc. VSD, ASD, valvular incompetence, eg. mitral or aortic incompetence.

Ventricular outflow obstruction: Systemic hypertension, aortic stenosis, pulmonary hypertension, and pulmonary stenosis.

Clinical features:

Symptoms: Infants may present with irritability, poor feeding, sweating, cough, and grunting. Older children may have cough, wheezing, dyspnea, peripheral edema and other features specific to cause; they may complain of chest pain and orthopnea, and productive of pink frothy sputum

Signs: Tachycardia (a sustained HR of more than 180 beats per min (bpm) in infants, 150 beats per minute in children upto 5 years and more than 130 bpm in children older than 5 years), 3rd heart sound/ gallop rhythm is typically seen with AHF. Heart of more than 220 – 240 bpm in infants and 150 – 170 bpm in older children raises the likelihood of supraventricular tachycardia.

Tachypnea as a result of pulmonary edema due to left ventricular failure is a common sign of acute myocardial failure in children.

Signs of poor CO and peripheral perfusion: cold extremities, poor quality of pulses, mottled or pale skin, prolonged capillary refill time, sweating, elevated jugular venous pressure, peripheral and sacral edema, basal inspiratory crackles; in severe cases may progress to widespread crackles and wheeze, hepatomegaly an indication of venous congestion (pulsatile in tricuspid regurgitation – transmitted V wave), ascites, and signs specific to cause, e.g., endocarditis, murmurs of valvular lesions.

Chest X-ray

The X-ray may show any of the following:

1. Pulmonary venous hypertension: vascular engorgement of the upper pulmonary vessels
   - Prominent pulmonary venous markings - Interstitial edema
   - Kerley B lines (fluid-filled peripheral pulmonary septae, seen laterally in the lower lobes),
   - Kerley A lines (edematous central septae) radiate towards the hila in the mid-and upper-lobes, much thinner than adjacent blood vessels.
   - Loss of distinction of blood vessels due to fluid collecting around them.
   - Edema fluid in lobar fissures.

2. Bat-wing edema indicative of left heart failure: bilateral, involving all lobes, maximal near the hilae and fading out peripherally

3. Cardiomegaly (i.e., cardio thoracic ratio more than 0.55 in infants and more than 0.5 in patients older than one year, on an inspiratory film). Dilatation of the right or left ventricle displaces the lower left border of the heart to the left, and therefore dose not allow easy distinction between right and left ventricular failure.

4. Globular cardiac dilatation is suggestive of pericardial effusion, particularly if the onset is rapid and if it is not accompanied by pulmonary edema

Electrocardiography

ECG can be normal in severe disease, but abnormalities may suggest the cause of heart failure such as QRS abnormalities in cardiomyopathy, arrhythmias. Sinus tachycardia, low-voltage QRS complexes (<5mm in any precordial lead), ST-T wave abnormalities, or prolonged QT interval may be indicative of myocarditis; sometimes conduction disturbance may be the only abnormal finding in myocarditis.

Echocardiography

Echocardiography can be used to measure ventricular EF at the bedside. The normal Ventricular Ejection Fraction (EF) of the right ventricule is 0.50 to 0.55, and the normal EF of the left ventricular is 0.4 to 0.50. The EF is normal in patients with diastolic heart failure and is reduced in patients with systolic heart failure. The estimated ejection fraction gives an indication of global ventricular function. Structural abnormalities (congential abnormalities, valvular defects, concentric hypertrophy, pericardial effusion) may indicate cause of heart failure.

Management of heart failure

Acute heart failure is a medical emergency, in which diagnosis of the cause and empirical treatment may have to be carried out simultaneously. Initial assessment should include peripheral perfusion and pulse, measurement of blood pressure, jugular venous pressure, and auscultation of lungs and precordium, drawing blood for investigations (electrolytes, glucose etc.), 12- lead ECG and saturation. Treatment strategies include the following:

General measures

Improving oxygenation by increasing FiO_2: Sit patient up and administer oxygen 45-60% through mask or CPAP, and if necessary by controlled ventilation.

1. Minimizing peripheral oxygen demand: sedation with morphine, control of fever with paracetamol.

In severe cases insert central venous cannula to assess filling pressure and allow administration of vasoactive drugs.

2. Optimise the ventricular preload, without overload. To relieve the systemic and pulmonary congestion if needed, a diuretics (Furosemide 1-2 mg/Kg IV) may be used cautiously. Furosemide can also be administered as a continuous infusion at 0.1 to 0.4 mg/kg per hour. However, diuretics are not the first line of management if blood pressure is low. If CVP is low fluid boluses should be given very cautiously in aliquots of 2-5 ml/kg while monitoring response in HR, perfusion, CVP, urine output.

Improving cardiac contractility by digitalization, and, if necessary, inotropic support.

3. Inotropic support is indicated if systolic blood pressure < 5th centile for age. particularly if there are signs of organ hypoperfusion (oliguria, confusion, metabolic acidosis). Dopamine (5-15µg/kg/min) is the first inotrope of choice in AHF if patient has hypotension. It may be give by peripheral vein. An alternative is dobutamine infusion, starting at 5µg/kg/min and increasing by 2.5µg/kg/min every 10 minutes until systolic blood pressure is within acceptable range, or when maximum dose of 20 µg/kg/min. It should be given into central vein. Dobutamine may cause vasodilatation aortic balloon pump counter-pulsation m ay be used to temporarily support a patient awaiting definitive surgical treatment

4. Reduction in ventricular afterload *i.e.* resistance to forward flow of blood) can improve ventricular function and peripheral perfusion.

Nitroprusside given by continuous infusion is most preferred vasodilator.

ACEIs (eg, captopril, 0.1 mg/kgtest dose, increasing to 0.3 mg per kg every 8-12 hours).
Initial test dose is necessary due to risk of severe hypotension particularly if patient is also treated with high doses of diuretics; Hyperkalemia may occur.

Inodilators, phosphodiesterase III inhibitors amrinone and milrinone are commonly used in low CO states as they optimize CO by altering afterload.

5. Treatment of cause:
   a) treatment of arrhythmias as appropriate
   b) antibiotics in bacterial endocarditis
   c) drainage of pericardial effusion
   d) surgical treatment: septal defect repair, valve replacement, transplantation.

6. The hemodynamic modulation of heart failure does not protect the myocardium from ongoing damage or decay. A focus on cardioprotection is now being recommended for the management of acute heart failure. Levosimendan is new inodilator that has ability to protect the myocardium from ischemic injury. Early clinical trials indicate that treatment of acute heart failure with levosimendan has survival benefit.

Management strategies based on type of heart failure

The treatment of decompensated heart failure in the ICU is best guided by the type of heart failure involved (systolic, diastolic, left-sided, or right-sided failure) and by invasive hemodynamic measurements.

Management strategies for left heart failure based on the Blood pressure

The management of decompensated left-sided heart failure is traditionally designed for a systolic - type heart failure even though some cases may involve diastolic failure.

Low Blood Pressure: Decompensated heart failure accompanied by hypotension is cardiogenic shock. This condition is most often associated with viral myocardiits and pulmonary embolus Hemodynamic drugs are notoriously unsuccessful in cardiogenic shock. Increasing blood pressure is a priority and dopamine is preferred because it acts as a vasopressor in high doses and retains some positive inotropic actions associated with lower doses. Dobutamine can be added to dopamine to further enhance cardiac output, but the combined effects of dopamine and dobutamine increases risk of tachyarrhythmia and increases myocardial 0_2 consumption, which can be detrimental in a failing heart.

Normal Blood Pressure: Use Inodilator therapy with dobutamine or milrinone, or vasodilator therapy with nitroglycerin. Both drugs augment cardiac output and reduce ventricular filling pressures. Blood pressure is usually unaffected in the usual doses, but dobutamine can increase blood pressure and milrinone can promote hypotension. Dobutamine can increase myocardial O_2 consumption. Milirinone may be preferred to dobutamine because of its lack of effect on myocardial O_2 consumption. Milrinone is also preferred to dobutamine in patients receiving beta-blockers drugs.

High Blood Pressure: Use vasodilator to augment cardiac output by reducing ventricular afterload. The overall effect is a decrease in arterial blood pressure and a increase in cardiac output. Nitroprusside is a more effective vasodilators that nitroglycerins, However, nitroglycerin is a safer alternative. Low infusion rates are usually required to produce effective arterial vasodilation; tolerance can appear after 16 to 24 hours of continuous drug admisntration.

Diuretic therapy with furosemide is indicate if vasodilator therapy does not reduce the pulmonary congestion. Although diuretic therapy with furosemide has been a cornerstone of management for chronic heart failure, diuretics should be used cautiously in the management of acute, decompensated heart failure. Intravenous furosemide often causes a decrease in cardiac output in patients with acute left heart failure. This effect is the result of a decrease in venous return and an increase in systemic vascular resistance.

Management strategies for Diastolic Heart Failure

There is no general agreement about the optimal treatment of diastolic heart failure. Positive inotropic agents have no role in the treatment of diastolic heart failure. Because ventricular filling is impaired in diastolic heart failure, diuretic therapy can be counterproductive and can further impair ventricular filling and cardiac output. Vasodilators have been a popularity used in treatment of diastolic failure. Vasodilator such as notroglycerin and Milrinone, also have lusitropic actions that promote ventricular relaxation during diastole and thus might be the preferred vasodilators for diastolic heart failure.

Management strategies for Right Heart Failure

Therapeutic strategies for right heart failure are similar in principle to those just described. Dobutamine is an effective agent in right heart failure. Nitroprusside has been used in right heart failure, but it is not as effective as dobutamine.

In conclusion, the management of acute, decompensated heart failure should augment cardiac output and reduce ventricular filling pressures while producing little or no increase in myocardial O_2 consumption. Diuretic therapy with intravenous furosemide can be counter-productive in acute, decompensated heart failure.

Chapter nine

Cardiac Arrhythmias

In infants and children life threatening cardiac rhythm disturbances more frequently are the result rather than the cause of acute cardiovascular emergencies. Primary cardiac arrest is uncommon in pediatric age group.

The Normal Electrocardiogram

The surface electrocardiogram (EGG) is a graphic representation of the sequence of myocardial depolarizaton and repolarizatign with each normal cardiac cycle consisting of a P, QRS and a T wave (Fig. 9.1). Electrical depolarization begins in sinoatrial node at the junction of the superior vena cava and right atrium and advances via atrial tissue and the internodal pathways to the atrioventricular (AV) junctional tissue. It then progresses via the bundle of His and its divisions to depolarize the ventricular myocardium. The normal PR interval and QRS' duration are given in Table 9.1.

Table 9.1: Average PR interval and QRS duration

Features	*0-1 mo*	*1-6 mo*	*6-12 mo*	*1-3 yr*	*3-8 yr*	*8-12 yr*
P-R Interval (sec)	0.1	0.1	0.11	0.12	0.13	0.14
QRS Duration (sec)	0.05	0.05	0.05	0.06	0.07	0.07

Rhythm Abnormalities

A rhythm disturbance in a child should be treated as a life threatening emergengy. It compromises cardiac output or has the potential to degenerate into a lethal (collapse) rhythm.

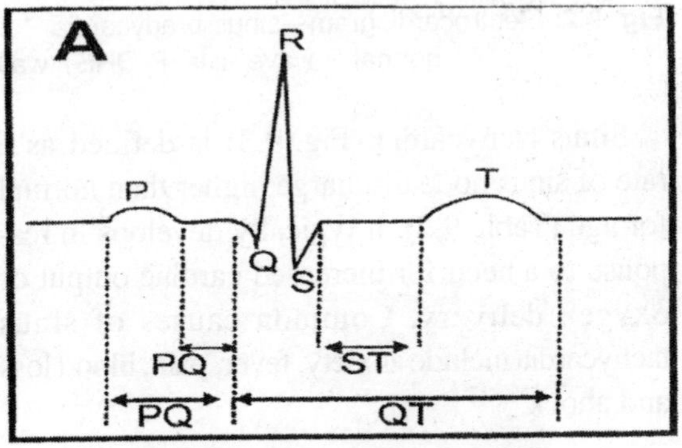

Fig. 9.1: Normal ECG tracings

In the setting of acute emergencies, cardiac rhythm disturbances should be classified according to their effect on central pulses:
Fast pulse rate = Tachyarrhythmia
Slow pulse rate = Bradyarrhythmia
Absent pulse =Pulseless arrest (Collapse rhythm).

Sinus Arrhythmias

Sinus arrhythmia represents a normal physiologic variation in impulse discharges with respiration. There is slowing of heart rate in expiration and an acceleration during inspiration. Sinus arrhythmia is exaggerated during febrile illnesses and by drugs that increase vagal tone, such as digitalis. It is usually abolished by exercise.

Sinus bradycardia (Fig. 9.2) is due to slow discharge of impulses from the sinus node. In children, a sinus rate less than 90 beats/min in neonates and less than 60 beats/min thereafter is considered to be sinus bradycardia. It is commonly seen in athletes and healthy individuals.

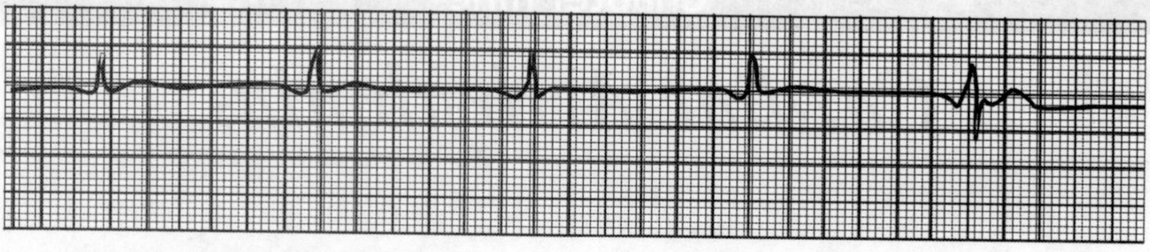

Fig. 9.2: Electrocardiogram—sinus bradycardia. * Rate is less than normal for age. Rhythm is regular with normal P wave axis, P-QRST wave sequence and normal QRS duration

Sinus tachycardia (Fig. 9.3) is defined as a rate of sinus node discharge higher than normal for age (Table 9.2). It typically develops in response to a need for increased cardiac output or oxygen delivery. Common causes of sinus tachycardia include anxiety, fever, pain, blood loss and shock.

Table 9.2: Heart rates in normal children

Age	*Range (per min)*	*Mean (per min)*
Newborn to 3 months	85-205	140
3 months to 2 years	100-190	130
2 years to 10 years	60-140	80
> 10 years	50-100	75

Extrasystoles

Extrasystoles are produced by discharge of an ectopic focus that may be situated anywhere in atrial, junctional or ventricular tissue. Usually isolated extrasystoles are of no clinical or prognostic significance.

Premature atrial complexes are common in children even in absence of cardiac disease. Atrial extrasystoles must be differentiated from premature ventricular complexes (PVCs). A premature P wave preceding the QRS that has a different contour compared with that of normal sinus P wave, is essential for diagnosis.

Premature ventricular complexes may arise in any region of the ventricle. Extrasystoles produce a smaller stroke and pulse volume than normal and if quite premature may not be palpable or audible with stethoscope. It is important to distinguish PVCs that are benign from those that are likely to degenerate into more severe dysrhythmias. The following are indications for further investigation of PVCs that could require suppressive therapy: (i) Two or more ventricular premature beats in a row (ii) Multifocal origin (iii) Increased ventricular ectopic activity with exercise (iv) R on T phenomenon (premature ventricular depolarization occurs on the T wave of the preceding beat) and (v) Presence of underlying heart disease.

An intravenous lidocaine bolus and drip is the first line of therapy. Amidorone is reserved for refractory cases or for patients with hemodynamic compromise.

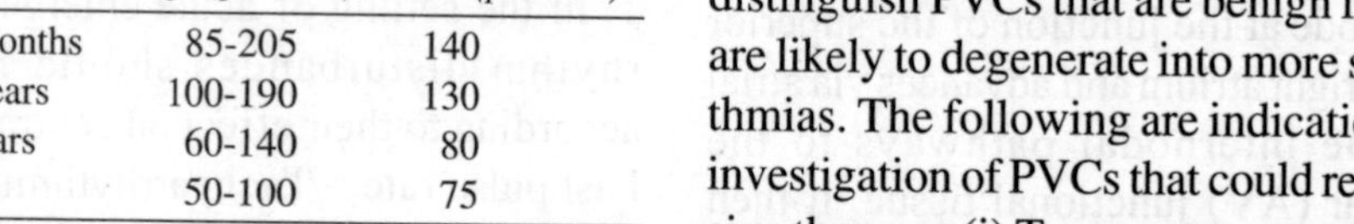

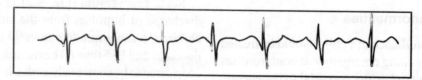

Fig. 9.3: Electrocardiogram (Sinus tachycardia)

* Rate is greater than normal for age. * Rhythm is regular with normal P wave axis, normal P-QRS-T wave sequence and normal QRS duration.

TACHYARRHYTHMIAS

Supraventricular Tachycardia

Supraventricular tachycardia (SVT) involve components of the conduction system within or above the bundle of His. It includes arterial tachycardia, and junctional tachycardia. Re-entry through an accessory pathway is the most common mechanism of SVT in infants. Re-entrant SVT (Fig. 9.4) is characterized by an abrupt onset and cessation; it may be precipitated by an acute infection, usually occurring when patient is at rest. The heart rate usually exceeds 180 beats/min in older children and >240/min in infants. If the attack lasts 6-24 hrs, the child may become acutely ill, restless and develop an ashen colour. SVT must be differentiated from other tachyarrhythmias as they may also be associated with poor systemic perfusion (Table 9.3).

Synchronized cardioversion (0.5 joules/kg) is the treatment of choice in unstable patients. In unstable patients with a readily available IV access, and a stable patients adenosine by rapid intravenous push is the treatment of choice. Adenosine has rapid onset of action and minimal effects on cardiac contractility. Verapamil may produce hypotension and cardiac arrest in infants younger than one year of age. It is contraindicated in this age group. Vagal stimulation maneuvers such as valsalva maneuver and ice-packs or cold water splashes on face may be tried in stable patients or while arranging for adenosine or cardioversion, but these are of unproven efficacy.

On ECG heart rate associated with SVT varies with age. The rhythm is usually regular. P wave is difficult to recognize or P wave axis is

Table 9.3: Diagnosis of tachyarrhythmia

Types	*Heart rate (beats/min)*	*P. wave*	*QRS duration*	*Regularity*
Sinus tachycardia	< 200	Always present Normal axis	Normal	Varies with respiration
Atrial tachycardia	180-320	Present: 50% cases Superior axis Common	Normal or RBBB pattern	Regular
Atrial fibrillation	120-180	Fibrillatory waves	- do -	Irregularly Irregular
Atrial flutter	Atrial:250-300 Ventricular:100-320	Saw toothed flutter waves	- do -	Regular ventricular response
Ventricular tachycardia	120-240	Absent or atrio-ventricular dissociation	Prolonged	Slightly irregular

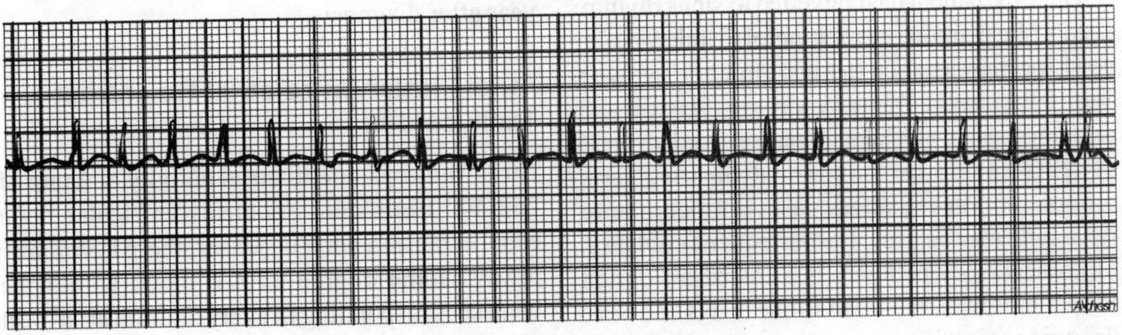

Fig. 9.4: Supraventricular tachycardia

Table 9.4: Commonly used antiarrhythmic drugs

Drugs	*Indication*	*Oral dose*	*Intravenous*	*Comments*	*Side effects*
1. Lidocaine	VPC, VT, VF		1 mg / kg may repeat q 5 min 3 times	Intravenous maintenance 20-50 µgm/kg/min	Confusion, convulsion, coma, parasthesia, respiratory failure
2. Propranolol	SVT, PVCs	1-4 mg kg/d q 6 hr	0.01–0.1 mg/kg	Long acting agents (atenolol) preferred for long term therapy	Memory loss, bradycardia, bronchospasm hypotension, CCF
3. Digoxin	SVT (non-WPW) arterial flutter, fibrillation	10 µg/kg/ 24 hr	IV dose = ¾ of oral dose	Oral total loading dose: Preterm: 20 µg/kg/ Term: 30 µg/kg/ > 6 months: 40 µg/kg	Nausea, vomiting anorexia, prolonged PR interval, AV block
4. Adenosine	SVT		0.1-0.2 mg/kg:	Very short half life	Increased heart block with Carbamazepine, causes transient bradycardia
5. Amiodarone	Drug resistant SVT, VT		5 mg/kg over 20-60 min.	Contraindicated in severe sinus Disease or AV	Asystole, hypo or hyperthyroidism, elevated Block triglycerides, Pulmonary fibrosis.

SVT = Supraventricular Tachycardia; VT = Ventricular Tachycardia
PVC = Premature ventricular complexes; VF = Ventricular fibrillation

abnormal (p') [the normal p **wave** is positive in leads I and aVF]. QRS duration is less than 0.08 sec in most (>90%) children; 10% have broad QRS complexes.

Once the patient has converted to sinus rhythm, agents like digoxin or propranolol (Table 9.4) are used for maintenance therapy. In children with Wolff-Parkinson-White syndrome, digoxin and calcium channel blockers should be avoided; these patients should be maintained on long term propranolol. In refractory cases amiodarone or flecainide may be used. Radiofrequency ablation of an accessory pathway is a treatment option for patients who require multiple drugs and have drug side effects or have refractory arrhythmias.

Infants presenting with SVT within first 3-4 months of life have a lower incidence of recurrence. Older patients have a 60% chance of recurrence and are treated for a minimum of one year after diagnosis.

Atrial Flutter (Intra-atrial Re-entrant Tachycardia)

Atrial flutter is due to atrial activity at a rate of 250-400 beats/min. As atrio-ventricular node cannot transmit such impulses, there is virtually always some degree of AV block within the ventricles responding to every 2nd-4th atrial beat (Fig. 9.5).

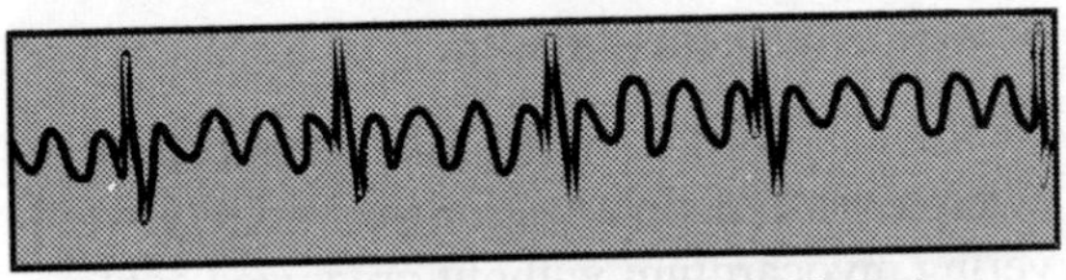

Fig. 9.5: Electrocardiogram (atrial flutter)

In older children, atrial flutter usually occurs in the setting of congenital heart disease while neonates with atrial flutter have normal heart. It usually converts to sinus rhythm by DC cardioversion, which is the treatment of choice. Vagal maneuvers (such as carotid sinus pressures or iced saline submersion) or adenosine usually produce a temporary slowing of the heart rate.

Neonates with normal heart responding to digoxin, are treated for 6-12 months.

Atrial Fibrillation

The atrial excitation is chaotic and more rapid (300-700 beats/min) producing an irregularly irregular ventricular response and pulse. It is rare in young and infants. Atrial fibrillation occurs more frequently in older children with rheumatic mitral valve disease. ECG shows loss of P wave with complete irregularity of QRS complex. The best initial treatment is digitalization, which restores the ventricular rate to normal, although the atrial fibrillation usually persists. Normal sinus rhythm may then be restored with digoxin, any type 1 agent such as quinidine or procainamide or by DC cardioversion. Amiodarone controls heart rate and cardioverts. Digoxin does not cardiovert.

Ventricular Tachycardia

Ventricular tachycardia (VT) is defined as at least 3 continuous PVCs at greater than 120 beats/min. ECG shows broad QRS complex (Fig. 9.6). The ventricular rate may vary from normal to more than 400 beats per minute. Slow ventricular rates may be well tolerated, but rapid ventricular rates compromise stroke volume and cardiac output and may degenerate into ventricular fibrillation. The majority of children who develop VT has underlying structural heart disease or prolonged QT syndrome. Other potential causes include acute hypoxemia, acidosis, electrolyte imbalance, drug toxicity (e.g. tricyclic antidepressants) and poisons.

VT without palpable pulses should be treated with defibrillation (2 J /kg). If VT is associated with signs of shock (low cardiac output, poor perfusion) but pulses are palpable; the indicated treatment is synchronized cardioversion (0.5 joules/kg). Ideally the patient should be intubated and ventilated with 100% oxygen, vascular access is established, and adequate sedation and analgesia are provided. If the underlying cause of the VT is determined (e.g. electrolyte imbalance or drug toxicity), it must be treated.

On ECG ventricular rate is >120 beats per minute and regular. The QRS is wide (greater than 0.08 second. P waves are often not identifiable. When present, they may not be related to the QRS. T waves are usually opposite in polarity to the QRS.

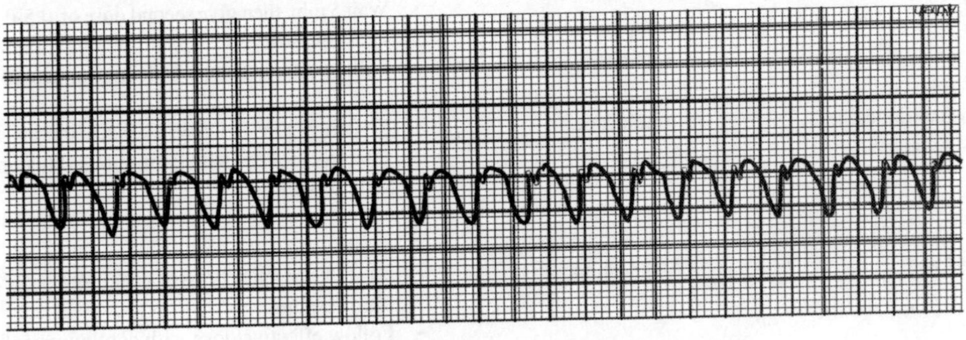

Fig. 9.6: Electrocardiogram: Ventricular tachycardia

Lidocaine is useful to raise the threshold for ventricular fibrillation and to suppress postcardioversion ventricular ectopy. It should be administered before cardioversion if vascular access has been established and the drug is readily available. A loading dose is administered, followed by an infusion. However, cardioversion should not be delayed in an unstable child if the drug is not readily available or if vascular access has not been achieved. Lidocaine infusion should be considered following return of spontaneous circulation if the ventricular arrhythmias are thought to be associated with myocarditis or structural heart disease. A staged approach to treatment of ventricular tachycardia is given in Table 8.5.

Torsade de Pointes: It is a variant of VT with alternating polymorphic broad complex tachycardia. Predisposing factors include prolonged QT interval, hypokalemia, hypocalcemia and hypomagnesemia. Class I antidysrhythmics, tricyclics, phenothiazines and antimony compounds toxicity may cause torsade de pointes.

Treatment: includes treatment of the cause. Drugs used are similar to those used for VT. Correction of hypomagnesemia and hypocalcemia should be undertaken.

Ventricular Fibrillation

Ventricular fibrillation (VF) is a chaotic, disorganized series of depolarization that results in a quivering myocardium without organized contraction. Ventricular systole does not occur, so pulses are not palpable. Ventricular fibrillation (Fig. 9.7) is an uncommon terminal event in the pediatric age group and is documented in only about 10% of children. Resuscitative outcome, however, appears to be considerably better if VF rather than asystole or electromechanical dissociation is the underlying rhythm in a pulseless patietns. The definitive treatment for VF is prompt defibrillation. Defibrillation is the untimed (asynchronous) depolarization of a critical mass of myocardial cells to allow spontaneous organized, myocardial depolarization to resume. If organized depolarization does not resume, VF will continue or will progress to electrical silence. At this point restoration of spontaneous cardiac activity may be impossible.

Bradyarrhythmias

Sinus arrest or sinoatrial block may cause a sudden pause in the heart beat. The former is sup-

Table 9.5: Staged approach to ventricular tachycardia

Stage	*Intervention*	*Recommended Dose*
Stage 1 Hemodynamically unstable	DC cardioversion	• Use shock sequence
Stage 2 No evidence of hemodynamic instability	Lidocaine	• 1-1.5 mg/kg as bolus injection • Wait 5 min, then give second dose of 0.5-0.75 mg/kg if necessary • Follow effective dose with continuous infusion
Stage 3 No response to lidocaine Q-Tc < 0.44 sec.	Amidorone	• 5-10 mg/kg IV in D5W, over 20-30 mins. If effective, follow with continuous infusion at 5-10 μg/kg/min.
Stage 3 Q-Tc < 0.44 sec.	Magnesium	• 50 mg/kg $MgSO_4$ IV over 1 min. Repeat in 10 min if no response • Follow effective dose with continuous infusion of $MgSO_4$

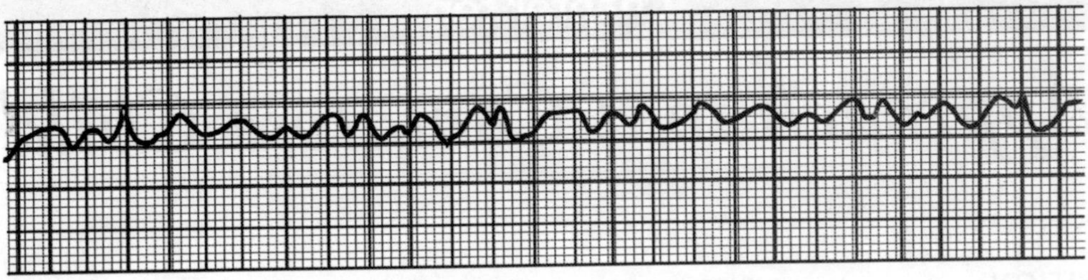

Fig. 9.7: Electrocardiogram: Ventricular fibrillation

posed to be caused by failure of impulse formation within the sinus node and the latter by a block between the sinus impulse and the surrounding atrium.

Sinoatrial block is rare in childhood except as manifestations of digitalis intoxication or in patients who have had extensive atrial surgery.

Atrioventricular (AV) block may be divided into three forms.

1st degree block: The P-R interval is prolonged (~0.16 sec), but all the atrial impulses are conducted to the ventricle.

2nd degree block: Some impulses are not conducted to ventricle.

3rd degree block (complete heart block): No impulses from atria reaches the ventricles. Congenital complete AV block is most often caused by autoimmune injury of the fetal conduction system by maternally derived IgG antibodies. Autoimmune diseases account for 60- 70% of all cases of congenital complete heart block and about 80% of cases in which there is a structurally normal heart.

A precise diagnosis of specific bradyarrhythmias is not important at the stage of resuscitation. Therapy can be determined once the clinical condition is stable.

Bradycardia (HR < 60 / mt) associated with poor systemic perfusion should be treated in any infant or child, even if blood pressure is normal. Adequate ventilation with 100% oxygen must be ensured, chest compressions performed if pulse is weak, epinephrine (0.01 mg/kg of 1: 1000 solution) and or atropine (0.02 mg/ kg/ max. dose of 1 mg) are administered as necessary.

Symptomatic patients with congenital complete heart block require permanent cardiac pacemaker implantation. It should also be considered in patients who have progressive cardiac enlargement, awake heart rates < 40 beats/min or Stokes Adams Syndrome.

Cardiac pacing is required in neonates with ventricular rates <50 beat/min, with hydrops, with congenital heart disease or heart failure after birth. Isoproterenol, atropine or epinephrine may be used to increase the heart rate temporarily until pacemaker placement can be arranged.

Electromechanical Dissociation

In electromechanical dissociation there is evidence of organized electrical activity on EGG but failure of effective myocardial contractions, as evidenced by the absence of a palpable pulse. The mechanism is not understood. Underlying causes, which must be looked for and corrected if present, include severe hypovolemia, hypoxemia, severe acidosis, tension pneumothorax, cardiac tamponade and hypothermia.

Chapter ten

Approach to a Comatose Child

DEFINITION

Coma is defined as a state of decreased consciousness from which the child cannot be aroused by ordinary verbal, sensory or physical stimuli. Consciousness involves awareness of self and environment. Both cognitive functions, and ability to respond to stimuli are impaired in coma.

Consciousness is maintained by the interaction of the reticular activating system (RAS) with the cerebral hemispheres. The cerebral cortex is stimulated by the RAS and reciprocally modulates the activity of the RAS. Coma occurs with dysfunction of either (i) both cerebral hemispheres or (ii) the RAS—the central core of the brainstem and midbrain or both.

MANAGEMENT

A child in coma must be regarded as a medical emergency. Management strategies involve (i) emergency measures (ii) diagnostic work up and (iii) definitive treatment.

Emergency Measures

These should be undertaken immediately even before a complete clinical examination. The physician should ensure that the child has stable airway, breathing and circulation (ABC). Measures to stabilize these should be instituted like in any emergency situation (Table 10.1).

An emergency neurologic assessment to evaluate the level of consciousness and signs of raised ICP and impending herniation should be performed during the stabilization period. The latter need immediate management (Table 10.2).

Table 10.1: Emergency measures to be taken in a comatose child

1. Check airway patency: Intubate if Glasgow Coma Score <8; or pooling of secretion.
2. Check breathing: Give 100% oxygen; use bag and mask/tube if respiratory depression.
3. Check circulation: Start IV N. Saline or Ringer's lactate 20 ml/kg to maintain BP and peripheral perfusion. Inotropic support if needed. Give antihypertensives if hypertensive encephalopahy.
4. If seizures-control with anticonvulsants: Diazepam 0.3 mg/kg IV.
5. If raised ICP/impending herniation: Head elevation 15-30°, measures to reduce ICP: manual hyperventilation
6. Metabolic support: Give 2 ml/kg of 25% glucose IV.
7. Consider specific antidotes in case of known poisoning.
8. Immobilization of cervical spine, emergency neuro-imaging and neurosurgical consulation in suspected traumatic coma.

Table 10.2: Impending herniation—suggestive signs and management

A. Suggestive signs:

1. Decorticate or decerebrate posturing
2. Abnormalities of vital signs: tachycardia or bradycardia, hyperventilation, Cheyne Stokes breathing or irregular respiration, hypertension or hypotension
3. Pupillary abnormalities: unilateral or bilateral fixed dilated pupils, unequal pupil

B. Treatment:

1. Hyperventilation: manual with bag and mask or ventilator if available
2. Mannitol: 0.5 g/kg, (2.5 ml of 20% soln/kg) IV, over 20 minutes, then 0.25 g/kg IV 4-6 hourly
3. Dexamethasone: 0.6 mg/kg
4. Thiopental or Pentobarbital if needed

This is essential to (i) plan the type of intervention measures needed according to the severity of the neurologic injury (ii) gather important baseline information before certain drugs are administered that may interfere with neurologic examination *viz* anticonvulsants, sedatives etc. The Glasgow Coma Scale (with its modification for children) is a simple and useful tool for clinical monitoring (See Table 3.1). If there is a suspicion of trauma—either by history or on examination, the child should also be evaluated by a neurosurgeon and general surgeon and managed appropriately.

DIAGNOSTIC APPROACH

The diagnostic approach involves answering of the following questions:

1. Where is the lesion?
2. *Is it progressive:* Is there any imminent life threatening event?
3. *What is the specific etiology:* Metabolic or structural?
4. What can be done about it?

A carefully taken history, physical and neurological examination, along with some important investigations are needed for answering the first three questions; the fourth can be answered accordingly.

History

To find cause of coma, the following points in history are often helpful:

1. *Onset:* A gradual onset indicates a slowly progressive cause *viz* metabolic or an inflammatory or destructive lesion, whereas a sudden onset indicates a vascular event. A tumor or an abscess may at times have a sudden onset of coma particularly if there is a bleed into the tumor or rupture of abscess into the ventricle.
2. *Fever:* Fever generally indicates an infectious cause *viz* meningitis, encephalitis, cerebral malaria etc.
3. *Associated symptoms:* A viral prodrome may suggest viral encephalitis. A biphasic illness with the child having vomiting and altered sensorium while apparently recovering from a viral illness suggests Reye's syndrome.
4. *Ingestion of toxic substances:* e.g. tablets, liquids lying at home. Direct history may not be available; circumstantial history e.g. an empty bottle found near the child may be helpful.
5. *Trauma:* History of trauma may at times not be forthcoming either because it went unnoticed or (ii) information is deliberately withheld for fear of 'charge of negligence' or 'abuse'.
6. *Bite/Sting:* e.g. snake bite, the history may again be circumstantial.
7. *Past illness:* Children with known illness e.g. diabetes, epilepsy, renal disease, heart disease etc. may develop coma because of associated complications.

The history is further supported by a meticulous clinical and neurological examination.

General Physical Examination

Some of the important physical findings that should be actively looked for include:

1. Signs of trauma: bruising, bleeding etc.
2. *Any peculiar odour:* e.g., fruity in diabetic ketoacidosis, typical smells in various poisonings.
3. *Jaundice and hepatomegaly:* may suggest a primary hepatic cause.
4. *Cardiac findings*: any arrhythmia, cardiac failure etc. may suggest a hypoxic-ischemic cause.

NEUROLOGICAL EXAMINATION

The neurologic examination is the keystone of diagnosis. The important aspects include examination of eyes, the breathing pattern and the motor response.

Examination of the Eyes: This gives some of the most important information in comatose patients.

i. *Position of the eyes:* Normally the eyes at rest are in midposition and looking ahead. In a comatose child also the eyes are often midposition or slightly divergent. Conjugate deviation of the eyes suggests either an ipsilateral cerebral hemispheric lesion or a contra-lateral pontine lesion. Dysconjugate deviation of the eyes either at rest or evoked by head turning or caloric stimulation indicates a brainstem lesion.

ii. *The pupils:* Pupillary size and reaction give valuable clues to diagnosis (Table 10.3). Pupils may be affected variably in metabolic coma, but generally remain reactive. Absence of pupillary reaction is strongly suggestive of structural disease.

iii. *The oculocephalic reflex (Doll's Eyes):* This is tested in the comatose child by holding the head with the eyes open, and then suddenly turning it to one side—if the eyes deviate to the opposite side, this is called the positive oculocephalic or Doll's Eye Reflex. *Positive reflex indicates an intact brainstem.* It is positive in diffuse hemispheric disease and supratentorial coma and absent in brain stem lesions. The reflex should never be tested in children with suspected cervical injuries (Fig. 10.1).

The same information can be got from the oculovestibular reflex (Cold Caloric response) which can be done even in patients with cervical injuries. Before starting the test, one must ensure that the tympanic membrane is intact. The head is positioned in midline and raised 30° from the horizontal. Ice cold water about 50 ml (max. 120 ml), is slowly injected through a catheter into the auditory canal. In an awake person, nystagmus is produced with the slow component in the opposite direction. With supratentorial lesions, and an intact brain stem, tonic deviation of the eyes towards the cold stimulus is seen. Absence of the reflex indicates brain stem damage.

iv. *Fundus:* Papilloedema with or without retinal hemorrhages occurs with raised ICP. Subhyaloid hemorrhage may occur with subarachnoid hemorrhage, subdural hematoma, and trauma particularly that caused by child abuse.

Table 10.3: Pupillary size and reaction in comatose patients

Pupils	*Lesion/ Dysfunction*
1. Pinpoint (<2mm)	Pontine, cerebeller
2. Small (2-3 mm)	Medullary Metabolic (opiates, Barbiturates phenothiazines)
3. Midsize (5-7 mm) midposition non reactive	Midbrain or below
4. Dilated non reactive	Diffuse damage, (Atropine, barbiturate)
Unilateral dilated	Uncal herniation non reactive

Motor response: The motor response, which is elicited often by a painful stimulus or deep pressure over supraorbital region, may be either appropriate, inappropriate or absent.

An appropriate response implies withdrawal away from the painful stimulus. Purposeful withdrawal and/or speech suggest preservation of cortical function.

Decorticate posture: Flexion and adduction of upper limbs and extension of lower limbs is associated with cortical or hemispheric dysfunction.

Decerebrate posture: Extension of upper limbs and lower limbs, occurs with high pontine and mid brain lesions, bilateral hemispheric lesions, or severe hypoxemia.

Flaccidity with absence of motor response suggests a pontomedullary or lower brain stem lesion.

Asymmetric responses occur with hemiplegia, and other focal deficits.

Respiration: The pattern of respiration forms an important part of the neurologic examination. The different patterns of respiration seen with different lesions are shown in Table 10.4.

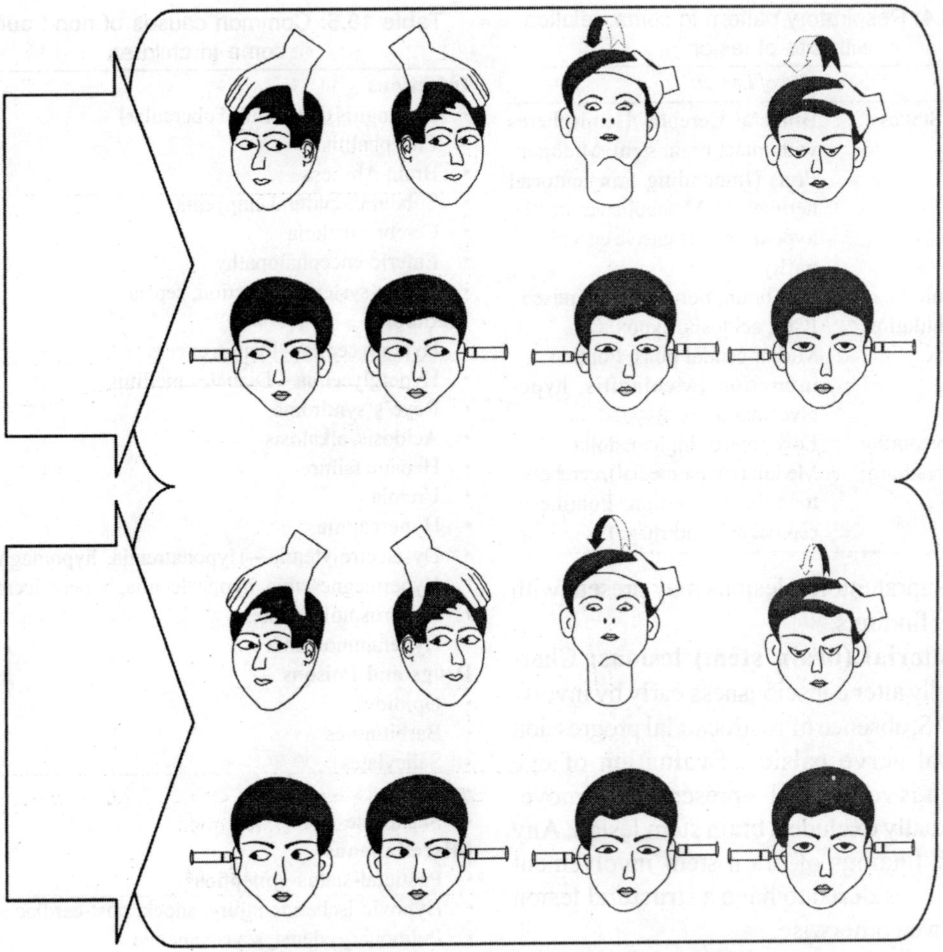

Fig. 10.1: Ocular reflexes in comatose patients

Meningeal Signs: If present, indicate meningitis, meningoencephalitis or subarachnoid bleed. Meningsmus may also be seen in enteric fever and cerebral malaria, and when associated with focal signs, may occur in brain abscess, epidural hemorrhage, cerebrovascular accidents, and tumors including tuberculoma and cerebellar herniation. Meningeal signs are often not seen in infants and may be lost in deeply comatose, children.

After a proper history, physical and neurological examination, one should be able to decide whether the comatose child has (i) a metabolic disorder or (ii) a structural lesion (supratentorial/ infratentorial).

Metabolic coma: is characterised by—(i) gradual progression (ii) symmetric neurologic findings (iii) preserved pupillary light reflex.

Structural lesions: may be supratentorial either bilateral, or if unilateral they either compress the contralateral hemisphere or the brain stem to affect the RAS. They are characterized by initial asymmetric findings e.g. hemiparesis, hemisensory deficit or aphasia. Deterioration occurs characteristically in a rostral-caudal manner with rapid changes in clinical findings.

Table 10.4: Respiratory pattern in coma, relation with site of lesion

Pattern	*Site of Lesion*
• Cheyne Stokes	: Bilateral Cerebral Hemispheres with intact brain stem, Midbrain, Pons (Impending transtentorial herniation), Metabolic *viz* uremia, hypoxia, hypertensive encephalopathy
• Neurogenic hyperventilation	: Mid brain, pons (Diffuse raised ICP), acidosis, hypoxia
• Apneustic breathing	: Mid or caudal pons, Pontine infarction (Meningitis, hypoglycemia, anoxia)
• Cluster breathing	: Low pons or high medulla
• Ataxic breathing	: Medulla (dorsomedial), cerebellar tonsillar herniation, Pontine or cerebellar hemorrhage)

At times, supratentorial lesions may present with symmetric findings.

Subtentorial (brain stem) lesions: Characteristically alter consciousness early by involving the RAS, absence of rostrocaudal progression and cranial nerve palsies. Evaluation of eye movements is very useful—preserved eye movements virtually exclude a brain stem lesion. Any child with findings of brain stem involvement should be considered to have a structural lesion unless proven otherwise.

The common causes of non-traumatic coma are shown in Table 10.5. The most important cause of non-traumatic coma in our country are CNS infections—meningitis (pyogenic and tubercular), and encephalitis. Cerebral malaria and other infections are the other frequent causes.

TREATMENT

Comatose children should be managed in a Pediatric Intensive Care Unit. The emergency measures have been outlined in Table 10.1. Further management and diagnostic workup must be approached simultaneously. (For more details of other management strategies see next chapter on Intensive Care Needs of Critically Ill Neurologic Patients).

Table 10.5: Common causes of non-traumatic coma in children

Infections
- Meningitis (Bacterial, Tubercular)
- Encephalitis
- Brain Abscess
- Subdural/epidural empyema
- Cerebral malaria
- Enteric encephalopathy
- Severe systemic infection, sepsis

Metabolic
- Hypoglycemia—Insulin excess
- Hyperglycemia—Diabetes mellitus
- Reye's syndrome
- Acidosis, alkalosis
- Hepatic failure
- Uremia
- Hypercapnia
- Dyselectrolytemia—Hyponatremia, hypomagnesemia,
- Hypermagnesemia, hypocalcemia, hypercalcemia.
- Hyperosmolar states
- Hyperammonemia

Drugs and Poisons
- Opioides
- Barbiturates
- Salicylates
- Sedatives
- Snake bite

Miscellaneous
- Postictal-status epilepticus
- Hypoxic-ischemic injury, shock, post-cardiac arrest
- Pulmonary edema, severe anemia
- Hypertensive encephalopathy

General Measures

i. Frequent monitoring of vital signs and neurological parameters to detect any life threatening events like raised ICP, or herniation syndromes.
ii. Management of oxygenation and airway.
iii. Optimal fluid intake and output management.
iv. Correction of acid base and electrolyte disturbances.
v. *Temperature control:* Management of fever, or at times hypothermia.
vi. *Nursing care:* Keeping the patient on side, turning regularly, maintenance of cleanliness

and hygiene, particularly care of mouth and skin, urinary catheterization and protection of eyes with pads.

vii. *Nutrition*: For children with prolonged coma, special attention has to be given to their nutritional requirements; parenteral or nasogastric feeding may be needed.

Specific Treatment

Specific management is dictated by the etiology of coma e.g.

1. *Antibiotics for meningitis:* If lumbar puncture is contraindicated, antibiotics should be started if there is a clinical suspicion of meningitis.
2. *Antimalarials (Quinine by IV infusion):* for proven or strongly suspected cerebral malaria
3. Anti-virals: Acylovir in suspected herps encephalitis
4. Anticonvulsants for status epilepticus.
5. *Antidotes:* for specific poisonings.
6. *Antihypertensives:* for hypertensive encephalopathy.

INVESTIGATIONS

Initial Diagnostic Workup

The usual laboratory studies include a complete and differential blood count, blood glucose, electrolytes, liver and renal functions, coagulation studies, toxicology and ammonia and an arterial blood gas (ABG) (Table 10.6). A lumbar puncture is indicated in suspected meningitis provided it is not contraindicated due to raised ICP or hemodynamic instability.

CT Scan

A CT scan is often needed as an emergency investigation particularly in children with suspected trauma, raised ICP and focal neurologic deficits. Whenever a structural lesion is suspected, a CT scan should be obtained at the earliest. The comatose chiid should be stabilized, and intubated before getting a CT scan. The CT scan reveals the site and often the nature of the lesion and helps in ruling out the lesions that are likely to cause cerebral herniation. In diffuse involvement with raised ICP the CT may show signs of cerebral edema. A normal CT does not however rule out underlying raised ICP.

Further Studies

Further studies would depend upon the suspected diagnosis based on history, physical examination and neuroimaging studies.

Electroencephalogram (EEG)

The EEG has a diagnostic as well as prognostic

Table 10.6: Value of routine laboratory investigations in a comatose child

Investigations	*Findings*	*Interpretation*
Blood Film	Malaria parasites	Cerebral malaria
Urine (catheter specimen)	Ketones	Diabetes mellitus
	Sugar	
	Protein	Renal hypertension
Dextrostix	Blood glucose	Diabetes, Diabetic ketosis hypoglycemic coma
Blood	Glucose,	Diabetic/hypoglycemic coma
Biochemistry	Electrolytes	Hypo-hyper-natremia,
	Urea	uremia
Gastric contents	Drugs/poisons	Poisoning
X-ray skull	Fractures	Trauma
Lumbar puncture	Cells, protein, blood	Encephalitis subarachnoid hemorrhage
Blood culture	If patient febrile	Sepsis

Table 10.7: EEG findings in certain conditions causing coma

EEG findings	*Interpretation*
• High voltage focal slow waves	Underlying supratentorial lesion
• Periodic lateralised epileptiform discharges (PLEDS)	Herpes encephalitis
• Paroxysomal seizure discharges	Status epilepticus
• Slowing of Alpha-rhythm	Metabolic coma
• Progressing to diffuse slowing	
• Triphasic paroxysmally waves 2-4 Hz/sec. bilaterally	Hepatic or other Metabolic coma

role in coma. Typical EEG findings in some conditions causing coma are shown in Table 10.7.

EEG patterns of burst suppression, monorhythmical alpha like activity, electro-cerebral silence or very low amplitude, and monotonous 0.5-3 Hz high voltage activity have been associated with poor outcome. EEG findings of poor outcome do not always correlate with the clinical assessment of deep coma. The appearance of sleep spindles is indicative of a good prognosis, even in the presence of delta waves.

Evoked Potentials

Somatosensory (SEP) and brain stem evoked potentials are immensely useful in monitoring and assessing brain stem functions in coma. The absence of all waveforms in these modalities is associated with severe neurologic residua or brain death. SEP are the most sensitive reliable method for evaluation of the neurologic outcome in the comatose child. Normal SEPs early during the course of coma predict a normal outcome in 93% cases and absent SEP(s) predict poor outcome in 100% cases; asymmetrical SEP(s) typically associated with sequelae such as hemiparesis.

Prognosis

The prognosis of coma mainly depends upon its etiology, duration and depth. Recovery is best in postictal coma, whereas that from anoxia has the poorest outcome. CNS infections have a mortality of about 40%. Longer the duration of coma, poorer is the outcome. Glasgow coma scale score 5 or less, fixed dilated pupils for more than 2 hours, decerebration, flaccidity and areflexia have been associated with poor outcome. Cardio-respiratory arrest occurring any time in a comatose child and absent brain stem reflexes have a grave prognosis.

Chapter eleven

Status Epilepticus

Status epilepticus (SE) is an emergency that requires early recognition and vigorous treatment. Any type of epileptic seizure can develop into SE but the most commonly associated syndrome is tonic-clonic or convulsive SE. The outcome depends mainly on the rapidity and adequacy of care. A skillful approach is mandatory to prevent mortality.

DEFINITION

The International League Against Epilepsy (ILAE) definition of status epilepticus as a condition characterized by an epileptic seizure that is so frequent or so prolonged as to create a fixed and lasting condition is difficult for practical application. Traditionally SE in children is defined as:

- Seizure lasting more than 30 minutes, or
- Recurrent seizures lasting greater than 30 minutes without full return of consciousness.

In practice, any child who continues to convulse even after arrival to hospital or physicians's office should be treated as a case of SE. Also a child with epilepsy should be considered in SE if the seizure persists for more than twice the usual duration of the previous seizures.

PATHOPHYSIOLOGY

Prolonged seizures cause an increase in metabolic rate, and cerebral oxygen extraction and consumption and subsequently neuronal injury. During the first 30 minutes of seizures there is sympathetic overactivity, the manifestations of which include tachycardia, hypertension, hyperglycemia and hyperpyrexia. If SE persists for more than one hour, hyperkalemia, hypoglycemia, hypotension and respiratory acidosis may ensue. Massive activation of both sympathetic and parasympathetic systems leads to severe autonomic disturbance including hyerpyrexia, excessive sweating, and salivary and tracheobronchial hypersecreation. CSF pleocytosis may occur. The complication of SE are listed in Table 11.1.

Table 11.1: Complications of status epilepticus

• **Cardiovascular:**	Bradycardia, arrhythmia, cardiac failure or arrest, hypertension, hypotension, shock
• **Respiratory:**	Hyperpnoea, apnoea, irregular or Cheyne stokes breathing, respiratory acidosis, aspiration pneumonia, pulmonary oedema
• **Renal:**	Oliguria, acute renal failure, acute tubular necrosis, myoglobinuria (from rhabdomyolysis)
• **Autonomic:**	Hyperpyrexia, excessive sweating, excessive secretions with airway obstruction
• **Metabolic:**	Hyperglycemia, hypoglycemia, Hyperkalemia, Hyponatremia, metabolic and lactic acidosis.

ETIOLOGY

The important causes of SE may be broadly divided into:

1. *Acute:* CNS infections (meningitis/meningoencephalitis), febrile convulsions, vascular episodes, trauma, metabolic and poisonings.
2. *Static:* SE occurring as first manifestation of or during the course of epilepsy, with or without an underlying neurologic disorder. In known

epileptics, non-compliance or withdrawal of antiepileptic therapy, intercurrent infections and stress may predispose to SE.

In our own experience, CNS infections are the commonest cause of refractory SE (Table 11.2).

Table 11.2: Causes of refractory SE among children admitted to Pediaric Emergency and Intensive Care Unit, PGIMER, Chandigarh

Causes	*Total Number*
Bacterial/ purulent meningitis	26
Encephalitis	11
Idiopathic epilepsy	10
Post-hypoxic encephalopathy	4
Reye's encephalopathy	2
Shigella encephalopathy	2
Others	5
Total	60

From: *Singhi S, Singhi PD, Banerjee S. Journal of Child Neurology 1998;13:23-26.*

MANAGEMENT

Prompt and aggressive treatment of SE is essential. The main goals of management are (i) supporting vital functions and (ii) terminating seizure activity as expeditiously as possible. A simplified management scheme is as follows:

A. Stabilization

Within first few minutes, ensure adequate cerebral oxygenation and perfusion by maintaining optimal respiratory and hemodynamic function.

Airway

Ensure airway patency by proper positioning of head and suctioning of pharyngeal secretions. Oral or nasal airways may be used, but forced opening of clenched jaw should be avoided. Early nasogastric decompression should be done to prevent vomiting and secondary aspiration.

Breathing

All patients should receive 100% oxygen by mask to ensure adequate oxygenation. Ventilation with bag and mask should be started if there are signs of inadequate oxygenation and ventilation; these include–inadequate chest movements, poor air entry on auscultation, tachypnoea, apnoea, poor respiratory effort, central cyanosis, oxygen saturation < 90%. If this is found unsatisfactory, the child should be intubated. Endotracheal intubation is also indicated if the child has signs of increased intracranial pressure (ICP) that requires controlled oxygenation and hyperventilation or refractory SE. For successful intubation, rapid sequence intubation (RSI) is the preferred method. In this procedure, after pre-oxygenation with 100% oxygen and premedication with atropine (0.01-0.02 mg/kg IV) a priming dose of muscle relaxant is given. This is followed by full dose of muscle relaxant and sedation with diazepam in rapid succession (See the Procedures section for details).

Circulation

Assess circulatory status and ensure its stabilization. Establish vascular access immediately for administration of (a) anti-convulsants and (b) fluids. In a convulsing child at times it may be difficult to establish an intravenous access. In such a situation one may use:

a. *Intraosseous (IO) route:* In children less than 6 years: All medications and fluids that are given IV may be administered by IO infusions.
b. *Per rectal (PR)/Intramuscular (IM) route:* Only few drugs are effective in controlling SE through these routes. Diazepam and Lorazepam can be given PR and Midazolam can be given IM. Phenytion prodrug (Fosphenytoin) is reportedly effective in SE when used by IM route.

B. Evaluation

Evaluation is done simultaneously to find out the underlying cause. This includes rapid history, physical examination and selected investigations (Table 11.3).

Table 11.3: Investigations in a patient with SE

Blood:	Haemogram, Glucose, Calcium, Magnesium, Urea, Electrolytes, ABG, Anti- epileptic drug levels, toxicology screen, Cultures if febrile
Urine:	analysis and toxicology
LP (CSF):	analysis in suspected meningitis
Continuous EEG Monitoring:	In refractory status epilepticus and SE in neonates
Neuro Imaging (CT/MRI):	If focal findings are present or in a case of suspected head injury or coma

C. Termination of Seizures

Step 1

Immediate control of seizures is attempted with ***intravenous (IV) benzodiazepine***. Either Diazepam 0.3 mg/kg (max. 10 mg) or Midazolam 0.2 mg/kg (at a rate no greater than 1 mg/min), or Lorazepam 0.05 to 0.1 mg/kg (max 4 mg.) is given over 2 min. It may be repeated after 5 minutes if seizure persists. The onset of action of these drugs is within 1-3 minutes of administration, the duration of action of Diazepam is 5-15 minutes, and of Lorazepam is 24-48 hrs. Many prefer Lorazepam over Diazepam, because it has a longer duration of action and lesser incidence of respiratory depression and hypotension. In case of difficulty in establishing intravenous access, diazepam can be given per rectum in the same doses. Midazolam has shortest duration of action.

Recent studies in adults favour lorazepam over diazepam as the preferred initial therapy as it has a longer duration of action and lesser incidence of respiratory depression and hypotension and intubation. However, in children use of multiple doses of lorazepam increases risk of respiratory depression.

Rectal Diazepam: Only if IV route is not available rectal diazepam should be used though rectal dizepam is considered as effective as IV diazepam. It aborted seizures in 96% of patients in one study, when given within 15 minutes of seizure onset. Diazepam gel is not available in our country as yet, but one can use the parental solution for the same purpose. It is given in a dose of 0.5 mg/kg up to a maximum of 10 mg and may be repeated after 5-10 minutes if seizure persists. It is given without dilution and by using a small syringe or a small catheter on the end of a syringe. It should be infused 4 cms into the rectum. The anal opening should be strapped after administration for about half an hour to prevent leakage of the drug.

Sublingual Lorazepam can be used in a dose of 0.1mg/kg up to a maximum of 4 mg and may be repeated after 10 minutes if seizure persists and then again once more. One has to actively look for hypotension and respiratory depression. Rectal lorazepam has not been extensively studied as rectal diazepam. In a study conducted in the pediatric population comparing rectal and intravenous diazepam and lorazepam, there were minimal differences in the mean time to seizure control for both the drugs with both types of administration.

Intramuscular (IM) Midazolam: Midazolam stands out in comparison to other benzodiazepines as it is water soluble and can be administered IM. IM midazolam has been used as first line drug for controlling SE and a dose of 0.2 mg/kg is reported to be clinically efficacious in >90% of children in SE. It is particularly valuable when there is difficulty in establishing an intravenous route.

Buccal midazolam was shown to be as effective as rectal diazepam if not more, in a randomized study conducted in children and young people with SE lasting for more than 5 minutes. Buccal midazolam stopped seizures in 75% of 40 and diazepam in 59% of 39 patients. Though some studies have shown that **intranasal midazolam** administration can also be used for control of SE, more extensive trials are yet to be carried out.

Step 2

Phenytoin is given intravenously, in a loading dose of 20 mg/kg, slowly (to avoid hypotension and cardiac arrhythmia). A supplemental bolus of 5 mg-10 mg/kg may be repeated after 10 mins if the seizure persists especially in neonates and young infants. Onset of action is 10-30 minutes after infusion and duration of action is for 12-24 hours. Phenytoin should be diluted only with normal saline, not with glucose solutions as it may precipitate and form micro crystals. If seizures do not recur, maintenance dose of phenytoin (5-8 mg/kg/day) should be given after 12-24 hours of the initial loading dose.

Fosphenytoin, a phenytoin prodrug, represents significant advances in treatment of children with convulsive SE. It is a water-soluble phosphate ester of phenytoin that gets rapidly converted to phenytoin. In contrast to phenytoin it can be administered IM with rapid and complete absorption. The dose of fosphenytoin is 15-20 mg/kg of Phenytoin equivalents/kg, infused at a rate of not more than 3 mg/kg/min, not to exceed 150 mg/min.

Step 3

If seizure activity persists or recurs despite benzodiazepines and phenytoin, phenobarbitone or paraldehyde may be used.

Phenobarbitone is preferred to phenytoin in neonates if there was no initial response to benzodiazepines. It is given in a loading dose of 15-20 mg/kg IV at a rate of 1.5 mg/kg/min. In neonates an additional dose of 5-10 mg/kg may be given. The maintenance dose is 3-5 mg/kg/day given in two divided doses, 12-24 hours later. Owing to the cumulative respiratory depressant effect of benzodiazepines and barbiturates, facilities should be available for mechanical ventilation.

Paraldehyde is given in a dose of 0.3 ml/kg up to a maximum of 10 ml (i.e., 30 kg patient). It is diluted with mineral oil in a glass syringe and infused per rectum about 4 cms into the rectum. The buttocks are then elevated and squeezed together for 5 minutes to avoid evacuation. One has to watch carefully for mucosal irritation.

Intravenous Valproate: Use of intravenous valproate has shown promising result in the management of refractory status epilepticus. Preliminary studies in adults and in children have shown that sodium valproate is effective and safe over a large range of doses as well as various rates of administration, including when given as a rapid bolus. In a recently concluded randomized trial on 40 children with RSE, we found that intravenous sodium valproate was as effective as diazepam infusion is controlling refractory status epilepticus in children and it was free of adverse effects such as respiratory depression and hypotension. Sodium valproate was given as an initial loading bolus of 30 mg/kg diluted 1:1 in normal saline over 2-5 min. If the status was not controlled within 10 minutes after the bolus dose, a repeat bolus dose of 10 mg/kg was given. This was followed by infusion at rate of 5 mg/kg/hr, which was continued until a seizure free period of 6 hours and then reduced at a rate of 1 mg/kg/hr every 2 hourly. After discontinuation of intravenous infusion, a maintenance dose of 10 mg/kg/dose 8 hourly I.V. was continued until the child could take oral anticonvulsants.

Step 4

If seizure activity persists even after the above-mentioned treatment, the child has to be treated as refractory status epilepticus—Consider use of diazepam or midazolam infusion, barbiturate induced coma, or inhalation anaesthetics. Before use of anaesthetic agents the patient should be put on a ventilator and continuous EEG monitoring regardless of the drug used. The purpose is to give sufficient dosage to produce either a flat EEG or a burst suppression pattern.

Diazepam infusion may be considered when there is an initial response to benzodiazepines and particularly when ventilatory support is not readily available. Diazepam is diluted in normal maintenance fluid (N/5 saline in glucose) to give a strength of 0.04 mg/ml. The starting dose is 0.01 mg/kg/min, which is increased gradually every few minutes until the seizures are fully controlled. Most children require 0.02 mg/kg/min, but can tolerate even higher doses if requires. We have sometimes used doses upto 0.1 mg/kg/min. Midazolam infusion may also be used as an alternative but it is associated with higher risk of seizure recurrence after initial control.

Pentobarbital coma: is preferred because of its relative short half life (11-23 hours) permitting rapid coma reversal. The loading dose is 10-15 mg/kg; the initial maintenance rate is 1 mg/kg/hr, which is increased every 5-10 min until SE is controlled or a flat EEG is attained.

Thiopental is used when short acting general anaesthesia is desired. Initial dose is 4-8 mg/kg IV given over 2 min, followed by a continuous infusion of 0.2 mg/kg/min. The rate is increased every 3-5 min by 0.1 mg/kg/min until SE is controlled or a flat EEG recording is attained. The major limitation of the drug is hypotension which often requires vasopressor support.

Inhalation anaesthetics are an alternative adjunct if barbiturate coma is not an option. Agents like halothane or isoflurane may be used. This needs involvement of anaesthetist and anaesthetic apparatus. All these agents may however, increase intracranial pressure, and are very rarely used in children.

Other Drugs

Propofol in high doses have been shown to be effective. The initial dose is 1-3 mg/kg IV followed by a continuous infusion of 2-10 mg/kg/hour as guided by EEG. However such patients invariably require intubation and mechanical ventilation because of hypoxia or inefficient ventilation. The other adverse effects are apnea, bradycardia, hypertriglyceridemia, rhabdomyolysis and unexplained metabolic acidosis. Propofol is not cleared for use in young children.

Lidocaine has a biphasic effect, as it can itself produce seizures at higher concentrations. It is generally not recommended but may be used when other proven drugs are not available or in children who become hypotensive from other drugs. The initial loading dose is 1-2 mg/kg IV given over 2 min; if seizures stop, continuous infusion of 20-50 μg/kg/min is given.

Etomidate infusion 20 mg/kg following a loading dose of 0.3 mg/kg, **ketamine infusion** and **chlormethiazole infusion** 0.08 mg/kg/min in incremental dose may also be used.

Electroencephalographic monitoring is essential in treatment of SE. In a recent study in adults, 48% of patients had persistent seizure activity and 14% had persistent non-convulsive status after clinical control of convulsive status.

OUTCOME AND PROGNOSIS

Complications of SE are shown in Table 11.1; some of these could be fatal such as cardiac arrhythmias and acute renal failure.

The mortality ranges from 3-10% in children and the morbidity is twice this. Neurological sequelae–motor or cognitive deficit–have been found in 9-28% and subsequent epilepsy in 23-30%. Very few children after SE were found to be normal on followup. We found that SE was the most important determinant of decrease in IQ of children with epilepsy. The outcome depends mainly on the age, rapidity of SE and adequacy of care. In the emergency department, the outcome is primarily a function of the underlying etiology. When there is nonidiopathic, nonfebrile etiology and no acute or progressive CNS insult, morbidity and mortality are low. On the other hand mortality and morbidity are highest with SE associated with CNS infections.

Table 11.4: Protocol and time table for the treatment of status epilepticus

(min)Time	*Drug treatment*	*Supportive treatment*
0		Ensure adequate respiration Intubation considered
2-3		Start low flow oxygen Start an intravenous line with D5W or normal saline Draw blood for glucose, hepatic and renal function, CBC with DLC, electrolytes, calcium, magnesium, blood gases and toxicology screen
		Obtain urine for routine examination
3-5	Diazepam: 0.3mg/kg or Lorazepam 0.1mg/kg-infused over 2 minutes	Start second IV line with D5W or normal saline for simultaneous administration of a second medication and IV fluids
7-8	Phenytoin- 20mg/kg dilute in saline and infuse at a rate of not more than 1 mg/kg/min	**D50W**- 1ml/kg IV push; Thiamine-100mg-IV push, Pyridoxine-100-200mg of IV push in children < 18 months of age Monitor blood pressure
10	Repeat Diazepam/Lorazepam	Bicarbonate depending on results of blood gases
15	Repeat Diazepam/Lorazepam	
20	IV valproate 30 mg/kg; 1:1 in saline	
30	Diazepam or Midazolam infusion (Diazepam: 0.01mg/kg/min, max 0.1mg/kg/min, Midazolam: 2μg/kg/min up to 12 μg/kg/min in increments of 1μg/kg/min every 5-10 minutes till seizure control.*)	Transfer to PICU, prepare for intubation, ventilation, get EEG
60	Thiopental-load with 3-4 mg/kg given over 2 minutes followed by an infusion at 0.2 mg/kg/min.increase the dose every 3-5 minutes by 0.1mg/kg/min (until seizure control and the EEG is isoelectric.	Start mechanical ventilation

*Continue for 6 hours after the last seizure then start tapering every two hours by 1μg/kg/min.

In conclusion, SE requires prompt and vigorous treatment. Uncontrolled seizure activity can result in progressive neuronal damage. All treating units, should establish a time framed treatment protocol. Protocol used in our emergency unit and PICU is shown in Table 11.4. Aggressive approach is a pre-requisite to improve the outcome.

Chapter twelve

Intensive Care of Critically Ill Neurologic Patients

Intensive care of patients with acute neurologic disorders is multifaceted. Many consultants, physical and respiratory therapists, nutritionist and neurologic critical care nurses are often involved Neurocritical care starts with airway, breathing and circulation and goes on to specifics of neurologic problems (Table 12.1). During daily rounds, it is pertinent to review nursing care, physical therapy, infection precautions, nutrition, and other prophylactic measures. Each of these require specific management in neurologic critical illness and are discussed here. Lack of attention to any of these may potentially result in a less favourable outcome.

MANAGEMENT OF AIRWAY

Adequate supply of oxygen can be given through nasal prongs or plastic facemasks. However, most neurologic patients in ICU require help with airway management. Diminished activity in the upper airway muscles is more common in patients with acute central nervous system lesions. The tongue significantly contributes to airway obstruction when there is loss of tone in oropharyngeal muscles in patients with impaired consciousness. Inappropriate securing of the airway may rapidly result in hypoxemia. If ignored, these events may add to the initial insult and lead to a worse outcome.

Securing the airway by head tilt and gentle lifting of the jaw upward to open the collapsed airway is required. A nasopharyngeal or oral airway can be placed. An oral airway has the added advantage of protecting tongue bite in patients with seizures. Bag and mask ventilation without intubation can be fairly easily given and can maintain the airway for at least 1 hour.

Table 12.1: Components of neurocritical care

1. Airway, oxygen,
2. General Care—Nursing
3. Postural & physical therapy
4. Maintenance of cerebral perfusion pressure & cerebral blood flow—through fluids, BP management
5. Analgesia and sedation
6. Control of Status epilepticus & Refractory Status epilepticus
7. Diagnosis and Control of Raised ICP
8. Infection control
9. Specific aspects of Mechanical Ventilation
10. Monitoring—clinical and electrophysiological

Endotracheal Intubation

It is indicated in patients who cannot protect the airway, may have aspirated gastric contents and in those who are hypoventilating because of neuromuscular disease. Elective intubation using RSI should be done by an experienced person. Though nasal intubation has several advantages in patients with head injury and potential cerebrospinal fluid leak, it may lead to contamination and in some cases transient bacteremia. It may also lead to nasal septal necrosis and perforation of the nasal plate. In patients with

Guillain-Barré Syndrome and in patients who need mechanical ventilation for several days, the overwhelming comfort of nasal tube placement with appropriate mouth care may prevail over the disadvantage. ***Nonetheless, oral intubation is the preferred route.***

Recognition of difficult airway is important. Cues for a difficult intubation include inability to visualize oral structures such as soft palate, tonsillar fossa, and uvula when the mouth is wide open, significant facial trauma, cervical spine fracture, mandibular hypoplasia, obesity, and short muscular, thick neck. (See the appendix for procedure of endotracheal intubation, and chapter 5, Airway Management).

Tracheostomy

Early tracheostomy should be considered when prolonged mechanical ventilation is anticipated. The timing of tracheostomy placement is controversial. The central issues in the decision to proceed with early tracheostomy are the comfort of the patient, more effective tracheal suctioning, and the considerable risk of tracheolaryngeal stenosis from prolonged intubation. The incidence of tracheal stenosis is nearly 10 percent within 2 weeks after endotracheal intubation. General guideline is to wait 3 weeks to assess the need for tracheostomy but to proceed with tracheostomy earlier in patients who may significantly benefit from the increased comfort. Tracheostomy should be considered earlier for deeply comatose patients and in patients with severe Guillain-Barré Syndrome characterized by severe quadriplegia and progressively abnormal results of electrophysiological studies. Many patients may be weaned from mechanical ventilation within 2 to 3 weeks, tracheostomy should be postponed in such patients.

GENERAL NURSING CARE

Neurologic evaluation should be directed at assessing the progress of primary disease and degree of CNS compromise. Evaluation for the latter should include assessment of respiratory pattern, heart rate, blood pressure (lability, hypertension), and gradation of sensorium changes. Glasgow coma scale (GCS) modified for children is commonly used for quick assessment of sensorium. Elevation of intracranial pressure should be anticipated in patients who have low GCS score, decerebrate or decorticate posture, or continuous seizure activity.

Routine evaluation (monitoring) of patients every hour to measure the level of alertness, detect new neurologic signs, and recognize seizure, agitation and pain is important. Changes in neurologic condition may be subtle, and in many instances no exact physiologic measurement is available to confirm a change in neurologic status.

Mouth, Skin and Eye Care

Important aspects of nursing care are attention to mouth, skin and eye; checking of Foley's catheters, nasogastric tubes, and intravascular catheters; dressing changes for monitoring devices and adequate body positioning and respiratory care. Equally important in intensive care is optimization of comfort and, if possible, sleep.

Skin care has a high priority in immobilized patients. Decubital ulcers, or more often patches of demarcated painful erythema indicative of developing ulcers may appear, in spite of meticulous care. The risk of ischemic damage over the sacral skin area is most prominent in the supine position and less in the 45° position. Frequent turning in bed, lanolin creams and dry patting of the skin are essential. Use of air-fluidized mattresses is critical when prolonged immobilization from coma or quadriplegia (Guillain-Barré Syndrome) is expected. Repositioning is performed every 2 hours but must be more frequent if erythema occurs.

Eye care is important in comatose patients. Daily application of methyl-cellulose drops with taping of the eyelids is important to reduce corneal abrasions. Positive pressure ventilation may cause severe conjunctival chemosis, resulting in inability to close the eyes.

Mouth care includes use of lip balm, repositioning of the oral tube to reduce pressure sores, and moistening of the gum and mouth.

Positioning of comatose patients: A neutral or side-lying position should be adopted, with a pillow between the legs to prevent internal rotation, adduction, and inversion of the upper legs. Patients with a flaccid paralysis from Guillain-Barré Syndrome should have footboards, splinting to prevent contractures, and trochanter towel rolls to prevent entrapment neuropathy of the peroneal nerve. It is important to avoid compression at the elbows to protect the ulnar nerve.

Comatose patients with marked extensor posturing are difficult to position. Footboards and splints are not useful, because they apply stretch and potentially further increase the tone.

In the properly "aligned" patient in a dorsal position, the head is in neutral position, arms are flexed at the elbow with the hands resting at the side of abdomen. The knees are extended or are slightly flexed, with trochanter rolls folded under the greater trochanter hip joint area to reduce pressure on the peroneal nerve at the fibula head, and the feet are ideally at 70° to 90° to the legs, with the toes pointing upward.

Positioning of patients with hemiplegia: The head and neck should be in midline. A pillow is placed in the axilla to counter the tendency of the arm to adduct and rotate internally. The paralyzed arm is supported on a pillow with the elbow partially flexed. Trochanter rolls are used to prevent external rotation at the hip joint. In the lateral position, patients should be turned on the unaffected side without flexion of the trunk spine. Extension, adduction, and internal rotation of the shoulder should be avoided.

In patients with flaccid quadriplegia (Guillain-Barré Syndrome) the frogline position (a modification of Fowler's sitting position) is favoured. The shoulders are supported with several pillows in the axilla and under the knees, and the hips slightly abducted, splinting of the hands and use of footboards are essential for preventing contractures.

PHYSICAL THERAPY

Physical therapy should begin virtually immediately; it includes passive range of motion and chest physiotherapy for postural drainage.

Initially, range of motion exercise are passive, consisting of abduction, adduction, flexion and extension motions. Passive movements of the limbs are focused on proximal limb muscles, with flexion and extension of the knee while the hip is extended and the foot is held in dorsiflexion. Range-of-motion exercise should ideally be done two times daily. Active exercises should be done gradually.

Chest physiotherapy is extremely important. It involves positioning for postural drainage, suctioning and if possible breathing exercises. Percussion and vibration are additionally effective in mobilizing retained secretions. Coughing must be stimulated in alert patients. Huffing (large inspiration followed by short expiratory blasts) may stimulate coughing (Table 12.2).

A flat position before tracheal suctioning may increase intracranial pressure. It is, therefore, important to assess the effect of position change on intracranial pressure. If intracranial pressure does not return to baseline value after a mild increase from change into a flat position, brief hyperventilation through a manual resuscitation bag is necessary. Marked intracranial pressure surges or plateau waves can be muted by an intravenous bolus of lidocaine (1 mg/kg).

Incentive spirometry is important in patients with neuromuscular respiratory failure. It may prevent mechanical ventilation in patients with Guillain-Barré Syndrome.

Table 12.2: Essentials of chest physiotherapy

- Percussion and vibration
- Coughing exercises
- Suctioning (preceded by hyperoxygenation, FiO_2 1.0 for 15 seconds)
- Mucolytic agents, bronchodilators, and nebulizers for humidification

MANAGEMENT OF AGITATION

Many patients with an acute, catastrophic intracranial neurologic illness are agitated and are often noticeably uncomfortable. Typical neurologic causes for severe agitation and confusion are bifrontal infarcts, infarction of the basal ganglia, large infarcts of the middle cerebral artery territory and involvement of the thalamus.

Agitation may also have its origin in borderline ventilation and gas exchange. Patients with aspiration pneumonia or early acute respiratory distress syndrome become significantly tachypneic and agitated, and oxygenation rapidly becomes insufficient. Mechanical ventilation is often only possible with some degree of sedation. Pulling of intravascular and bladder catheters, endotracheal tubes, and nasogastric tubes may be a danger to the patient.

Traditionally, neurologists have opposed the use of any form of sedation to counter agitation. This reluctance can be overcome if recovery from sedation is rapid or sedation can be reversed with an antidote. Current examples are—propofol and midazolam.

Pharmaceutical Agents for Sedation

Propofol

The major distinguishing feature of propofol is the speedy rate of recovery, within minutes, in almost all patients. Brain stem reflexes may become abolished and only pupil size and light response may remain preserved. It is contraindicated in rapidly evolving neurologic catastrophies. Propofol may also have a place in the management of increased intracranial pressure. It is given as an infusion at a low-dose rate of 0.1 mg/kg per minute, with incremental doses at 5-minute intervals until reasonable sedation occurs. Even after high-dose propofol infusion for almost a full day, awakening after discontinuation is comparatively rapid. Antidote for propofol is not available. Propofol may reduce blood pressure. Its use in very young children usually is not recommended.

Midazolam

Midazolam is a short-acting benzodiazepine. It has an antidote and causes complete amnesia of unpleasant events. The clearance of midazolam is significantly reduced in hepatic or renal failure *Dose:* bolus of 0.2 mg/kg, followed by infusion at rate of 1 to 2 μg/kg per minute (max upto 18 μg). The effect can be rapidly reversed with flumazenil 0.2 to 0.4 mg intravenously given over 15 seconds. Repeat doses at 1-minute intervals may be needed for maximal effect.

Lorazepam

IV 0.05 mg/kg slowly may be used as an alternative.

PAIN MANAGEMENT

Pain is highly prevalent in patients with acute neurologic disorders. Disturbance of sleep from pain is extremely detrimental in patients with early diaphragmatic failure from acute Guillain-Barré Syndrome and may lead to premature endotracheal intubation and mechanical ventilation. Immediate relief of pain not only results in visible comfort but also reduces potentially threatening physiologic responses.

Pain is signalled not only by moaning, crying, grimacing, and extreme restlessness but also by profuse sweating, sustained tachycardia, blood pressure fluctuations, and dilated pupils. One should be sensitive to the fact that lack of expression of pain does not mean lack of pain.

The decision to use pain medications depends greatly on whether simple nursing measures (e.g., adequate positioning, catheterization) or use of distraction techniques (music, television, family visits) can reduce pain. When no other obvious cause is apparent, analgesics should be administered. Increased agitation with any type of stimulation and change in physiologic parameters such as tachycardia, blood pressure surges are at times helpful indications. Pain may appear in several forms, including hyperalgesia, sciatica, muscle pain and cramps, and joint stiffness. Typically there is nocturnal aggravation. Positioning, splinting, and use of bed cages, gloves, or cotton socks may reduce burning, needle-like pain and a feeling of skin tightening. Hot or cold packs may also be useful.

Opioid analgesics remain the mainstay of pain management in patients with critical neurologic illness.

Opiates

Opiates are invariably effective. Fear of addiction after prolonged hospital use is vastly exaggerated. Morphine is the prototype narcotic. Intravenous administration is preferred for acute pain management. Alternative (but weaker) narcotic analgesics are codeine and pethidine. They have less severe potential side effects in particular, less sedation. They must be used preferentially in patients with acute central nervous system injury in whom sedation is unacceptable.The doses and route of administration of opiate commonly used in PICU are shown in Table 12.3.

Nausea and vomiting occur in 30 percent of patients treated with repetitive doses of narcotics but are rapidly reversible. Narcotics are also known to cause water retention from secretion of antidiuretic hormone. Combined with excessive vomiting this may potentially lead to profound hyponatremia. Respiratory depression (detected by relative hypercapnia because of hypoventilation) occurs in susceptible patients but is dose-dependent.

Naloxone reverses opioid toxicity. Repeated doses of 0.2 mg every 3 minutes are needed to obtain an effect.

Table 12.3: Opiates for pain management in the PICU

Agent	*Route*	*Dose (mg/kg)*	*Peak effect, hr*	*Duration hr*
Codeine	IM	0.5-1	0.5-1	4-6
Dose	p.o.	0.5-1	1.5-2	3-4
Morphine	IM	0.1	0.5-1	3-5
Pethidine	IM	1.0	0.5-1	2-3

Nonsteroidal Anti-Inflammatory Agents

NSAIDs are promising in patients with acute neurologic illness and severe headaches because they have a minimal effect on the level of consciousness. Use of NSAIDs is potentially associated with major side effects such as mucosal damage, gastrointestinal bleeding, and perforation, but these side effects are less common with brief exposure. Cimetidine and sucralfate are ineffective in protection against gastric ulcers from NSAIDs. NSAIDs are contraindicated in patients with intracranial hemorrhage.

Seizure Control

Seizure control is necessary to prevent cerebral damage. It must be achieved as early as possible (For details see chapter on status epilepticus). Briefly, Diazepam bolus (0.2-0.3 mg/kg IV) is used for controlling seizures. A repeat dose may be used. If diazepam is ineffective, intravenous phenytoin (20 mg/kg diluted in saline, at a rate of 0.75 mg/kg/min) is the recommended drug. IV phenytoin may cause bradycardia and other arrhythmias, depress myocardial contractility, cause peripheral vasodilatation and hypotension. It should therefore be used with caution in cases with unstable hemodynamic status. If seizures are still uncontrolled we use IV valproate 30 mg/kg bolus diluted 1: 1 with normal saline, and if needed diazepam by continuous IV infusion (0.01–0.05 mg/kg/min) and if necessary thiopental (loading dose 2-8 mg/kg IV) followed by infusion at a starting rate of 0.2 mg/kg/min, increasing every 3-5 min by 0.1 mg/kg/min till seizure are controlled. Both the drugs cause marked respiratory depression, esp. thiopental therefore facility for mechanical ventilation must be available if these drugs are used. Thiopental may also cause cardiac depression and severe hypotension, and compromise cerebral perfusion, which could be deleterious in patients with raised intracranial pressure. Blood pressure must be monitored in such patients and inotrope support should be instituted at the earliest to maintain normal blood pressure. (for details see ch-10 Status Epilepticus).

MANAGEMENT OF VOLUME STATUS

Hypovolemia is an important potential clinical concern in virtually all patients with acute central nervous system injury. Once common, orders by physicians for fluid restriction in patients with acute catastrophic events have now been modified into skillful limitation of free water and maintenance of euvolemic fluid status. Coincident with this diametrical change in patient fluid management has been a change in the management of acutely increased blood pressure. In many instances simply completely ignoring of acute hypertension has become a standard approach in the immediate management of acute neurologic disorders.

Critically ill patients often have a marginal fluid balance and disproportionately increased risk of dehydration. This may be because of several factors. First, the inability/ failure to recognize the thirst signal in comatose patients after acute catastrophic events may lead to rapid deficits in volume. Second, insensible losses associated with fever are invariably underestimated. Also, profound emesis may contribute to dehydration and hypovolemia, which is often unveiled when these patients are placed on mechanical ventilators. Sudden introduction of positive pressure ventilation in previously hypovolemic patients results in a marked decrease in blood pressure. Hypotension is a consequence of a decrease in cardiac output, primarily because of decreased venous return.

An initial fluid bolus of 20 mL/kg/hour is appropriate. The preferred fluid is 0.9 percent sodium chloride; glucose-based solutions are avoided. The next step in computation of maintenance fluid is calculation of the insensible losses from lungs and skin; it is often underestimated. Hyperventilation, sweating, dysautonomia in Guillain-Barré Syndrome with episodic diaphoresis may increase insensible losses.

Urine output must total at least 1 mL/kg per hour. Urine output greater than 2 mL/kg/hour may indicate over intake of fluids, at urine flow > 5 ml/kg diabetes insipidus should be excluded.

As indicators of volume status in patients with acute neurologic illness one should monitor, serum sodium, creatinine, blood urea, serum glucose, plasma osmolality, pH, PCO_2, PO_2, base excess, urine osmolality (optional) and urine specific gravity.

Fluid Replacement

Use of crystalloids is generally preferred in patients with acute neurologic disorders (Isotonic saline, Ringer lactate solution). Major drawback of using isotonic saline and Ringer's solution is redistribution. These fluids remain intravascular for a maximum of 2 hours, barely enough time to have a major effect on volume status, and are clearly insufficient when a sustained effect is warranted. The effect of hypertonic saline is much more significant as it recruits fluid from the intracellular space but again it is transient. Colloid replacement is more effective in situations requiring rapid correction of intravascular volume. The disadvantages of colloids are greater expense, reduction in ionized calcium and a small risk of anaphylactic reactions and clinically relevant coagulopathy

The effect of fluid challenge is determined by changes in blood pressure (increases), heart rate (decreases), and urine production (increases). Lack of a persistent effect in hypovolemic patients warrants infusion of 3 percent hypertonic saline, given at a rate of 4 mL/kg over 3 minutes. Response can be prolonged when saline is combined with 5 percent albumin. Judicious use of small, incremental quantities may reduce the risk of pulmonary edema in patients.

BLOOD PRESSURE MANAGEMENT

Increase in blood pressure is common in acute central nervous system lesions. Causes for increase in blood pressure may include pain, agitation, and frequent bucking of the ventilator. Hypertension after acute CNS injury has historically been attributed to the "Cushing response". Classic explanation is increased intracranial pressure associated with a decrease in cerebral perfusion pressure resulting in brain stem ischemia. Distortion of the brain stem is likely explanation. Unfortunately there is often a tendency to immediately control acute hypertension, which is theoretically linked to the fear of progression of brain edema in a lesion with an acutely opened blood brain barrier, extension of the volume of intracerebral hematoma and possible clinical deterioration from hemorrhagic transformation. These basic premises can be challenged. A study of patients with untreated very high systolic blood pressure could not identify an increased risk of progression of symptoms in acute stroke. Until results of prospective studies become available, increased blood pressure after acute brain injury probably should be left alone.

When hypertension accompanies an acute encephalopathic illness, it must be determined as to whether the high BP is the cause of coma or a reflex response to a primary brain injury and increased intracranial pressure. Fundoscopy to look for signs of chronic hypertension ECG chest X-ray and a CT Scan may be helpful. In patients with hypertensive encephalopathy the goal of therapy is to reduce mean arterial BP by 25% over period of minutes to one hour. The treatment is directed at reducing fluid overload, cardiac output, reducing peripheral resistance or at inactivating the hormonal system which has been stimulated. Hypertensive crisis may be managed by infusion of sodium nitroprusside, or stat dose of diazoxide (1-3 mg/kg IV), Labetalol (1-3 mg/kg/hour) or hydralazine. Sodium nitroprusside (0.5 to 8.0 μg/kg/min) by continuous IV infusion at a rate titrated to achieve desirable BP is the drug of choice in PICU. The vasodilator used most frequently is hydralazine hydrochloride, at a dose of 0.1 to 0.2 mg/kg, IV push with a maximum of 20 mg every 4 to 6 hourly. Nifedepine, oral or sublingual, 0.25 mg-0.5 mg/kg 4-6 hourly may be used for in the emerency room management of hypertensive urgencies and emergencies where IV infusion is not feasible. Unexpected sudden decrease in blood pressure may occur sometimes, hence BP should be continuously monitored. Alongwith vasodilation, diuresis should be induced by means of loop diuretics. (Furosemide 1 to 2 mg/kg by slow IV administration). Oral antihypertensive drugs that have been used successfully in PICU patients include labetolol (maximum 5 mg/kg), captopril (maximum dose 8 mg/kg/d in two to three doses per day, onset of action in 15 to 90 minutes), clonidine hydrochloride (maximum dose 2-4 mg/d in two divided doses, onset of action in 30 to 60 minutes), and propranolol hydrochloride (maximum dose 10 mg/kg/d in two to three doses, onset of action in two to 72 hours).

Treatment of hypertension is a reasonable consideration in pediatric patients with impending congestive cardiac failure, those who have computed tomography scan evidence of rapidly worsening brain edema and those with persistent extreme surges in blood pressure.

Agents with combined α-and β-adrenergic receptor blocking properties are preferred in the management of acute hypertension. Labetalol is relatively easy to use, and an unexpected decrease in blood pressure does not occur. Labetalol is not recommended for patients with asthma, and chronic or severe left ventricular failure. In these patients, an angiotensin-converting enzyme inhibitor or calcium channel blocker should be the preferred agent.

MANAGEMENT OF RAISED INTRACRANIAL PRESSURE

Raised Intracranial Pressure

Normal intracranial pressure (ICP) is less than 15 mmHg. An increase in ICP may be accompanied by disruption of autoregulation, hence maintenance of adequate cerebral perfusion pressure (CPP) becomes important.

CPP = MAP – ICP (or CVP if greater)

where MAP is mean arterial pressure.

Relationships of cerebral blood flow, cerebral blood volume, cerebral perfusion pressure (CPP), ICP, and mean arterial blood pressure to one another are complex. Monroe-Kellie doctrine states that although intracranial volume relationships may vary, the total intracranial volume remains constant. The intracranial volume is determined by the sum of the volumes of brain tissue (90%), cerebrospinal fluid (CSF) (5%) and blood (5%). This volume is constant because the skull is rigid. The introduction of an additional volume (e.g., a mass or swollen brain tissue) must, by necessity, be compensated for by changes in the blood or CSF compartments for intracranial volume to remain stable. Failure to do so results in increased pressure in the intracranial compartment and tissue shift.

Causes of raised ICP include:

1. Increased brain tissue: tumor, cerebral edema.
2. Increased CSF: hydrocephalus.
3. Increased cerebral blood volume: hyperemia, drug-induced vasodilation, hypercapnia, coughing, venous hypertension, hematoma.

The major mechanisms that compensate for an increase in ICP are movement of CSF into the spinal subarachnoid space and decrease of blood from the cerebrovascular bed. CSF absorption, is largely caused by the low outflow resistance of the arachnoid villi. If the limits of these compensatory mechanisms are exceeded, the ICP begins to rise. The end result is brain tissue protrudes through opening or lining of intracranial cavity, causing brain herniation syndromes. The herniation may occur under the falx cerebri, or central or diencephalic transtentorial herniation, uncal herniation over the lateral edge of the tentorium (Fig. 12.1), and, in a number of cases, herniation through a craniotomy defect.

Clinical Features

Usual early features are headache (classically worse in the morning) and vomiting (typically without nausea), followed by visual disturbance,

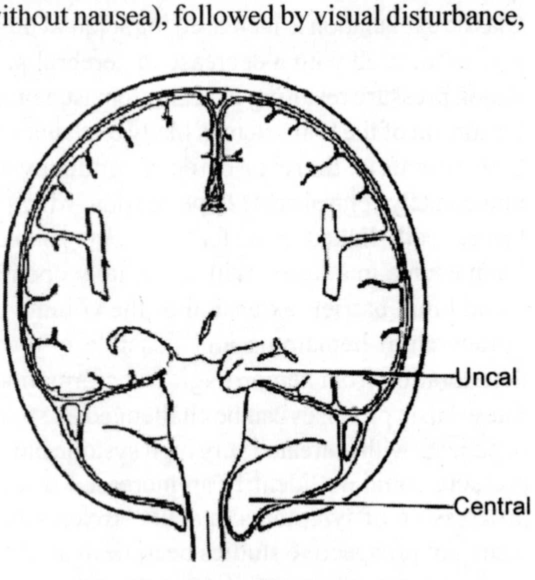

Fig. 12.1: Sites of brain herniation

Table 12.4: Syndrome of brain herniation

Cingulate (Lateral) Herniation

A lesion in one cerebral hemisphere causes lateral displacement across the midline of the intracranial cavity under the flax cerebri and may lead to compression of the internal cerebral vein and ipsilateral anterior cerebral artery. It may be asymptomatic. Compression of blood vessels may contribute to cerebral ischemia and increased intracranial pressure and transtentorial herniation.

Central Downward (Transtentorial) Herniation

Downward displacement of the cerebral hemispheres pushes the diencephalons and midbrain through the tentorial notch, compressing branches of the basilar artery and causing deterioration of the brain stem. With progression it causes lethargy, decreased purposeful movement, ipsilateral weakness or paralysis, up-going plantar reflex, Cheyne-Stokes respirations or normal pattern, small (1-3mm), equal and reactive pupils and increasing blood pressure, stupor, coma and decorticate posturing;

Once Midbrain is affected the patient has decerebrate posturing, bilateral weakness or paralysis, central neurogenic hyperventilation and fixed mid-dilated (3-5mm) pupils

Progression involving Pons results in absent oculocephalic and oculovestibular reflexes (Doll's eye movements) and cluster respirations (slow to absent).

Finally when Medulla is affected, the patient has absent motor responses, ataxic respirations (gasping), fully dilated pupils and hypotension.

Uncal Herniation

An expanding mass in the temporal lobe or middle fossa pushes the uncus toward or over the edge of the tentorium, compressing the oculomotor nerve, midbrain, and brainstem.

The physical findings initially are related to compression of third cranial nerve on the same side as mass. There is ipsilateral dilation of pupil with sluggish or no reaction. The major difference between central and uncal herniation is the initial pupil changes in uncal herniation.

Irreversible damage to III cranial nerve (late third nerve sign) and dysfunction of midbrain results in stupor, opposite side extension posturing and same side weakness and paralysis, and same-side fixed and dilated pupil. Infarction of midbrain causes bilateral extension posturing, central neurogenic hyperventilation, progressing to bilateral fixed and dilated pupils.

Downward Cerebellar (Tonsilar) Herniation

There is rapid descent of the contents of the posterior fossa into the foramen magnum and onto the medulla. This results in acute dysfunction of lower pons and medulla, rapid deterioration in level of consciousness, acute flaccid quadriplegia, and terminally cardiopulmonary arrest.

depressed consciousness level and coma. Signs of brain herniation (Table 12.4), and cardiorespiratory changes are seen in preterminal stages (e.g., Cushing's response of hypertension and bradycardia, respiratory arrhythmia).

In an intact pressure regulation system, cerebral blood flow is constant with a CPP between 50 and 150 mm Hg or mean arterial blood pressure between 60 and 160 mm Hg. Autoregulation is often impaired in patients with acute brain injury, but impairment is highly variable in different regions of the brain. Marginal decrease in blood flow may cause ischemia, this can be compensated for by increased oxygen extraction from the blood. Further reduction in cerebral blood flow leads to ischemia and infarction. The goals of ICP management are shown in Table 12.5.

Table 12.5: Raised intracranial pressure: Goals of management

1. Reduction in ICP *to prevent herniation.*
2. Maintenance of *optimal CBF*- to prevent further hypoxic ischemic injury.
3. *Reduction in cerebral metabolic rate* - to prevent demand-supply mismatch.

Therapeutic Options

A reduction in increased ICP may be achieved through CSF withdrawal by ventricular drain, reduction of the cerebral tissue volume by osmotic dehydration, reduction of the cerebral blood volume by reduction of cerebral blood flow or by promotion of cerebral venous drainage, and removal or decompression of a mass (Table 12.6).

Table 12.6: Intracranial pressure reduction: Methods

1. ***Reduction of the cerebral blood volume*** by reduction of cerebral blood flow (Hyperventilation) or by promotion of cerebral venous drainage (head-positioning)
2. ***Reduction of the cerebral tissue volume***—osmotic dehydration
3. ***CSF withdrawal*** by ventricular drain
4. Removal or decompression of a mass

Use of different modalities to treat raised ICP depends on the cause and speed of onset. Acute raised ICP should be treated as follows:

1. Intubation and manual hyperventilation to reduce $PaCO_2$ to 30-35 mmHg and thus achieve a reduced cerebral blood volume.
2. Mannitol (20%) 0.25-0.5 g/kg to reduce cerebral water content.
3. Dexamethasone for edema associated with tumors.
   These should be followed by maintenance of CPP at more than 70 mmHg, mannitol 0.25 g/kg every 4-6 hours. Furosemide may be added but one should be beware of a sudden fall in CPP because of hypovolemia. Controlled ventilation should be instituted if respiratory failure is present.
4. Intravenous thiopental may be used in refractory/unresponsive patients to reduce cerebral metabolic rate and therefore cerebral blood volume. The dose used is dose: 1.5 to 5 mg/kg by slow bolus infusion; followed by continuous infusion of up to 5 mg/kg/ hour to produce burst suppression on EEG. This should be given with full resuscitation facilities at hand; a reduction in MAP occur.
5. **Ventricular drainage** remains a very rational solution to increased ICP in patients with acute hydrocephalus, in closed head injury, however, its use is very controversial.

CT scan should be obtained to exclude surgical lesions such as hematoma, tumor, hydrocephalus.

Reduction of mean arterial blood pressure reduces cerebral blood flow, but in a defective auto-regulatory system, it produces ischemia. Conversely, an increase in mean arterial blood pressure increases blood flow and blood volume, and may result in an increase in ICP. Oxygenation and normal mean arterial blood pressure should therefore be maintained. High levels of positive end-expiratory pressure (10-12 mmHg) may not markedly influence cerebral venous return. However, it may interfere with systemic arterial pressure.

The head position should be neutral to reduce any possible compression of the jugular veins that could lead to a decrease in intracranial venous outflow. The head should be elevated 15°-30°. Elevation of the head, however, may cause a reduction in arterial pressure, particularly if patient has marked hypovolemia or orthostasis. Trendelenburg's position should be avoided except in overt life-threatening shock. ICP should be monitored closely in patients.

Sedation: Any patient with increased ICP should be comfortable and rested. For endotracheal and bronchial suctioning number of passages through the endotracheal tube should be limited to one. A bolus of lidocaine should be administered endotrachealy (3 mg/kg/dose) to mute this response.

A euvolemic state should be maintained; fluid restriction is no longer recommended as treatment of increased ICP. Dehydration associated with fluid restriction causes hypotension and hemoconcentration with increased viscosity, which may have deleterious effects on cerebral perfusion.

Seizure prophylaxis and control: Seizures may greatly increase ICP. Prophylaxis with antiepileptic drugs is desirable. Intravenous loading with phenytoin should be strongly considered in patients with marginally compliant brain parenchyma and in patients at high risk for seizures.

In general, antihypertensive agents should be avoided, particularly vasodilators, such as hydralazine and nitroprusside, which may increase ICP to unacceptable levels.

Hyperventilation

Acute hyperventilation remains a very effective way of reducing intracranial pressure. It causes a reduction in ICP by cerebral vasoconstriction, which in turn reduces cerebral blood flow. Vasoconstriction is mediated by a change in the pH of CSF, and a narrow response to hyperventilation exists. Cerebral blood flow decreases 40 percent approximately 30 minutes after reduction of $PaCO_2$ by 15 to 20 mmHg. The effects of hyperventilation on cerebral blood flow and ICP are therefore not significant after several hours.

When hyperventilation is instituted, the change in ventilation should be derived largely from a change in respiratory rate. The respiratory rate can be increased while a normal tidal volume of 12 ml/kg is maintained. Increasing minute ventilation by changing both components may potentially lead to high airway pressures, barotraumas, and at the extreme, pneumothorax. End-tidal carbon dioxide can be used to monitor $PaCO_2$ but arterial blood gas is more reliable.

Sudden reduction in $PaCO_2$ may cause very significant hypotension. There is no evidence to suggest that patients with a recent severe impact to the brain need to be treated with prophylactic hyperventilation. There is a growing consensus that osmotic agents should be used first and that hyperventilation should become a second method of treatment only if brief, rapid reduction of ICP is necessary.

Weaning the patient from hyperventilation should be gradual; ventilation is reduced by two breaths per minute during careful monitoring of ICP. A rebound of ICP occurs in some patients but in many instances is simply not distinguishable from an increase due to progressive clinical neurologic deterioration.

Short-term hyperventilation remains an almost ideal method to reduce ICP in acute raised ICP. Neither prophylactic nor prolonged use is recommended. Hyperventilation is possibly best used as an adjunct to osmotic therapy. It can be introduced several times when needed rather than be used without interruption for prolonged periods.

Osmotic Diuresis

The basic principle of osmotherapy is to decrease brain water. Osmotic agents mostly shrink brain tissue that has not been damaged. The available agents include mannitol, hypertonic saline, albumin, glycerol and urea. In most institutions either mannitol or hypertonic saline is used to decrease ICP. Mannitol induces movement of brain water into the vascular space, increases cerebral blood flow from transient hypervolemia and hemodilution and results in a decrease in blood viscosity. Mannitol also probably increases CSF absorption.

The dose is 1.25-2.5 ml/kg of 20 percent solution (0.25 to 0.50 g/kg). Reduction in ICP with mannitol administration should be apparent after 15 minutes. Failure of ICP to respond to mannitol should be considered a poor prognostic sign. The goal for serum osmolarity should be 310 to 320 mOsm/L. A rebound to higher ICP values after administration of mannitol was discontinued was found in 12 percent patients. The ICP-reducing effect of mannitol diminishes over time and becomes ineffective once serum osmolality exceeds 320 mOsm/L.

Furosemide with albumin or hypertonic saline 3 percent, 50 ml in 10 minutes, can be given.

Barbiturate therapy is useful in reduction of ICP and may certainly decrease mortality in patients with uncontrollable ICP refractory to all other standard medical and surgical treatments. Treatment with barbiturates is highly complex.

Myocardial depression and hypothermia are major concerns. There is an increased risk of nosocomial infections particularly pneumonia, approximately 50 percent of the patients treated with barbiturates need inotropic agents to control hypotension. In many dobutamine and epinephrine are needed as well as additional fluids. These patients require regular hemodynamic monitoring. Barbiturate treatment is started with pentobarbital, 10 mg/kg intravenously over 30 minutes. The maintenance dose is generally 1 to 3 mg/kg hours by constant intravenous infusion. A higher dose (5 mg/kg per hour) can be used initially for several hours to obtain adequate loading. Thiopental may be used as an alternative. Blood pressure can be maintained with dopamine infusion (5 to 20 μg/kg per minute). Suppression of the electroencephalogram is usually seen when serum barbiturate levels are around 30 to 40 μg/dL. Common practice is to maintain barbiturate treatment for 2 to 3 days. When computed tomography scanning does not show any new findings or progression of findings and ICP is well controlled, barbiturate therapy can be withdrawn slowly by reduction of the infusion rate by 50 percent each day.

Miscellaneous Options: Use of corticosteroids has been futile in patients with severe head injury, high-dose dexamethasone and methyl prednisolone (30 mg/kg) do not improve outcome.

Moderate hypothermia (core temperature, 32°C to 33°C) for 24 hours by use of cooling blankets above and below the patient has been shown to reduce ICP and increase CPP without an increase in risk of bacterial infections.

MECHANICAL VENTILATION

Management of mechanical ventilation is different in neurologic critical illness for several reasons. First, many patients have normal baseline pulmonary function. Second, mode of ventilation in acutely ill neurologic patients is often intermittent mandatory or assisted control. Third, ventilator dependency is less common, and most acutely ill neurologic patients can later be successfully weaned from the ventilator.

Indications

Indication for mechanical ventilation are impairment of respiratory drive or mechanics of the respiratory system or intrinsic pulmonary disease. ***Depression of level of consciousness is not absolute indication for mechanical ventilation. Also, there is no rationale to prophylactically intubate and hyperventilate patients to produce hypocapnia*** when there is a risk of brain swelling.

Central Nervous System Dysfunction (Impaired Respiratory Drive) – ***As a general rule, patients with abnormal breathing patterns that result in inadequate oxygen delivery and hypercapnia need to be mechanically ventilated.*** Many patients, particularly in the first hour, have marked spontaneous hyperventilation. There is a tendency to assume that the most prominent factor in hyperventilation is sustained resetting of the feedback loops in the respiratory centers. Patients with prolonged hyperventilation are probably better served by assisted mode of ventilation with mild sedation.

Hyperventilation may signal development of diencephalic herniation. Pathologic flexion or extension may emerge. Pupils usually remain in mid-position and become fixed. Ataxic and cluster breathing, recurrent apnea may indicate a high probability of progression to brain stem death. Cheyne-Stokes breathing patterns are relatively frequent but occasionally these occur in association with hypoxemia (PaO_2 below 60 mm Hg). Oxygen delivery through a nasal tube is sufficient to circumvent this problem.

In many patients, vigorous treatment with anticonvulsants to counter focal or generalized seizures results in hypoventilation and a need for airway protection and mechanical ventilation. Brain swelling with further impairment of consciousness probably remains the most common reason for intubation and mechanical ventilation.

Impaired Mechanics (Neuromuscular failure): Clinical features that should alert one to the possibility of neuromuscular respiratory failure are shown in Table 12.7. The first signs are subtle and are typically not detected by bedside measurements of respiratory mechanics or by pulse oximeter.

Patients with signs of diaphragmatic failure invariably have tachycardia and tachypnea. These clinical warning signs are usually associated with some sense of discomfort and anxiety. Hallmark of diaphragmatic fatigue is dysynchronous movement of the chest cage and abdomen. Dyspnea is much more significant when the patient is supine rather than sitting upright. An outward movement of the chest and inward movement of the abdomen characterize paradoxical breathing during inspiration.

Table 12.7: Clinical features of imminent neuromuscular respiratory failure

Dyspnea at low levels of work
Restlessness
Tachycardia
Tachypnea
Use of sternocleidomastoids
Forehead sweating
Staccato speech
Asynchronous (paradoxical) breathing

An important finding on examination is weakness of the trapezius and neck muscles. Progressive weakness of these muscles should alert one to imminent respiratory failure and may parallel diaphragmatic weakness.

In the daily monitoring of patients with a potential for respiratory failure, monitoring tongue and pharynx mobility is as important as following vital capacity and inspiratory pressure; forced vital capacity remains a very useful bedside test. The maximum inspiratory pressure (MIP, PI_{max}) and the maximum expiratory pressure (MEP, Pe_{max}) are clinically useful.

A frequent harbinger of respiratory failure is transient oxygen desaturation (70s to 80s) during monitoring with a pulse oximeter. Hypercapnia is a late manifestation of acute neuromuscular respiratory failure and corresponds with vital capacity of less than 5 mL/kg, a life-threatening situation that mandates immediate intubation and mechanical ventilation. Mechanical ventilation is indicated when clinical deterioration is associated with a vital capacity of 15 mL/kg or less, the MIP is less than –25 cm H_2O and respiratory rate exceeding 30 breaths/minute.

Interstitial Pulmonary Disease: Primary pulmonary causes that lead to mechanical ventilation are comparatively common. Aspirations frequently occur in patients with acute bulbar dysfunction, in patients who had a series of seizures, and in patients with vomiting and diminished pharyngeal reflex. Aspiration is rarely witnessed, but usually after an interval of 6 to 12 hours the patient becomes breathless with a productive cough, because of aspiration pneumonia. Chest radiography may show alveolar opacities in the most dependent part of the lungs, typically including the superior parts of the lower lobes and the posterior segment of the right upper lobe. Mechanical ventilation should be considered if profound hypoxemia develops.

Neurogenic pulmonary edema is rare in clinical practice. Its clinical presentation is similar to that of acute respiratory distress syndrome, and mechanical ventilation with positive end-expiratory pressure (PEEP) is invariably indicated.

In patients with trauma, pulmonary injuries should be strongly considered. Patients with associated flail chest are at considerable risk for hypoxemia and are best served by mechanical ventilation.

In occasional patients, underlying pulmonary disease such as asthma or emphysema worsen at the time of an acute brain injury. Inability to cough frequently results in mucus plugs that may cause significant oxygen desaturation. Mechanical ventilation, sufficient rest, and mild sedation are often needed for a short period.

Settings

When the decision to mechanically ventilate is made, proper settings must be selected. Initial tidal volume delivered by the ventilator is usually set to be relatively large, ranging from 12 to 15 mL/kg based on ideal, not actual, body weight. Patients with underlying pulmonary disease may need smaller tidal volumes (9 to 10 mL/kg). The respiratory rate must be chosen at the lowest possible setting to reduce the phenomenon of intrinsic PEEP or gas trapping; intrinsic PEEP is created when the time for expiration is less. This phenomenon is deleterious because it increases work of breathing and proximal airway pressure, and may cause hypotension. Commonly, the inspiratory time is set at 20-33 percent and the pause time for 5 percent, with the remaining allowed for expiration (inspiration-expiration ratio, 1:2 to 1:3). An important setting is the fraction of inspired oxygen (FiO_2). There should be a continuous incentive to decrease FiO_2. If reduction in FiO_2 is not tolerated, adequate gas exchange can also be achieved with increasing PEEP. Most often, PEEP is indicated when the PO_2 remains less than 60 mmHg despite a FiO_2 of 0.6. PEEP is often added to ventilation in cardiogenic pulmonary edema, acute respiratory distress syndrome, and diffuse bilateral pneumonia.

Modes of Ventilation

The most frequently used modes are controlled mechanical ventilation or assist-control and synchronized intermittent mandatory ventilation, with or without pressure support.

Controlled mode ventilation is used in patients with acute neurologic catastrophes and inability to breath, herniation, brain death, severed high cervical cord, status epilepticus, therapy-refractory increased intracranial pressure, patients with multitrauma and significant respiratory distress. Controlled mechanical ventilation has many disadvantages, largely related to use of sedation and neuromuscular blockade that eliminate respiratory drive. CMV modes are not responsive to the patient's needs and therefore may rapidly lead to inadequate ventilation.

Pressure Support Ventilation: This mode essentially decreases the work of breathing, but the tidal volume and respiratory cycle remain controlled by the effort of the patient. This mode is often used in overcoming the resistance of the endotracheal tube and in combination with the SIMV mode.

Continuous Positive Airway Pressure: This mode assists in spontaneous breathing, in patients with neuromuscular weakness the continuous positive airway pressure varies from 5 to 15 cmH_2O.

Weaning

Studies of weaning criteria in patients with central nervous system injury and neuromuscular weakness are virtually not available, and the published determinants in critically ill patients with long mechanical ventilation may not apply to the vast majority of patients with acute brain injury.

The practice of weaning may differ, but no method should be entertained unless several clinical and laboratory criteria are fulfilled. Weaning should not be entertained in patients who still require PEEP for adequate oxygenation and patients who have significant chest X-ray abnormality. Important adjunctive measures, such as correction of electrolyte imbalance, adequate hydration and nutrition, nursing in upright position, adequate clearing of secretions, and perhaps most important, adequate sleep must be ensured. It is critical that during weaning efforts, patients have effective rest at night. Weaning should be gradual, because a sudden transition may be stressful in most patients who have been intubated for short time, weaning can be accomplished by gradual T-tube weaning. Next to looking for obvious signs of discomfort, one should watch for an increase in respiratory rate, a decrease in tidal volume, a change in blood pressure (either way), an increase in heart rate (increase of more than 20 beats/minute). A T-piece can remain in place for 30 minutes with incremental increases in duration twice a day. Common practice is to begin with a trial of 30 minutes, rapidly increased to 1 and to 2 hours. Extubation is performed when the arterial blood gas values remain satisfactory and no rapid shallow breathing is observed.

Another approach is to use the SIMV mode. The SIMV mode is reduced in gradual steps. SIMV weaning is fairly simple, consisting of gradual reduction with 3 breaths/ minute starting two to three times a day. It is prudent to add pressure support at low levels (10 cm H_2O) for further patient comfort.

Pressure support weaning with SIMV may be preferred to other weaning regimens: Pressure support is set at a level that is comfortable for the patient, usually 15 to 25 cm H_2O followed by decrements of 2-3 cmH_2O, 2-3 times a day – depending on the patient response and stability. When the pressure support level of 5 cmH_2O is tolerated and the laboratory criteria are fulfilled, extubation can be undertaken.

Extubation should be well tolerated, but inspiratory stridor may develop virtually immediately within an hour, after extubation. Topical adrenaline (2 ml, 1:1000 solution) by nebulisation into the hypopharynx is a reasonable option, but reintubation is often necessary.

OTHER ISSUES

Isolation and Infection Precautions

Strict hand-washing between visits to patients, limitation of the use and duration of devices, proper isolation of infected patients, and aseptic technique reduce nosocomial infections. The isolation categories are shown in Table 12.8. Body substance isolation implies gloves should be worn for anticipated contact with blood, secretions, and any moist body substances. Gloves should be changed before another patient contact.

Table 12.8: Neurological diseases that require isolation

Disease Requiring Strict Isolation

(i) Rabies (ii) Varicella (iii) Hemorrhagic fever

Precautions:

- Separate room
- Negative pressure ventilation
- Masks, gowns and gloves
- Hand-washing after glove removal

Diseases that need Contact Isolation

- Adenovirus
- Herpes simplex (disseminated)
- Major staphylococcal infections

Diseases that need Respiratory Isolation

- Infectious mononucleosis

Diseases that need Enteric Precautions

- Hepatitis A,E
- Salmonella
- Shigellosis
- Campylobacter
- Giardia
- Rotavirus

Gowns, goggles and mask should be worn when secretions, blood, or body fluid is likely to soil or splash on clothing, skin or face (See Appendix-1). The type of soap or disinfectant probably is less important than the technique of hand washing (See Appendix-2). Adequate hand washing should ideally last 20 seconds, and a large volume of soap should be used.

To check device-specific nosocomial infections current recommendations are:

a. Maintenance of a sterile close drainage system for urine and no breaking in to obtain urinary samples or to irrigate the bladder
b. Replacement of intravenous catheter every 2 or 3 days

c. Replacement of central lines if infected or every 3 weeks
d. Proper handling of condensate in respiratory tubing, dispensing and storage of nebulized solutions, and changing of the tubing.

Intra Hospital Transport

Patients often need to be moved to radiology department for neuroimaging. It is important to assess possible change in vital signs after several minutes of manual bagging. Adverse events during transport that tentatively may lead to secondary insults to the brain are arterial oxygen saturation of less than 90 percent, hypoventilation in mechanically ventilated patients, severe hypocapnia by too frequent manual bagging; cardiovascular changes induced by sudden alteration in the mode of ventilation, and surges of intracranial pressure. Catheters and tubes may be pulled, most often during transfer.

It is important to have mannitol and antiepileptic drugs prepared.

Precautions Before In-hospital Transport

- Stable vital signs for 1 hour
- Perform tracheal suctioning before transport
- Check patency of intravenous sites
- Ensure stable vital signs and manual bagging of the patient for several minutes
- Ensure $SpO_2 > 90\%$
- No recent seizures
- Mannitol infusion prepared if needed
- When indicated, supplies such as antiepileptic drugs (diazepam, 5 mg) albumin 5% solution
- Monitor connected for arterial blood pressure tracings and ECG
- Pulse Oximeter connected.

Management of Nutrition

Nutritional support of critically ill patients with neurologic disorders has distinctive characteristics. Daily care is more often focused on countering the effects of hypermetabolism and acute gastro paresis and on treating complications associated with enteral nutrition than it is in other critically ill patients.

Outcome studies suggest that when nutritional support is prompt, mortality is reduced and the number of nosocomial infections is significantly lower.

Physical Signs of Malnutrition: Generalized muscle wasting, easily plucked, thin, dyspigmented hair (zinc def), nasolabial seborrhea, fissuring of eyelid corners, angular stomatitis, cheilosis (Vit B_2), periodontal disease, mottled enamel, and caries, raw and swollen tongue (niacin and folate), spoon-shaped nails (iron), hyperkeratosis and petechial hemorrhages of the skin (Vit C or K). Hypoalbuminemia is an important marker for malnutrition at the initial presentation. A significantly higher mortality is seen among patients with serum albumin levels below 3.0 g/L from malnutrition.

The main goals of nutritional support are to preserve muscle mass, provide adequate vitamins, minerals, fats and fluids (see chapter nutrition).

Reduction of Aspiration Risk

Swallowing mechanics may be disturbed in patients with a brain stem or hemispheric stroke and in patients with acute neuromuscular disease producing rapid deterioration. *Impaired level of consciousness, vomiting, seizures, obesity, nasogastric feeding are other risk factors. Aspiration is markedly increased in patients requiring emergency intubation. Similar risk occurs with extubation.* Aspiration pneumonia can possibly be prevented if patients with abnormal swallowing mechanisms are identified early. Features suggesting abnormal swallowing mechanism are abnormal laryngeal rise, poor throat clearing, weak or absent, gag reflex, poor pharyngeal sensation, oral motor rapid movement, poor vocal clarity and delay in swallowing. The gag reflex has a low predictive value and is absent in at least one-third of the normal population. Pharyngeal sensation may be more useful and recent studies have confirmed increased risks of aspiration in patients with pharyngeal sensory deficits.

An H_2-antagonist (cimetidine or ranitidine) should be administered to patients at high risk of aspiration. Omeprazole may be more effective than an H_2 antagonist. Both agents may reduce gastric volume and increase pH. Positioning at 45° head elevation is an important additional measure.

Chapter thirteen

Monitoring of a Patient in the Intensive Care Unit

WHAT IS MONITORING

The goal of pediatric critical care is to monitor and support and eventually restore vital system function in critically ill children. Repeated observations of the physiologic data over time in a critically ill child for diagnostic, therapeutic and prognostic purposes is termed as monitoring. The goals of monitoring are as follows:

1. *Diagnostic:* For diagnosis and assessment of the severity of the underlying condition that causes physiologic derangements.
2. *Therapeutic:* Indicates need for therapeutic intervention and assessment of response to the intervention.
3. *Prognostic:* Trends can indicate likelihood of survival and prediction of outcome.
4. *Warning:* Sudden physiologic derangement can be picked up by the alarms of a monitoring system.

An ideal monitoring system must have following characteristics:

Prerequisites of a Good Monitoring System

- Minimal risk to patient
- Painless, patient friendly
- Non-invasive as far as possible
- Continuous visual/ auditory display
- Data should be accurate, specific, reproducible and relevant to the patients underlying condition.
- Should track rapid changes in the physiological parameters monitored.
- Recording and storage facility to be available "Trends" give more information than individual data points.

What Can be Monitored?

The list of physiological variable that can be monitored is growing. The following is a partial list:

Respiratory

Respiratory rate, breathing pattern, arterial blood gases (PaO_2,pH), arterial oxygen saturation (SpO_2), mixed venous oxygen saturation (SvO_2), and transcutaneous oxygen tension ($TcPO_2$), respiratory mechanics (vital capacity, thoracic compliance), end-tidal CO_2 tension ($PEtCO_2$), and respiratory muscle function (maximum inspiratory and expiratory pressures).

Cardiovascular

ECG, electrical axis, arrhythmias, blood pressure, arterial pressure, venous pressure, cardiac output, ejection fraction, ventricular pressure–volume loops. Pulmonary artery pressure.

Nervous System

Level of consciousness, neuro-deficits, EEG, evoked potentials, intracranial pressure, cerebral perfusion pressure, jugular venous bulb saturation.

Gastrointestinal

Esophageal pH, esophageal sphincter tone.

Metabolic

Temperature, blood chemistry, glucose, urea, creatinine sodium, potassium, calcium, magnesium, oxygen consumption, CO_2 production, urine output.

Musculoskeletal System

Intra abdominal pressure, muscular compartment pressure, skin pressures.

Equipment Monitoring

Monitoring is a repetitive, fatiguing job that machines do extremely well and people do poorly. The same signals have to be sampled over and over again, often more frequently than is possible for a person.

Thus the usage recognizes the delegation of an activity (to monitor) to a machine (the monitor). The machine monitor must give a signal when dangerous deviations occurs because people are unsteady observers of machine signals collected so accurately, quickly, frequently and monotonously. We might monitor with the help of the machine.

Advantages

Storage facility, Graphic Representation, Visual/Auditory display, Reproducibility, Alert/alarm, Rapid data assessment.

Disadvantages

Expensive, Needs maintenance, Analysis not possible.

Human Monitoring

Advanced technological monitoring is an important aspect of pediatric critical care but it should serve as an adjunct to and not a substitute for clinical monitoring. The most efficacious and probably most cost-effective monitoring of a patient is the frequent assessment by a bedside nurse or a physician. Neurologic status, heart rate, respiratory rate, adequacy of air exchange, movements of the chest wall and breath sounds, temperature of the extremities, capillary refill, quality of the pulses, hourly urinary output, etc. are better assessed by a nurse or physician. A well-trained nurse/physician team can check these parameters several times in a reproducible form, document them, and integrate all this information to assess the overall status of a patient. Human monitoring is also necessary even after equipment monitoring for analysis of the parameters in the context of the patient, understanding the physiology and take diagnostic and therapeutic decisions. This type of "technology" is not available for purchase. It is the product of a dedicated and specialized education process, which can receive periodic backups and unlimited upgrades, and is available in any country. Without a doubt, human monitoring is the most valuable monitoring system in existence in critical care.

Both, human beings and equipment, are required for good monitoring of critically ill patients.

RESPIRATORY MONITORING

Monitoring of the respiratory system is aimed at assessing integrity of airway, efficacy of breathing; oxygenation and ventilation, and work of breathing.

Physical examination continues to have a great clinical relevance and is often the deciding factor between monitor-error and true change in patient status. However, non-invasive techniques to assess gas exchange and pulmonary mechanics supplement physical examination. These provide a continuous data system with alarms to identify changes in patient status and alert care givers.

Patency of airway is best assessed by clinical methods and may be categorized as normal, maintainable by positioning, suctioning, airway insertion, non-maintainable, requiring intubation.

Assessment of oxygenation and ventilation must be carried out separately. While assessment of oxygenation implies assessment of oxygen content in the arterial blood, ventilation implies assessment of CO_2 elimination by lungs. Respiratory parameters that need to be monitored, therefore, may be grouped as those reflecting oxygenation, and those showing ventilation (i.e. CO_2 removal). Oxygenation can be assessed by clinical monitoring from arterial blood gas analysis (PaO_2,pH), arterial oxygen saturation (SpO_2) by pulse oximetry, mixed venous oxygen saturation and transcutaneous oxygen tension ($TcPO_2$). Ventilatory function may be monitored from respiratory rate, breathing pattern, chest movements and air entry, respiratory mechanics (vital capacity, thoracic compliance), end-tidal CO_2 tension ($ETCO_2$) by capnography, and assessment of respiratory muscle function (maximum inspiratory and expiratory pressures) and CO_2 on blood gas analysis.

1. **Respiratory rate:**
   Respiratory rate can be monitored by physical counting or continuously by an impedance technique measuring electrical changes between a pair of ECG electrode placed on either side of the chest. The counting of respiratory rate must be done for a full minute, without disturbing the child. An elevation of respiratory rate is often the earliest danger sign, and degree of elevation is proportional to severity of the underlying disease.
2. **Assessment of the work of breathing** at the bedside is achieved by taking into account the rate of breathing, the respiratory pattern and use of accessory muscles. Abdominal-thoracic asynchrony is a useful sign of severe fatigue and impending respiratory failure.
3. **Arterial blood gases (ABGs):**
   Direct measurement of PaO_2 and $PaCO_2$ is the most common and accurate method of measuring gas exchange, and remains the main stay of monitoring oxygenation and ventilation. The disadvantages are invasive nature of the procedure, intermittent sampling (which may miss sudden change), and time lag between sampling and result. The changes in ABGs may occur relatively late in the evolution of respiratory failure. An indwelling arterial cannula may simplify the repeated sampling and reduce errors from direct arterial puncture.
   Some change in arterial PO_2 and CO_2 on routine blood gas analysis may not necessarily be abnormal if clinical condition has not changed. Blood gas measurements may vary considerably. In a study of adults, the arterial PO_2 varied by as much as 36 mmHg, whereas the arterial PCO_2 varied by as much as 12 mmHg. *Routine monitoring of ABGs, without a change in clinical condition of the patient, is therefore not needed, and may be misleading.*
   The gold standard for monitoring ventilation is measurement of $PaCO_2$ and pH in arterial blood. $PaCO_2$ reflects the balance between the alveolar ventilation and the CO_2 output of the body. However, accurate evaluation of ventilatory function requires simultaneous consideration of blood pH. Ventilatory failure is commonly defined as a combination of $PaCO_2$ greater than 50 mmHg and arterial pH less than 7.30 (For details see Chapter 13, Acid Base Disorders).
   Even when blood gas analysis is readily available, clinical assessment of the patient must not be overlooked. Some patients with developing respiratory failure maintain blood gas values within the normal range for a long time. Laboratory evidence of ventilatory failure then appears rapidly commen-

surating with overt respiratory exhaustion.

4. **Pulse oximetry:**

Pulse oximeter provide non-invasive continuous monitoring of oxyhemoglobin contents i.e. O_2 saturation of hemoglobin (SpO_2) in the arterial blood. A light probe placed on ear lobe or finger, measures the light absorbance of oxygenated and non-oxygenated hemoglobin with each pulsatile signal generated by arterial blood flow.

An oximeter reading >92% generally represent a PaO_2 of 60 mmHg and above. Most of the commercially available pulse oximeters measure arterial oxygen saturation within 95% confidence limit of $\pm$4%, when the SpO_2 is above 70%. The lag time between respiratory or ventilatory changes and pulse oximetery recording of the changes in O_2 saturation vary between instrument to instrument (range 7-20 seconds). In general, ear probes have a faster and more accurate response than finger probes.

Pulse oximetery may not provide accurate SpO_2 data in the presence of carboxyhemoglobin, methemoglobin, jaundice, low perfusion states and hypothermia. However, it provides accurate and reliable measure of oxygen saturation in children with cyanotic heart disease.

SpO_2 is most useful in the clinical situation where the objective of monitoring is to detect at the earliest hypoxemia, as SpO_2 is more sensitive to changes in the lower range of PaO_2. Thus, pulse oximetery is routinely indicated in patients with critical airway, tracheostomy, those on oxygen therapy, on assisted ventilation, and those undergoing a diagnostic procedure that may compromise airway and cause hypoxia (e.g. bronchoscopy).

Oximetery is not useful during cardiopulmonary resuscitation, in monitoring hyperoxia, hypovolemia, and in fine tuning of mechanical ventilation. The use of pulse oximetery has definitely reduced the need for invasive ABG monitoring in critically ill patients.

5. **Transcutaneous blood gas measurements:**

Transcutaneous arterial oxygen tension ($TcPO_2$) and carbon dioxide ($TcPCO_2$) can be measured continuously with help of skin electrodes. There is a good agreement between direct arterial and transcutaneous measurement of gas in most older infants and children. $TcPO_2$ is sometimes inaccurate in critically ill children with low cardiac output and shock, because of poor skin perfusion. Also, at high PaO_2, $TcPO_2$ tends to underestimate PaO_2. Despite this, $TcPO_2$ monitoring remains a useful clinical tool, particularly in normoxemic or hyperoxic range where large changes in PaO_2 are accompanied by small or undetectable changes in SpO_2.

$TcPCO_2$ generally follow the trend of $PaCO_2$, but the gradient increases disproportionately in presence of shock. Nonetheless transcutaneous monitoring provides a noninvsive, continuous, real-time estimate of arterial blood $PaCO_2$ that would be useful for monitoring ventilation. The disadvantages of transcutaneous monitors are problems of reliability, need for repeated calibrations, maintaining a temperature of skin electrode in the range of 43-45°, fragility of electrodes, and need to cross check the data against arterial blood gases.

6. **Mixed Venous PaO_2:**

The oxygen in arterial blood represents the sum of the oxygen in mixed venous (pulmonary artery) blood and the oxygen added from alveolar gas. When gas exchange is normal, the PO_2 in alveolar gas is the major determinant of the arterial PO_2. However when gas exchange is impaired, the contribution of the alveolar PO_2 declines and the contribution of the mixed venous PO_2 rises. The influence of the mixed venous PO_2 on the arterial PO_2 is determined by the degree of intrapulmonary shunt. In the normal lung, decreases in venous PO_2 have relatively little effect on the arterial PO_2. However, as shunt fraction increases, changes in venous PO_2 begin to affect the arterial PO_2. If shunt fraction is increased to 100%, the venous PO_2 is the sole determinant of the arterial PO_2. Thus, *in pulmonary conditions associated with a high shunt fraction, such as pulmonary edema or pneumonia, the mixed venous PO_2 is an important consideration in the evaluation of hypoxemia.*

7. **Mixed Venous O_2 Saturation (SvO_2):** Mixed venous and central venous oxygen saturation represent the oxygen remaining in venous blood after tissue oxyen extration. Their values are function of combined arterial oxygen content (Hb, PaO_2), cardiac output and tissue oxygen consumption (VO_2). Hence SvO_2 has been used as a sensitive variable of the overall balance between oxygen supply and demand. Continuous SvO_2 monitoring is possible with the help of special pulmonary artery catheters containing fiberoptic filaments. The catheter can also measure all the indices measured by a regular pulmonary artery catheter. SvO_2 can be measured intermittently by withdrawing blood sample from tip of a central venous catheter (CVC). The advantage of the SvO_2 measurement over SpO_2 measurement is that SvO_2 values fall on the steep portion of oxyhemoglobin dissociation curve; where relationship between SvO_2 and mixed venous oxygen pressure (PvO_2) is linear. Of the normal arteiral saturation of close to 100%, about 25% is off loaded at tissue level to meet tissue O_2 demand. The blood returning to heart is about 75% saturated. *In the healthy subjects SvO_2 values may vary between 70%-85%; a decrease below 70% indicates impaired systemic oxygen delivery and a values less than 50% reflect globally impaired tissue oxygenation.* SvO_2 can be affected by alteration in distribution of blood flow between organs with high and low ratio of oxygen consumption to perfusion.
   SvO_2 is reduced in states of decreased cardiac output, decreased arterial oxygen saturation, decreased hemoglobin concentration and increased tissue oxygen consumption. It is increased when oxygen consumption or tissue oxygen extraction is decreased. However, *in shock, a reduction in tissue oxygenation may be associated with a high SvO_2.* This is because of perfusion of some vascular beds in excess of their metabolic demands, local A-V shunting, and reduction in O_2 extraction and consumption due to cell injury.However, individual values of SvO_2 have no predictive value concerning *regional* oxygen transport.

8. **End tidal carbon dioxide tension ($ETCO_2$):**
   $ETCO_2$ is the CO_2 measured at the end of an exhalation. It correlates well with $PaCO_2$ (usually 1-5 mmHg less than $PaCO_2$). The monitoring device that measures $ETCO_2$ continuously by infrared analysis is reliable and sturdy. Changes in $ETCO_2$ may provide an early warning of acute cardiopulmonary changes. $ETCO_2$ is very useful in children with cerebral edema where maintaining $PaCO_2$ within a desired range is critical. It underestimates $PaCO_2$ in children with lung diseases because of poor mixing of gas in the lungs. A sudden increase in $ETCO_2$ occurs with sudden increase in cardiac

output or injection of sodium bicarbonate, while a gradual increase suggest hypoventilation, partial airway obstruction or increased CO_2 production. A sudden decrease in $ETCO_2$ occurs as a result of sudden hyperventilation, decreased cardiac output, massive pulmonary or air embolism, obstruction of endotracheal tube and leakage in the circuit. A gradual decrease in $ETCO_2$ suggests either decreased oxygen consumption, decreased pulmonary perfusion, or hyperventilation (Fig. 13.1).

End-tidal Carbon Dioxide ($EtCO_2$) during mechanical ventilation

In the usual case, the airway pressure pattern and expiratory volumes that correspond well to the patient's size and pulmonary function are associated with adequate alveolar ventilation. However, these variables measures the mechanical functioning of the respiratory apparatus and do not reflect gas exchange in the lung. Therefore, when respiratory support is administered, it is advisable to directly monitor its endpoint variables: removal of CO_2 and oxygenation of arterial blood. On-line measurement of $EtCO_2$ allows breath-by-breath, noninvasive assessment of the adequacy of ventilation.

Since CO_2 diffuses rapidly through the alveolar-capillary membrane, the alveolar and end-capillary partial pressures are nearly equal in an ideally perfused and ventilated lung unit. When the lung empties, the composition of the exhaled gas changes from that of dead-space gas toward that of alveolar gas. Hence, carbon dioxide concentration at end-exhalation ($EtCO_2$) reflects the $PaCO_2$ in the alveoli and end-capillary blood. However, even end-tidal expired gas is contaminated by a contribution from poorly perfused alveoli that constitute the alveolar dead space. Therefore, an average gradient of upto 5 mmHg exists between $EtCO_2$ and $PaCO_2$. The gradient depends primarily on the amount of alveolar dead space relative to alveolar ventilation.

Ventilatory modalities used in the ICU frequently combine spontaneous and mechanical ventilation in variable proportions. This results in a changing dead space to VT ratio, which will alter the relationship between $PaCO_2$ and $EtCO_2$. Changes in the patient's pulmonary pathology often have a similar effect. When the ventilator rate is high and VT is small, as in infants and small children, it may be difficult to get an appropriate end-tidal gas sample. Consequently, $EtCO_2$ may underestimate $PaCO_2$ considerably. It is therefore necessary to periodically compare blood gas $PaCO_2$ values with $EtCO_2$ values. Notwithstanding the need to compare end-tidal values to blood gas values, $EtCO_2$ provide a noninvasive on-line method of quickly detecting changes in the patient's respiratory status (Fig. 13.1). The fact that the respiratory dead-space volume affects $ETCO_2$ makes it useful in diagnosing conditions that lead to an increase in wasted ventilation such as pulmonary embolus, air embolus, and acute pulmonary hypertension. All of these conditions affect a sudden decrease in $EtCO_2$ relative to $PaCO_2$ (Fig. 13.1).

9. **Maximum inspiratory and expiratory pressures:** These are measures of respiratory muscle strength, and help determining possibility of weaning of a patient from mechanical ventilation. These are monitored in ventilated patients routinely.
10. **Indices of pulmonary gas exchange**
    Dead space (V_D/V_T): The determination of dead space ventilation (V_D/V_T) is based on the difference between the PCO_2 in

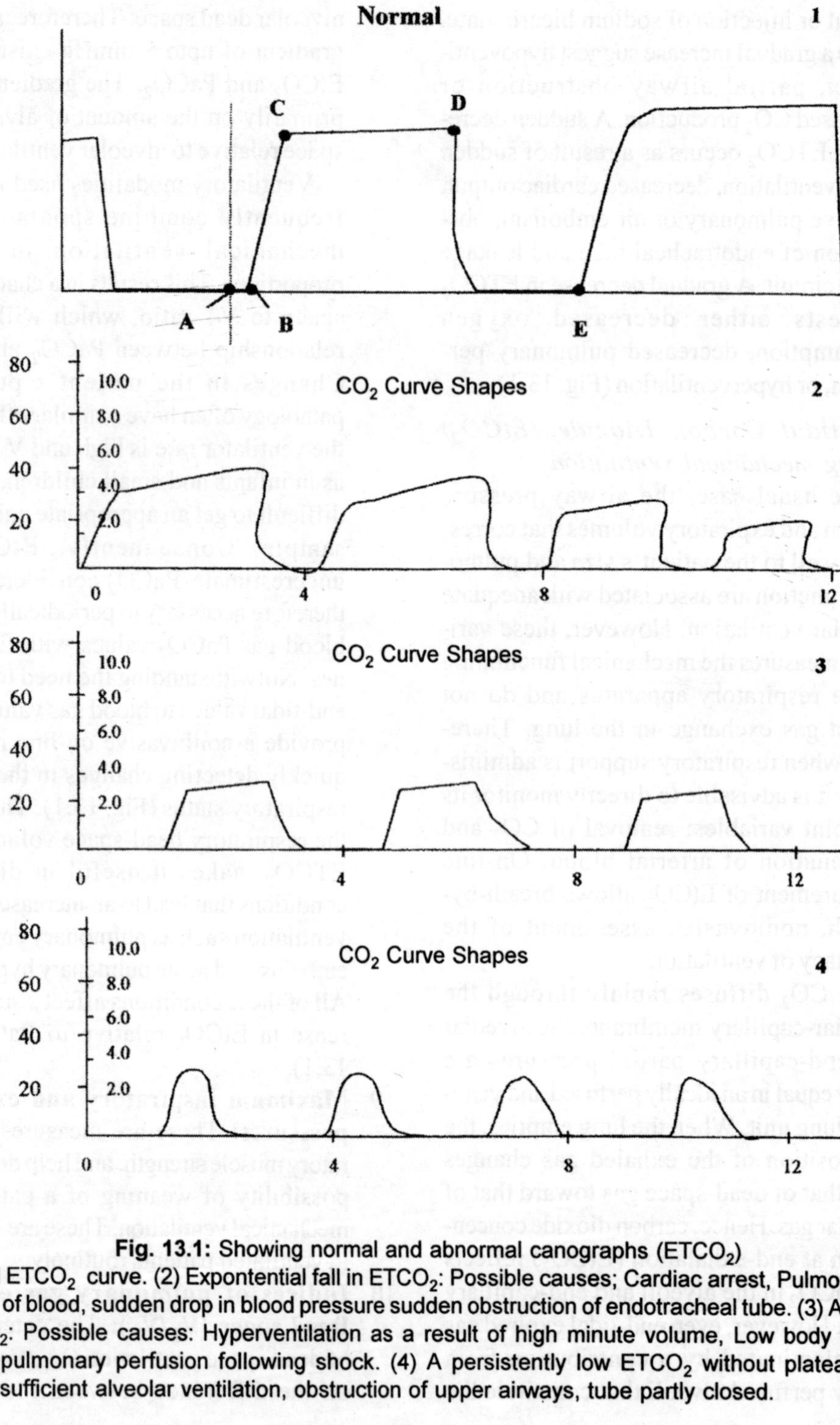

Fig. 13.1: Showing normal and abnormal canographs ($ETCO_2$)
(1) Normal $ETCO_2$ curve. (2) Expontential fall in $ETCO_2$: Possible causes; Cardiac arrest, Pulmonary emboli, Large loss of blood, sudden drop in blood pressure sudden obstruction of endotracheal tube. (3) A persistently low $ETCO_2$: Possible causes: Hyperventilation as a result of high minute volume, Low body temperature decreaed pulmonary perfusion following shock. (4) A persistently low $ETCO_2$ without plateau: Possible causes: Insufficient alveolar ventilation, obstruction of upper airways, tube partly closed.

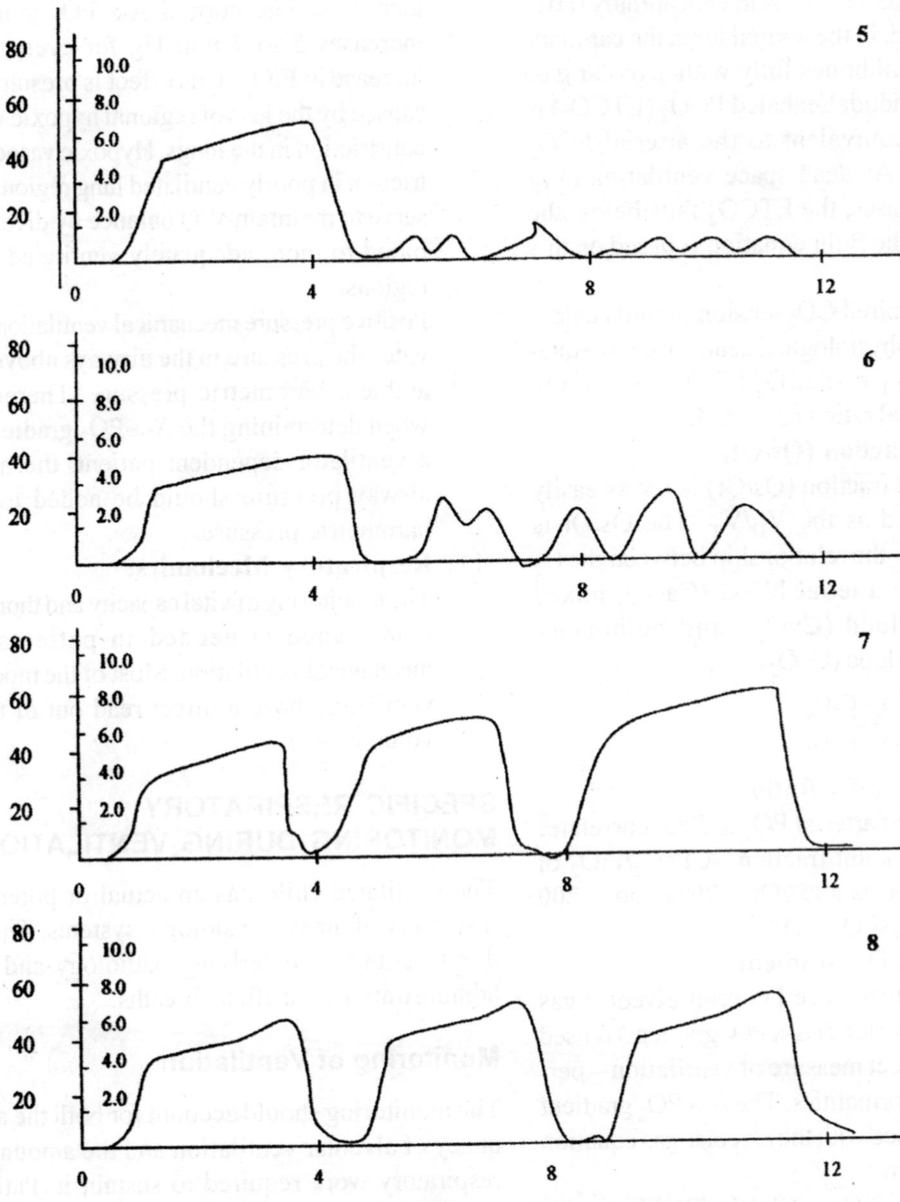

Fig. 13.1: Showing normal and abnormal capographs ($ETCO_2$)

(5) Sudden drop in $ETCO_2$ to around zero: Possible causes: Accidental extubation, Complete airway stenosis, Disconnection, oesophageal intubation (drop after 1-2 tidal volumes). (6) Drop in $ETCO_2$, but still above zero: Possible causes: Leaks tube, partial airway stenosis, Tube in laryngopharynx. (7) Gradual incresae in pCO_2: Possible causes: Increase in metabolism and body temperature (with MV = const.), Beginning of hypoventilation, Reduction in effective alveolar ventilation. (8) $ETCO_2$, plateau not horizontal: Possible causes: Asthma, ventilatory distribution problems (asynchronous emptying).

exhaled gas and PCO_2 in endcapillary (arterial) blood. In the normal lung, the capillary blood equilibrates fully with alveolar gas, and the endtidal/exhaled PCO_2 ($ETCO_2$) is roughly equivalent to the arterial PCO_2 ($PaCO_2$). As dead space ventilation (V_D/V_T) increases, the $ETCO_2$ falls below the $PaCO_2$. The Bohr equation is based on this principle.

Mixed expired CO_2 tension permits calculation of physiological dead space by equation $V_D/V_T = (PaCO_2\text{-}ETCO_2) \div PaCO_2$. The normal ratio is 0.33-0.45.

Shunt Fraction (Qs/Qt)

The shunt fraction (Qs/Qt) is not as easily determined as the V_D/V_T. The Qs/Qt is derived by the relationship between the O_2 content in arterial blood (CaO_2), mixed venous blood (CvO_2), and pulmonary capillary blood (CcO_2).

$$Qs/Qt = \frac{CcO_2 - CaO_2}{CcO_2 - CvO_2}$$

The PaO_2/FIO_2 Ratio

The ratio of arterial PO_2 to FiO_2 correlates well with shunt fraction. A PaO_2/FiO_2 of <200 suggests a Qs/Qt > 20% and > 200 suggests Qs/ Qt < 20%.

The A-a PO_2 Gradient

The PO_2 difference between alveolar gas and arterial blood (A-a PO_2 gradient) is used as an indirect measure of ventilation – perfusion abnormalities. The A-a PO_2 gradient is determined with the alveolar gas equation shown below:

$$P_AO_2 = PiO_2 - (PaCO_2/RQ)$$

$PiO_2 = FiO_2\,(PB - P_{H_2O}) = FiO_2\,(760 - 47)$, where PB is barometric pressure, and P_{H_2O} is partial pressure of water vapour. $PaCO_2$ is arterial carbon dioxide and RQ is respiratory quotient = 0.8. Normal gradient is 10-15 mmHg.

The A-a PO_2 gradient increases as the FiO_2 increases. The normal A-a PO_2 gradient increases 5 to 7 mm Hg for every 10% increase in FiO_2. This effect is presumably caused by the loss of regional hypoxic vasoconstriction in the lungs. Hypoxic vasoconstriction in poorly ventilated lung regions can serve to maintain V/Q balance by diverting blood to more adequately ventilated lung regions.

Positive pressure mechanical ventilation elevates the pressure in the airways above the ambient barometric pressure. Therefore, when determining the A-a PO_2 gradient in a ventilator-dependent patient, the mean airway pressure should be added to the barometric pressure.

11. **Respiratory Mechanics:**

The monitoring of vital capacity and thoracic compliance is needed in patients on mechanical ventilation. Most of the modern ventilators have a direct read out of tidal volume (V_T).

SPECIFIC RESPIRATORY MONITORING DURING VENTILATION

The ventilated child has an actual or potential instability of many physiologic systems. This is due to both the underlying pathology and the administration of artificial breaths.

Monitoring of Ventilation

The monitoring should account for both the adequacy of alveolar ventilation and the amount of respiratory work required to sustain it. Patient may be able to sustain adequate spontaneous ventilation under normal conditions but will develop ventilatory failure when CO_2 output rises. Respiratory work lacks a defined "gold standard" endpoint variable. Therefore, the work of breathing can only be monitored through repeated clinical assessment.

The best way to assess ventilatory function is

by direct observation of breathing and auscultation of breath sounds. No monitor provides information that is provided by the trained eye and ear. Observation of symmetry and amount of volume change in the chest, inspiratory and expiratory time, and the quality of breath sounds in the different lung fields gives an estimate of tidal volume (V_T), amount of location of airway obstruction, and distribution of ventilation. Additional measurement of respiratory rate, observation of suprasternal, intercostal, and subcostal retractions, assessment of the use of accessory inspiratory and expiratory muscles provide an estimate of minute ventilation and respiratory work. Appearance of erratic alterations in respiratory depth and frequency indicates impending respiratory fatigue. Clinical examination of the respiratory system is reasonably reliable and the only readily available method for evaluating respiratory work. It is however, notoriously inaccurate in estimating the adequacy of alveolar ventilation with regard to CO_2 output which requires analysis of $PaCO_2$ and pH from an arterial blood sample.

Monitoring of Oxygenation

Mechanical ventilation per se corrects hypoxemia when it is secondary to hypoventilation or increased tissue oxygen extraction. However, it may impair arterial blood oxygenation by depressing cardiac output or by inducing ventilation-perfusion abnormalities. In supine spontaneously breathing patient, the posterior-dependent-portion of diaphragm has a much greater excursion than anterior-non-dependent portion. The majority of the blood flow also is dependent and V/Q relationships are well matched. Ventilatory physiology is significantly changed when positive pressure is applied to respiratory tract. The dependent portion moves very little, majority of ventilation occurs in nondependent portion and central and upper airway. This is detrimental to V/Q mismatching and gas exchange; both venous admixture (the physiological shunt) and the proportion of "dead" space ventilation (V_D/V_T) get increased.

Clinical assessment of oxygenation depends on the detection of cyanosis, tachypnea, and secondary cardiovascular changes, such as hypertension and tachycardia. Pulse oximetery is the most appropriate method for monitoring oxygenation during mechanical ventilation. It provides a noninvasive estimate of arterial blood oxyhemoglobin saturation continuously. The advent of pulse oximetry has virtually eliminated the routine use of transćutaneous oxygen ($PtCO_2$) monitoring and on-line arterial PaO_2. Saturation values should be read only if a good plethysmographic pulse contour is seen. The probes should be appropriate for the measurement site. Inappropriately large probes may give erroneous saturation values. Pulse oximeter saturation values inconsistent with the patient's clinical status should be verified by arterial blood gas analysis.

Monitoring of arterial blood oxygenation assures adequate oxyhemoglobin saturation. Hypoxemia may be caused either by defects in pulmonary gas exchange or imbalance between oxygen delivery and use in the peripheral tissues. Estimation of the adequacy of oxygen delivery with respect to oxygen use requires simultaneous monitoring of mixed venous oxyhemoglobin saturation. Integrated monitoring of arterial and mixed venous oxygenation also allows evaluation of origin of hypoxemia.

Monitoring Oxygen Supply to the Breathing Circuit

In most ventilators there is inbuilt provision to monitor FiO_2, and the oxygen supply alarm is sensitive to a fall in the oxygen line pressure. Oxygen analyzer can also be added as separate monitor to the circuit. An erroneously low inspired oxygen concentration must always be considered and ruled out when encountering a patient with hypoxemia.

Airway Pressure

Airway pressure is the most commonly used variable in continuous monitoring of ventilatory function. Alterations in the phasic pressure pattern give warning of several potentially deleterious events. Airway pressure should always be displayed during mechanical ventilatory support. A low airway pressure limit may be set to sense the presence or absence of positive pressure breaths and to calculate ventilator rate.

A low-pressure alarm in a ventilator should always be assumed to indicate inadequate ventilatory support.

A high-pressure limit in a breathing circuit is intended to serve a dual function. It provides an indicator of elevated peak airway pressure and simultaneously vents off excess volume and pressure to protect the airway from over distension and barotrauma. The high-pressure limit of a ventilator should always be preset before connecting the patient to the breathing circuit. The appropriate level is approximately 5-10 mm Hg above the patient's expected peak airway pressure. *Either a decrease in lung compliance, increase in airway resistance, or a combination of these may produce an increase in peak airway pressure. Peak airway pressure is a function of both compliance and resistance, while plateau pressure only reflects compliance. A fall in lung-thorax compliance will elevate the plateau pressure and peak airway pressure simultaneously. However, increase in airway resistance will widen the difference between peak pressure and plateau pressure, and elevate only the former* (Fig. 13.2).

Common causes of abruptly elevated peak airway pressure include airway occlusion by accumulated secretions or a kinked endotracheal tube, endobronchial intubation, acute bronchoconstriction, and pneumothorax. A more gradual rise is seen during worsening of the patient's parenchymal pulmonary disease, such as pulmonary edema.

Airway pressure may also be used to detect the presence or absence of spontaneous respiratory cycles. The triggering event is a drop in circuit pressure during a spontaneous inspiration. The trigger sensitivity must be set meticulously to assure error-free detection of spontaneous breaths with minimum increase in the work of breathing. Airway pressure are without doubt very simple and useful monitoring tools. However, airway pressure prov ides more information about the functioning of the breathing circuit than about pulmonary ventilation.

End-inspiratory Peak Pressure

The peak pressure at the end of inspiration (PIP) is a function of the inflation volume, the flow resistance in the airways, and the elastic recoil force of the lungs and chest wall. At a constant inflation volume, the peak pressure is directly related to airflow resistance and to the elastic recoil (elastance) of the lungs and chest wall:

$$PIP \sim Resistance \times Elastance$$

Therefore when the inflation volume is constant, an increase in peak inspiratory pressure indicates an increase in either airway resistance or elastance of the lungs and chest wall, or both.

End-inspiratory Plateau Pressure

When the inflation volume is held in the lungs by occluding the expiratory tubing at the end of inspiration the proximal airway pressure decreases initially and then reaches a steady level, which is called the end-inspiratory plateau pressure. Because no airflow is present when the plateau pressure is created, the pressure is not a function of flow resistance in the airways. Instead, the plateau pressure (P_{plat}) is directly proportional to the elastance of the lungs and chest wall.

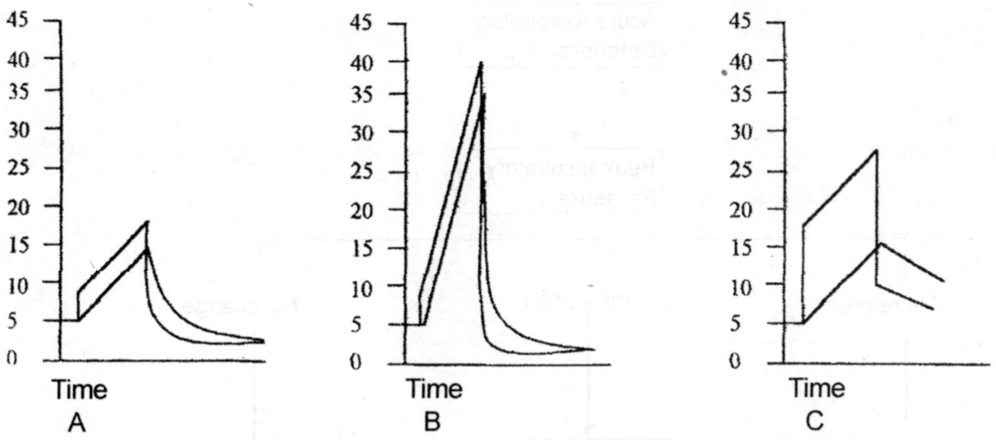

Fig. 13.2: Airway pressure wave forms with constant flow (A) Good compliance (B) Compliance—Reduced to half of A (C) Resistance—increased to 20 in both situations peak airway pressure increases

Therefore, the difference between end-inspiratory peak and plateau pressures is proportional to the flow resistance in the airways.

$$PIP - P_{plat} \sim \text{Airflow resistance}$$

If the peak pressure is increased but the plateau pressure is unchanged, the problem is an increase in airways resistance. In this situation, the major concerns are obstruction of the tracheal tube, airway obstruction from secretions and acute bronchospasm (Fig. 13.3). Therefore, airways suctioning is indicated to clear secretions, followed by an aerosolized bronchodilator treatment if necessary. If an aerosol bronchodilator treatment does not produce a decrease in peak inspiratory pressure (indicating bronchodilation), there is little justification for continuing the aerosol treatments (Fig. 13.3).

If the peak and plateau pressures are both increased, the problem is a decrease in distensibility of the lungs and chest wall. In this situation, the major concerns are pneumothorax, lobar atelectasis, acute pulmonary edema, and worsening pneumonia or ARDS. Active contraction of the chest wall and increased abdominal pressure can also decrease the distensibility of the thorax.

If the peak pressure is decreased, the problem may be an air leak in the system. A decrease in peak pressure can also be due to hyperventilation, when the patient is generating enough of a negative intrathoracic pressure to "pull" air into the lungs.

Expiratory Volume and Flow

Many ventilators are equipped with a flow probe or a volume gauge in the expiratory limb of the circuit. Measurement of expiratory volumes provides useful information regarding the patient's ventilatory status and the functioning of the breathing circuit. Comparison of set inspiratory tidal volume and minute ventilation with the reading of the expiratory spirometer allows evaluation of volume delivered into the patient's lungs. Monitoring of expiratory minute ventilation is particularly useful in adjusting ventilators for children who have an obligatory gas leak around uncuffed endotracheal tubes. It also allows estimation of the effectiveness of spontaneous respiratory efforts during intermittent mandatory ventilation and unassisted spontaneous breathing.

Thoracic Compliance

The compliance, or distensibility, of the lungs and chest wall can be determined quantitatively as the ratio of a change in lung volume (i.e., inflation

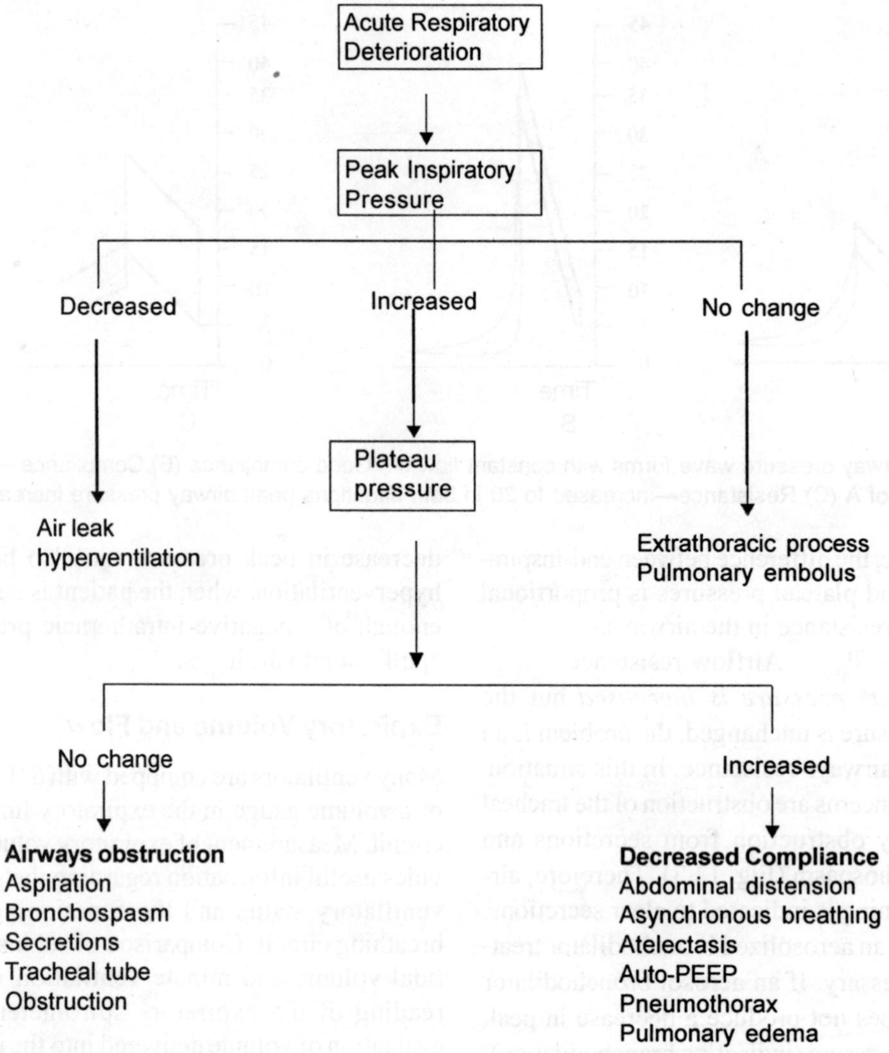

Fig. 13.3: Use of proximal airway pressure to evaluate an acute change in ventilatory status at the bedside

volume) to a change in plateau pressure.

$$C = VT/P_{plat}$$

The thoracic compliance in intubated patients with no known lung disease is between 0.05 to 0.08 L/cm H_2O (or 50 to 80 mL/cm H_2O). In patients with stiff lungs, the thoracic compliance is much lower at 0.01 to 0.02 L/cm H_2O. The compliance determination provides an objective measure of the severity of illness in pulmonary disorders.

While assessing compliance in a ventilated patient, one should remember the factors that influence static compliance. Condition of zero gas flow is necessary to measure the pressure. This can be achieved by "inspiratory hold" option on the ventilator. The level of PEEP (either externally applied or auto-PEEP) should be subtracted from the plateau pressure for the compliance determination. Volume is lost in ventilator tubing during each inspiratory phase because of inherent compliance of tubings. The usual compliance of connector tubing is 3 mL/cm H_2O, which means that 3mL of volume is lost for every 1 cm H_2O increase in inflation pressure.

Effective dynamic compliance is calculated by dividing ventilator-delivered volume by the peak airway pressure minus PEEP. The normal value is 50-80 mL/cm H_2O. The dynamic compliance may be decreased by disorders of airway, lung parenchyma or chest wall. If the fall in dynamic compliance is greater than total thoracic compliance it indicates an increase in airway resistance (bronchospasm, mucous plugging, kinking of endotracheal tube or excessive flow rate).

Pulmonary Graphics

Signals of Respiration

Respiratory cycles are described by three signals: volume (V), driving pressure (P), and time. The change in the V and the amount of time required to effect that change define the flow. Thus, the usual mode of evaluating the physiological changes in respiration is by studying the interrelationships of V, flow, P, and time. The fundamental act of spontaneous breathing requires the generation of P, which thereby initiates a flow that overcomes the elastic, flow resistive, and inertial properties of the entire respiratory system.

The interrelationships between the components may be easily visualized using two dimensional graphic plots of its variables, i.e., pressure versus volume (P-V), flow versus volume (Flow-V), and pressure- flow (P-flow). Such simple x-y plots provides valuable insight into the pattern of breathing. Physiological interpretations of pulmonary mechanics may be further enhanced by mathematical evaluation based upon assumptions such as the calculations of compliance (inverse of elasticity) and resistance.

Mechanics of Airflow

The flow of air into the respiratory tract results from the generation of a driving pressure.

The pattern of airflow is affected by the physical properties of the gas molecules, nature of airflow, and the dimensions of the airway, as well as elastic properties of the airway, the transmural pressure on the airway wall, and structural features of the airway wall. In infants and children the airways are narrower, the resistance to airflow is higher. The decreased airway compliance increases the propensity to airway collapse, whereas the predisposition to distensibility increases dead space ventilation.

Lung Compliance

The elastic properties of the lung parenchyma are related to surface tension, pulmonary tissues, gas exchange spaces, smooth muscle, connective tissue, and the vascular tissue. These forces are interdependent, maintain a complex balance and change with respiratory cycle.

The elastic behavior of the lung is characterized by the pressure-volume curve. More specifically, the ratio of change in lung volume to change in distending pressure defines the compliance of the lungs. Although the pressure- volume relationship of the lung is not linear over the entire range, the compliance is linear over normal range of tidal volumes beginning at FRC. Thus, for a given change in P tidal volume will increase in proportion to lung compliance. As lung compliance is decreased, the lungs are stiffer and more difficult to expand. When lung compliance is increased, the lung becomes easier to distend and is more compliant. Lung compliance and pressure-volumes relationships are determined by the interdependence of elastic tissue elements and alveolar surface tension. A typical value for lung compliance in a young healthy infant is 1.5-2.0 mL/cmH_2O/kg.

Flow (F) v Volume (V) Graphics

The tidal flow-volume relationship describes the pattern of airflow during tidal breathing. It is characterized by the tidal volume, peak inspiratory and expiratory airflow. The objective evaluation of tidal flow-volume loops includes peak inspiratory flow rate, peak expiratory flow rate, tidal volume, timing of peak inspiratory-expiratory flow, airflow at mid-inspiration and mid-expiration and airflow limitation at different points. Generally, any inspiratory, expiratory volume discrepancy should be <± 10%. Airflow limitation is described as abrupt downward deviation of the flow signal towards baseline and away from its normal direction. A complete flow limitation is defined as an 80% or greater reduction of the airflow signal. Evidence of expiratory flow limitation is also best evidenced from flow-volume loops. Flow volume loops under various abnormal condition are shown in Figure 13.4.

Pressure (P) v Volume Graphic

The pressure-volume relationship describes the pattern of tidal volume as a function of driving pressure. The *slope of the P-V loop represents the elasticity of the lung* (Fig.13.5). The inspiratory and expiratory portions of the P-V loop describe a hysteresis, which represents the resistive work of breathing. Based upon the location of P-V loops on the total respiratory P-V relationship, the configuration of the P-V loop may be altered and indicate either pressure or volume overdistension (Figs 13.5 C,D). In children with air trapping or obstructive airway disease, the expiratory component of the hysteresis is excessively increased (Fig. 13.5 B).

Pressure (P) v Flow (F)

The P-F loop describes the relationship between the driving pressure and the airflow. When the elastic component of pressure is substracted from the measured transpulmonary pressure signal, the sigmoidal resistance pressure-flow curve is obtained. This curve gives a visual representation of the respiratory resistive characteristics during a respiratory cycle. Throughout most of a typical respiratory cycle this relationship is linear except at peak flow rates where a sigmoid relationship evolves. The characteristics of P-F loops are altered with turbulent flow and airway disease. The shape and slope of the P-F relationship provides insight into the changes in resistance in patients with airway disease, the effects of bronchodilators and bronchoconstrictors.

CARDIOVASCULAR MONITORING

The adequacy of circulation and perfusion may be assessed by several means as shown in Table 13.1.

Table 13.1

Non Invasive	*Invasive*
• Heart rate	
• Clinical indices of systemic perfusion	• CVP
• ECG, BP • Chest X-ray	• Intra arterial Pressure monitoring
• Lab: blood gases, Lactate levels,	• Pulmonary artery wedge pressure
• Capnography • Echocardiographic assessment of cardiac function	Cardiac catheterization

Pulse Rate/Heart Rate

Heart rate/ Pulse rate can be determined by palpating over brachial or femoral arteries but it is essential to have a continuous display of heart rate in critically ill children. An increase in heart rate is often the earliest sign of shock, hypovolemia or sepsis. Pulse oximeters or ECG monitors, both display heart rate continuously.

ECG

Continuous display of ECG is essential to monitor cardiac rate and rhythm. Stray currents can interfere with ECG and after tracings. Burns have been reported from ECG electrodes in children with reduced skin integrity or perfusion, therefore their site should be changed periodically.

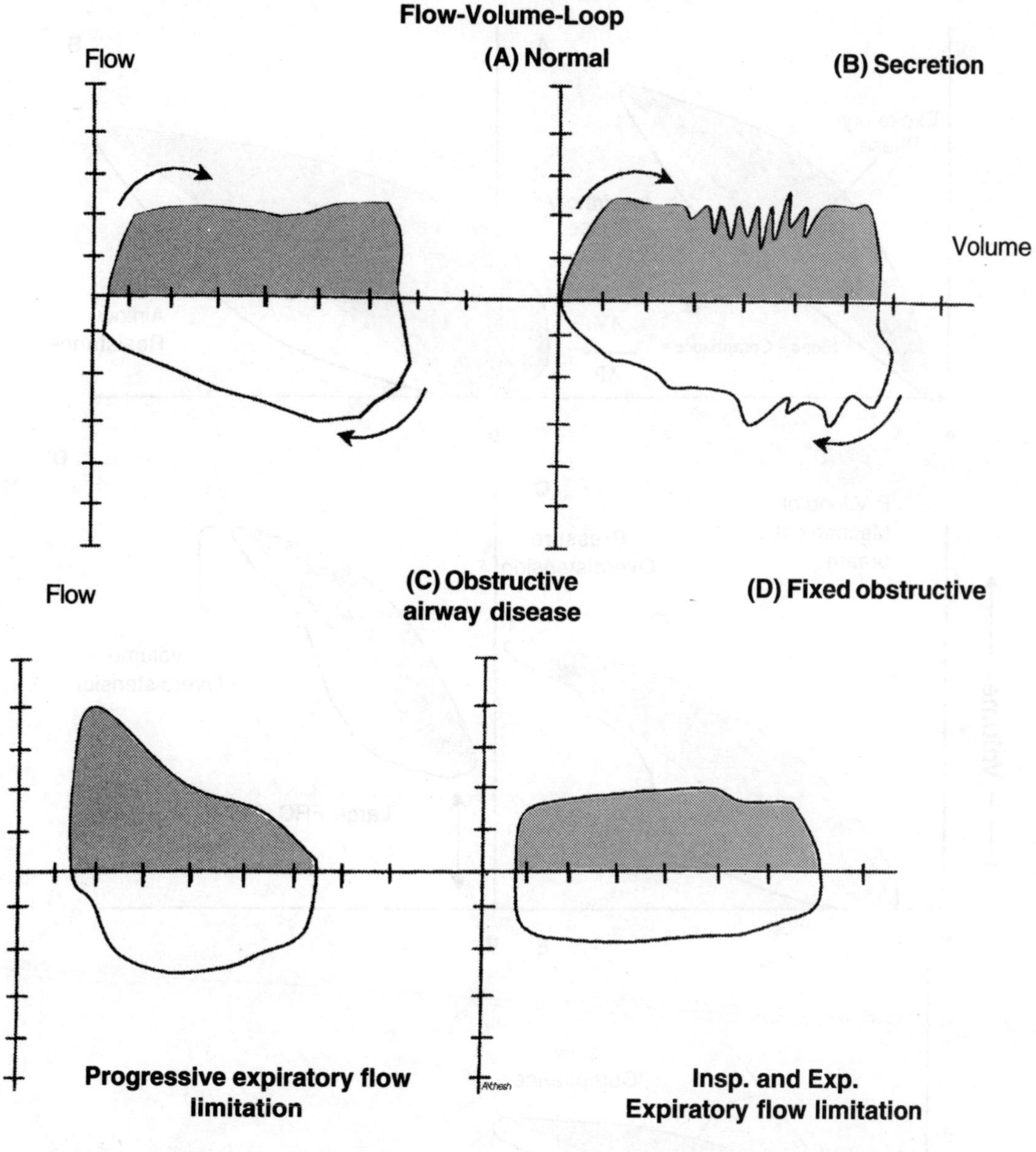

Fig. 13.4: Interpretation of flow-volume loops under different condition (A) Normal (B) Presence of secretions (C) Obstructive airway disease (D) Fixed obstruction

Blood Pressure (BP)

BP can be measured by cuff and auscultation, Doppler flow, oscillometery or direct arterial line. BP determined by palpation and auscultation using appropriate size cuffs is adequate in majority of patients. Continuous electronic monitoring of BP is needed whenever hemodynamic instability is present or when inotropic support is required to maintain BP. The automatic oscillometeric BP monitors are comparable in accuracy to auscultatory BP measurement, and are satisfactory for routine use. However in settings where signifi-

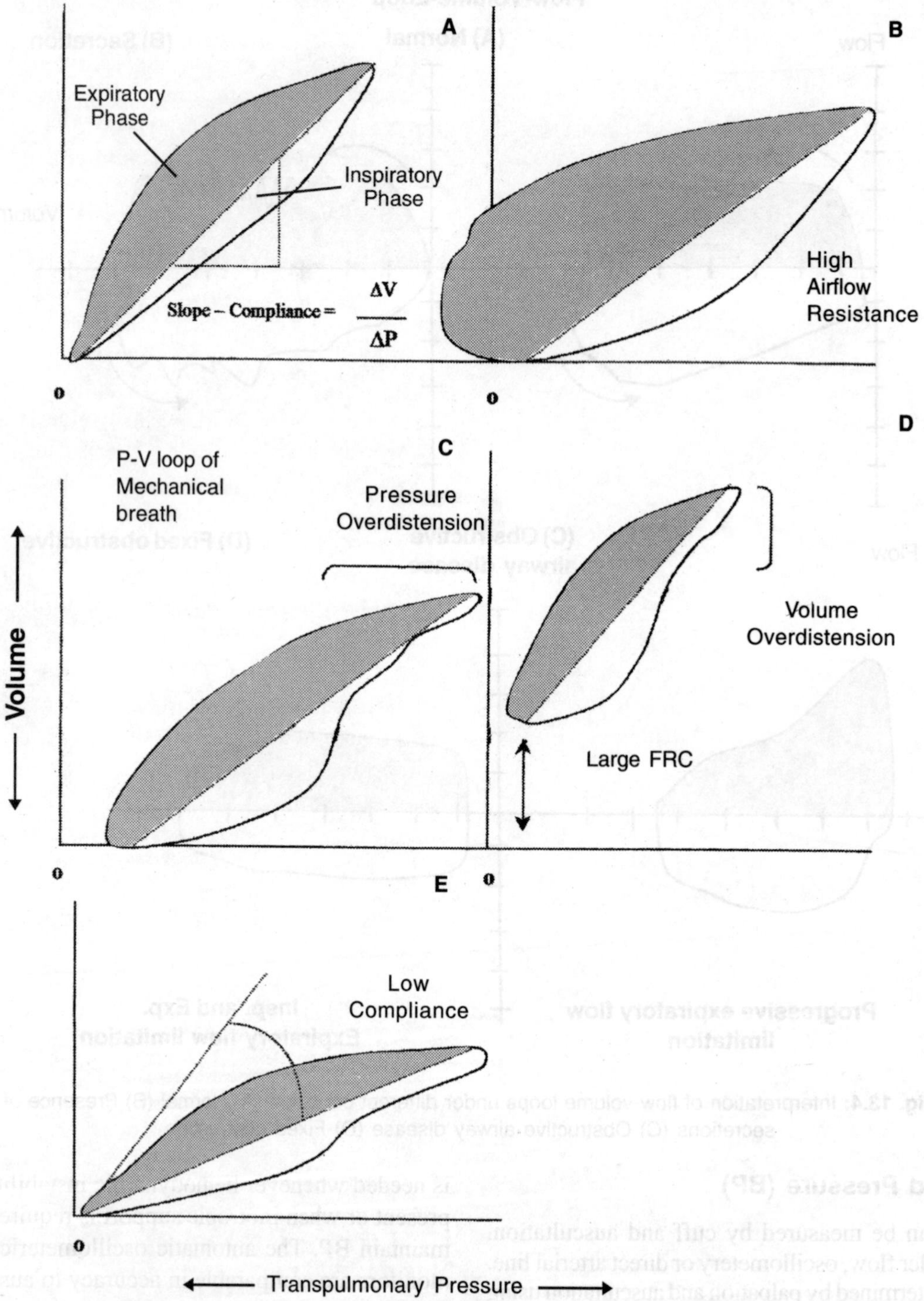

Fig. 13.5: Pressure volume (P-V) graphics (A) Normal (B) High air flow resistance (C) Pressure-overdistension (D) Volume overdistension (E) Low compliance

cance is attached to individual BP readings rather than to trends or where a high degree of accuracy is required these are not a satisfactory alternative to direct arterial BP.

Clinical monitoring of systemic perfusion may be carried out by assessment of mental status, heart rate, blood pressure, evaluation of peripheral pulses, capillary refill time, respiratory rate and urine output. An hourly monitoring of urinary output can be a very good indicator of the hemodynamic and fluid status as well as renal function. The daily input and output is of extraordinary help to understand the overall fluid balance in pediatrics.

Invasive Monitoring

Invasive methods of assessing the patient's hemodynamic status may be carried out by insertion of central venous lines (CVP), arterial cannulation, pulmonary artery wedge cannulation and cardiac catheterization. Of these, central venous catheters and invasive arterial lines are frequently placed in hemodynamically unstable patients when initial measures of stabilization are unsuccessful. CVP lines may be inserted either in the neck (internal jugular or subclavian route) or via the femoral route in which event, the tip of the catheter must lie at the junction of right atrium and inferior vena cava.

Invasive arterial lines are the gold standard for measuring arterial blood pressures and may be very useful in monitoring response to treatment in a patient with shock. Arterial lines also facilitate frequent blood sampling. All invasive lines, as their name implies carry a significant complication rate and hence must be used only in centres with considerable expertise and experience in the insertion and care of these lines.

Invasive BP monitoring through an arterial line is desirable but not mandatory when cardiovascular support is given. Direct pressure is 5-20 mmHg higher than the indirectly recorded BP. This difference is important in children with raised intracranial pressure to calculate cerebral perfusion.

Noninvasive monitoring using ultrasonic devices is accurate and may be used as an alternative to direct arterial blood pressure measurement in majority of children.

Central Venous Pressure (CVP)

The aim is to measure the pressure of blood within the intrathoracic portion of the superior/inferior vena cava. CVP (average 5-8 cmH_2O) may be measured directly or by using electronic monitors connected to a CVP line through a pressure transducer (Table 13.2). Clinically, this is usually done by an externally placed measuring device, the pressure being transmitted to it by a column of fluid within a centrally placed catheter. The pressure is measured relative to a reference point. Traditionally the point used is the intersection of the mid-axillary line and the 4th intercostals space with the patient in the supine position.

A CVP gives an indication of filling pressure of the right side of the heart, and right ventricular end-diastolic volume (RVEDV), which is an important determinant of stroke volume and cardiac output. CVP is used as an indirect estimate of RVEDV and also is an indirect measure

Table 13.2: Methods of central venous pressure measurement

Fluid-filled U-tube manometer	Pressure expressed as cmH_2O ($1 cmH_2O = 0.76$ mmHg) Requires no expressive monitoring or consumables Discrete rather than continuous measurement No waveform Inadvertent air embolism risk Prone to zero errors
Electronic transducer	Pressure expressed as mmHg (1 mmHg $= 1.3\ cmH_2O$) Real-time continuous measurement Waveform available Requires monitoring hardware Consumable costs Prone to zero errors

of myocardial dysfunction. In simple words CVP or right arterial pressure, in a child with normal cardiac contractility is a reliable measure of circulatory hemodynamics and preload to right ventricle. However, in children with pneumothorax, pericardial fluid collection, impaired cardiac function or in those on high PEEP, it is unreliable for monitoring hemodynamic status. Misleading and inaccurate information may be provided in patients with pulmonary arterial hypertension.

Cardiac Output

Clinical signs of poor peripheral perfusion such as cool extremities, and hypotension, decreased urine output are clear indications of low cardiac output. **The difference between core (rectal) and peripheral (skin) temperature** (DT) is a good measure of adequacy of tissue perfusion, and is also a simple and useful method to assess adequacy of cardiac output.

In pediatric intensive care, continuous dual temperature monitoring is commonly done by a rectal probe and a skin sensor on toes with a temperature sensor at its tip. Children respond to a decrease in perfusion with increased vasoconstriction and this produces a decrease in the temperature of the extremities.

Higher the difference, less is peripheral perfusion. Several commercial models of intensive care monitors have the facility for continuous measurement of two temperatures.

Capnography gives an indirect estimation of decreased cardiac output if the gradient between the arterial to end tidal CO_2 is increased.

Direct measurement of cardiac output is required in shock or in conditions associated with impaired myocardial contractility to monitor response to vasoactive drugs. The simplest and most practical method is the thermodilution technique, using a thermister-tipped Swan-Ganz catheter in the pulmonary artery. In the recent years, Doppler technology has been combined with echocardiography to allow for intermittent noninvasive measurement of cardiac output. Aortic flow velocity determined by Doppler technique permits calculation not only of cardiac output, but also of vascular resistance in many instances according to the formula: Vascular resistance = Perfusion pressure flow.

The technique of impedance cardiography has also been successfully used as a safe, noninvasive method to assess stroke volume and cardiac output in pediatric population. The values measured by this technique compare favorably with those measured by pulsed Doppler technique, and thermodilution method.

Pulmonary artery capillary wedge pressure (PCWP): A pulmonary artery catheter can be used to measure of PCWP, (also known as pulmonary artery occlusion pressure – PAOP). The normal value of PCWP is 4-12 mmHg, which is about the same as left atrial pressure. Same catheter may be used for measuring right ventricular and pulmonary artery pressures (normal systolic 20-30 mmHg, diastolic 5-15 mmHg) and calculation of pulmonary vascular resistance.

Echocardiography

Bedside assessment of myocardial dysfunction may be carried out by echocardiography which can quantitate both systolic and diastolic function of the heart and may also provide a clue to the cause of low cardiac output if significant pericardial fluid is present.

Monitoring of Circulation during Ventilation

Mechanical ventilation has marked direct and indirect effects on circulatory function. Alterations in airway and intrathoracic pressure change the loading conditions of the heart by altering venous return, transmyocardial pressure, and pulmonary vascular resistance. These complex cardiopulmonary interactions warrant monitoring of circulatory function during ventilatory support. Normovolemic patients usually have some decrease in blood pressure and cardiac output which is well tolerated. Circulatory function in these patients is adequately monitored using continuous electrocardiography and intermittent measurement of blood pressure. In hypovolemic patients hypotension and hypoperfusion get worsened by administration of positive pressure ventilation as venous return is further diminished by increased intrathoracic pressure. In such patients continuous monitoring of arterial pressure and central venous pressure is recommended upon initiation and during administration of ventilatory support. Patients with significant cardiac or pulmonary disease may have an unpredictable response to mechanical ventilatory support. Low lung compliance and congestive, after load-dependent heart failure usually are not associated with serious adverse circulatory effects. Compliant, emphysematous lungs, a stiff chest, and relatively low blood volume potentiate adverse circulatory effects of mechanical ventilation. Invasive monitoring of circulatory function, continuous arterial pressure monitoring and pulmonary artery catheterization with measurement of cardiac output and mixed venous oxyhemoglobin saturation are usually very valuable in such patients.

Circulatory assessment should always be performed while the patient is connected to the ventilator. Disconnecting the patient from the ventilator for hemodynamic studies not only undermines the value of the assessment but also subjects the patient to potentially serious derangement in cardiopulmonary function.

MEASUREMENT OF TISSUE HYPOXIA

The expanded concept of tissue oxygen deficit include accompanying CO_2 excess, and increase in anerobically generated lactic acid. Profound increase in venous and tissue PCO_2 value are quantitatively related to the severity of perfusion failure. Using this concept, the estimation of severity of low flow or tissue hypoperfusion has been based on measurement of dual defects of oxygen deficiency and CO_2 excess.

1. **Arteriovenous pH Difference:** Simultaneous estimation of both arterial and mixed venous blood gases may be used to indicate tissue hypoxia, hypercapnia and acidemia in patients with hemodynamic compromise. However, in patients with multiorgan failure and sepsis there may exist profound peripheral shunting. Blood, therefore bypasses the hypoxic tissue in functional shunts with the consequence that pulmonary artery blood probably reflect an 'effective' arteriovenous mixture.
2. **Oxygen Flux Test:** Infusion of a microvasodilator prostacycline (PGI_2) (5 mg/min/kg for 30 min) may be used to uncover covert tissue hypoxia. A significant increase in tissue oxygen uptake consumption index (VO_2) following the infusion suggest tissue hypoxia. VO_2 can be measured from measurement of arterial SaO_2, PO_2, Hb, cardiac output, and derived values of venous and arterial oxygen content.

   Oxygen content = (hemoglobin × 1.34 × % saturation) + (PO_2 × 0.0031)

   Oxygen delivery to tissues (DO_2) = Cardiac index × arterial oxygen content

   VO_2 = Cardiac index × Arteriovenous oxygen content difference

   $$O_2 \text{ extraction index} = \frac{\text{Arteriovenous oxygen content difference}}{\text{Arterial oxygen content}}$$
3. **Gastric mucosal pH:** A decrease in splanchnic blood flow with associated decrease in gut perfusion can result in tissue hypoxia, anaerobic glycolysis, and tissue acidosis. These alterations are reflected in the intestinal and gastric mucosa by increase in the tissue concentration of H^+ion and CO_2. The latter freely diffuses along its concentration gradient until an equilibrium is reached between luminal and intramucosal pCO_2. It is possible to measure gastric intramucosal pH by applying Henderson-Hasselbach equation, to simul-

taneously determined arterial plasma bicarbonate and CO_2.

It has been shown that intramucosal pH drops much earlier than the changes in VO_2 become evident. Gastric mucosal pH has also proven superior to global measure of oxygenation for predicting outcome of critically ill patients.

NEUROLOGICAL MONITORING

Monitoring of CNS functions is not as exact or simple as respiratory or cardiac monitoring. Clinical assessment of cognition, consciousness, motor capabilities, posture and reflexes and any lateralising signs indicate fairly well the neurological status. Pediatric adaptation of Glasgow coma scale scoring may be useful in overall assessment of CNS functions.

Central nervous system physiologic monitoring modalities include:

a. The clinically-apparent function,
b. Physical and mechanical variables,
c. Circulation or perfusion,
d. Bioelectrical measures, and
e. Biochemical measures.

Patterns of neurologic signs and the trend of the examination, are the most important factors to follow. Intracranial pressure monitoring provides information about cerebral perfusion pressure and risk of secondary cerebral injury. Cerebral blood flow is not easily quantified in the ICU, but Transcranial Doppler sonography is a reliable bedside technique. Neurophysiologic monitoring with electroencephalograph (EEG) and evoked potential (EP) can be used as a supplement to the neurologic examination and can provide an early indication of clinically relevant change due to evolving disease or in response to therapy.

All methods to monitor nervous system have their specific advantages and problems. An understanding of the information provided by each of the modalities is therefore, important.

Clinical Monitoring

It is oriented toward monitoring the course of the illness and in particular, towardsk detecting early signs of a decline in the patient's condition. It can reveal changing function in virtually every part of the nervous system when properly performed with an awake, cooperative patient. However, the sensitivity of the neurologic examination declines in patients with altered levels of consciousness and coma. Its utility can be obscured or obliterated when sedatives and paralyzing agents are used. It is advisable to suspend the sedatives and paralyzing agents briefly two or three times daily in order to correlate true neurologic function with other modalities.

Given that patient's neurologic outcomes are measured in terms of neurologic function (as opposed to ICP, EEG, or EP), monitoring strategies in the ICU must incorporate and emphasize the response of the patient's neurologic function to ICU interventions. ICU physician should establish the patient's baseline condition based on initial diagnostic examination, and perform a focused neurologic examination for comparison for monitoring the progress. For monitoring examinations, the ICU physician should choose a few pertinent, objective, measurable parts of the examination that can be performed rapidly and can be reproduced.

Clinical monitoring is useful wherever possible: Although a formal neurological assessment is not always feasible in the critical care unit, 5 features of the neurological assessment need special emphasis.

- Degree of altered mental status: the Glasgow Coma Score (GCS)
- Pattern of respirations
- Pupillary response
- Extra ocular movements
- Motor examination.

The Glasgow Coma Scale (GCS) is a commonly used scoring system in which three aspects of the neurobehavioral response are ascribed points—eye opening, best verbal response and best motor response to stimuli (See Table 3.1, Chapter 3). Charting of the serial GCS scores are useful in following the course of disease in-patients requiring neurocritical care.

In conscious patients, specific cortical functions can be tested. These may include language/aphasia, naming, calculations, right-left orientation, stereognosis or graphesthesia to name a few. In the ICU the trend in level of consciousness or the level of complexity of cortical functions is generally more significant than any specific level of consciousness. A patient who fails to improve or who is progressively worsening is worrisome.

The examination of the motor system can provide evidence of nervous system dysfunction regardless of the patient's level of consciousness. Understanding the normal vascular territories and associated motor function is important. The motor examination is an exercise in pattern recognition. Asymmetry of spontaneous movements can provide a clue to a hemiparesis as can asymmetry of the face or muscle tone. If there is no spontaneous movement, apply painful pressure on the trunk or proximally on the limbs. A localizing limb response, in which the patient moves the limb toward the stimulus as if to remove it, implies integrity of the cortical motor neurons and the corticospinal tract. Withdrawal from pain applied to the fingers or toes may represent either a spinal reflex or a localizing response, and thus is less helpful in determining the integrity of the corticospinal tract than proximally applied stimulation is. Abnormal posturing either spontaneously or in response to painful stimulation is seen in the unconscious patient. Abnormal extension of the limbs, abnormal extensor posturing carries the graver prognosis.

Patterns of weakness help to localize the site of injury. A lesion above the level of the cortico-medullary junction produces contralateral weakness. Occlusion of the anterior cerebral artery produces paresis of the leg, and ischemia of the middle cerebral artery produces weakness of the face and limbs and is associated with higher cortical function deficits. A lesion within the brain stem produces contralateral limb weakness and may cause ipsilateral cranial nerve palsies as well as altered consciousness and abnormalities in respiration. In particular, hemiparesis associated with a contralateral third cranial nerve palsy and a progressive decline in consciousness indicates midbrain injury from herniation. As with the level of consciousness, a change in the motor examination is more significant than any particular degree or pattern of weakness, particularly for disease for which there are therapeutic options. Functions of the brain stem can be tested. This includes the visual and occulmotor examination (cranial nerves II, III, IV, VI); cranial nerves V, VII, IX, X and XII ; and patterns of respiration.

There is no single sign or symptom which forecasts impending disaster.

Electroencephalography and Evoked Potentials

Electroencephalography (EEG) and EP testing can be used as a supplement to the neurologic exam. Continuous monitoring is a window into the ongoing neurologic functioning of patients. This window can provide an early indication of clinically relevant change due to evolving disease or in response to therapy, which is especially helpful when the neurologic examination is limited to severe coma, or neuromuscular blockade. EEG and EP can also provide important diagnostic and prognostic information.

EEG and Somatosensory evoked potentials (SSEPs) change predictably with cerebral ischemia, and recognition of these changes may allow intervention before frank tissue infarction. Additional roles include identification of sub-clinical or nonconvulsive seizures, identification of metabolic coma; and identification of compression of neural tracts due to expanding hematoma, edematous tissue, or hydrocephalus. The early identification of ischemia or significant edema allows for ICU intervention and minute-to-minute evaluation of response to therapeutic intervention.

Electroencephalography record ongoing summated electrical activity produced by neurons in the cerebral cortex. Activity is seen as low amplitude waves. EEG can identify cortical abnormalities (often before CT changes are evident), it cannot reliably identify subcortical disease. Specific EEG patterns can be used to identify ischemic changes and predict severity of injury. For typical EEG findings in some conditions causing coma (see Chapter 10).

EEG patterns of burst suppression, monorhythmical alpha like activity, electrocerebral silence or very low amplitude, and monotonous 0.5-3 Hz high voltage activity have been associated with poor outcome. EEG findings of poor outcome do not always correlate with the clinical assessment of deep coma. The appearance of sleep spindles is indicative of a good prognosis, even in the presence of delta waves.

Evoked potentials are produced by stimulating a sensory system and recording the electrical activity that follows. EPs can follow somatosensory auditory stimulation, brainstem auditory evoked responses (BAER), or visual stimulation (visual EP). The target EP activity occurs at a reproducible time after the stimulus. All EP responses are characterized and defined by latency and amplitude criteria. These responses occur sequentially.

Amplitude of EEG activity or the amplitude of EP responses, are of limited usefulness as strict criteria for defining disease because of high variability among normal subjects. The large range of patient-to-patient variability becomes less of a concern when EEG or EP are used for continuous monitoring in the ICU. An important premise for such monitoring is that the amplitude and latency of responses for a single patient are expected to remain relatively constant over short periods of time (hours to day), provided that those areas of the nervous system responsible for the responses are unaffected by disease. If the data change significantly, then a significant clinical change (for better or worse) is expected.

Disappearance of evoked potentials is associated with severe reduction in cerebral perfusion pressure and indicate a bad prognosis. Occasionally evoked potentials may be misleading in acute stages of the disease and may not predict the prognosis. The display of small changes in latency and aptitude are to subtle for most of the observers. However, dramatic changes especially in the brain stem potentials are often too late to allow therapeutic intervention before catastrophe occur. Thus, while evoked potentials are useful as predictors of prognosis, they are of little value as a guide to therapy.

The identification of seizures, especially non-convulsive seizures (NCSE), is a clear benefit of continuous EEG monitoring. NCSE can manifest as coma, and signs of seizure (nystagmus, or twitching of facial or upper limb muscles) may be asbent or subtle. Outcomes after ICU stays are worse if NCSE occurs, especially if the NCSE is prolonged or the diagnosis is delayed. It is expected, but not proven, that early recognition of NSCE would reduce the chance of further cerebral damage. Continuous EEG is more capable of distinguishing NCSE patterns from coma patterns in toxic/metabolic coma than in routine, intermittent EEG.

In summary, EEG and EP monitoring can be powerful tools for identifying neurophysiologic changes.

Intracranial Pressure Monitoring

Placement of an intraventricular catheter through a burr-hole and direct measurement of ICP through a transducer and a recording device remains the standard method. This method also offers a therapeutic option of withdrawing CSF to reduce raised ICP. Other methods are insertion of a subarachnoid bolt, and a subdural catheter.

Risk of cerebral injury posed by ICP elevation depends on the cause, acuity, severity, and duration of the elevation. ICP elevation that develops chronically, such as from tumor or some forms of hydrocephalus, can be well tolerated. On the other hand, in traumatic brain injury, acute ICP elevation in the range of 15 to 25 mm Hg is poorly tolerated and portends a poor outcome unless it is quickly controlled.

The ICP is a critical determinant of cerebral perfusion pressure (CPP), which is operationally defined as mean arterial pressure (MAP) - ICP (or jugular venous pressure if it is higher). The relationship between CPP and CBF is approximately linear when CPP is <50 to 60 mm Hg. Between CPP values of 50 and 150 mm Hg, there is very little increase in CBF, and at >150 mm Hg,CBF again increases as a function of CPP. The nearly plateau level of CBF when CPP is between 50 and 150 mm Hg represents autoregulation of CBF.

When CPP is below the autoregulatory range, the risk of cerebral ischemia is high, as in intracranial hypertensive crisis (high ICP) or syncope and cardiovascular collapse (low MAP). Other determinants of CBF regulation under normal circumstances include PaO_2, $PaCO_2$, arterial oxygen content, cerebral metabolic rate for oxygen consumption, and viscosity, all of which can be measured or manipulated in the ICU.

The purpose of ICP monitoring is prevention of secondary cerebral injury or ischemia, often based on the patient's relative risk of secondary cerebral injury. The indicators of this risk are clinical and radiologic evidence. When the GCS score is < 8 and the risk of ischemia is high, ICP monitoring is nearly always indicated.

When the patient is critically ill and comatose, and brain resuscitation or protection is the primary treatment objective, it is often much wiser to insert an ICP monitor and discover the raised ICP rather than wait and discover the consequences of elevated ICP later. If the ICP is normal, the monitoring device can be removed after a 24 to 48-hour observation period.

Cerebral Blood Flow (CBF)

Bedside measurement of CBF remains a long-standing goal of neuro-intensivists. CBF monitoring can gauge the presence or risk of cerebral ischemia, determine whether therapeutic interventions have restored adequate CBF, and provide useful informaton regarding the state of cerebral autoregulation. CBF monitoring can also identify cerebral hyperemia, which may potentially exacerbate increased ICP, cerebral edema, or hemorrhage. Transcranial Doppler sonography (TCD) is currently the most versatile and widely available quantitative technique of assessing CBF. Other currently available techniques include the xenon 133 scanning, positron emission tomography, and diffusion-weighted magnetic resonance imaging. Laser Doppler flowmetry can measure relative CBF changes.

Neurological Monitoring of ventilated patient

1. Clinical
   a. GCS, but affected by sedation, neuromuscular blockade
   b. Pupils—only definite sign in sedated patients
2. Intracranial pressure monitoring
   a. Ventricular—'gold standard' , allows CSF withdrawal, higher risk of infection
   b. Parenchymal—lower infection rate, recalibration difficult
   c. subdural—lower infection rate, less accurate
3. Cerebral oxygenation

Jugular bulb oximetry—retrograde placement of catheter in jugular vein allows intermittent or continuous measurement of oxygen saturation of blood leaving brain ($S_{jv}O_2$):

$S_{jv}O_2 = CBF/CMR\text{-}O_2$

where CBF= cerebral blood flow and $CMR\text{-}O_2$ = cerebral metabolicrate for O_2. if $CMR\text{-}O_2$ is constant then jugular saturation is dependent on cerebral blood flow. $S_{jv}O_2$ 60-80% is normal. $S_{jv}O_2 > 90\%$ indicates hyperemia, and $S_{jv}O_2 < 50\%$ suggests ischemia

Near-infrared spectroscopy is non-invasive transcranial measure of regional cerebral oxygenation; it is unreliable and experimental. Indwelling blood-gas electrode are invasive, measures local tissue pH, PaO_2, $PaCO_2$.

4. Transcranial Doppler provides non-invasive measure of cerebral blood velocities. Its role is established in the monitoring of vasospasm following spontaneous and traumatic subarachnoid hemorrhage.
5. Processed electroencephalogram (EEG) allows detection of seizure activity in paralysed patients, and is useful to guide therapies aimed at reducing cerebral metabolism.

OTHER SPECIFIC MONITORING DURING VENTILATION

Radiological Assessment

Ideally an X-ray should be obtained at the start of the ventilation and then after each tube change, after a sudden deterioration and after extubation. It should be looked for: position of endotracheal tube, gastric tubes and central lines. Position of the tube—should be between T2-T4, overall lung volume–inflation of the lung, over-inflation is seen as wide intercostal spaces and flat diaphragms, presence and severity of atelectasis, progress/ improvement of the primary pathology, size of the cardiac shadow, presence of air leaks: pneumothorax, pneumomediastinum, pneumopericardium, pulmonary interstitial emphysema (PIE)/ the hilar areas, development and pneumonia, pulmonary oedema and pulmonary congestion.

Bacteriological Monitoring

Routine cultures of ET tube secretions is controversial as it is difficult to differentiate between colonization of a chronically instrumented airway and actual ventilator associated pneumonia (VAP) based on cultures alone. Sudden change in the quantity and quality of endotracheal secretion associated with new fever or infiltrates on the chest X-ray be an indication of VAP and tracheal cultures may be warranted. Blood culture – may be done as clinical indicated.

CONCLUSION

Monitoring plays an essential role in the management of critically ill children, continuous observation using electronic monitors along with frequent clinical examination re ins the best readily available monitor. The basic minimum monitoring is summarised in Table 13.3.

Table 13.3: Basic minimum monitoring in PICU

Clinical monitoring

1. Vital Signs: Continuous display, record atleast 1-2 hrly
2. Level of consciousness, tone, responsiveness, pupil size —4 hourly
3. Intake, Output, Weight – daily
4. Urine flow – every hourly record, assess 8 hrly
5. Other relevant systemic examination.

Bedside continuous electronic monitoring

1. Heart rate, ECG, Blood pressure
2. Peripheral and core-temperature
3. CVP
4. Respiratory rate and wave form
5. Oxygen saturation.

Laboratory

1. Blood: Hematocrit (Hb), Coagulation parameters-daily
2. Blood biochemistry, electrolytes, urea and creatinine, glucose, Ca, Mg, PO_4^- daily; more frequently if needed
3. X-ray chest daily in acute phase, on ventilator, after intubation or extubation or repositioning of the tube
4. Cultures: Urine, blood, oropharyngeal/tracheal secretions, twice a week.

Chapter fourteen

Acid Base Disorders

Blood gas abnormalities form an integral part of management of critically ill patients and deserve important place in their care. Fear of proper analysis of blood gases is universal and this is an attempt to simplify the approach to blood gas analysis.

Acid is a substance, which can donate H ion. H ion is also known as a proton. Hydrogen atom is made of a proton and an electron revolving around it. Loss of electron from this atom result into proton (H+).

Base is defined as a substance that can accept a proton e.g. OH ions can combine with H ions to form water, thus substance that can donate OH ions is called as a base. NaOH is a base.

$NaOH = Na^+ + OH^-$

CONCEPT OF pH

Concentration of H ions in a solution can be conveniently mentioned in two forms, in the form of nanomoles/lit or in the form of pH (pH is negative log of H ion concentration)

$$pH = -\log \frac{1}{\text{H ion concentration}}$$

As is obvious from the above equation, if the concentration of H ion increase the pH will decrease. (When H ions increase the product of one upon H ion concentration will decrease). Normal H ion concentration is 40 nanomoles/ L; this corresponds to pH of 7.40. The range compatible with life is 20-160 nanomoles/L, equivalent to a pH of 6.8 – 7.7. Metabolic alkalosis is known to vary in response from no compensation to almost near normal compensation.

Buffer is a substance that has the capacity to minimize the pH change that addition of an acid or base would otherwise produce. The most important biological buffers are bicarbonate/CO_2, intracellular phosphate, proteins and hemoglobin. Of these the most important extracellular system is bicarbonate/CO_2, the activity of which is described by Henderson-Hasselbatch equation.

pH as a ratio: The essence of understanding acid base lies in realization of the fact that pH is a ratio between acid and base. Henderson-Hasselbach equation states the same thing in more complex mathematical form. Normal pH means normal ratio between acid and base in the body. Bicarbonate buffer system in the body will illustrate the above statement. $pH = 6.1 + \log 10 ([HCO_3^-]/ [CO_2])$. The ratio between bicarbonate and carbonic acid is 20:1, at this ratio the pH is normal. Addition or deletion of acid or alkali will alter the ratio and thus the pH; body tries to normalize the ratio and thus the pH.

Metabolic and Respiratory Components

Any change in pH that occurs primarily because of bicarbonate is called as metabolic change; the change occurring because of CO_2 is called as respiratory. Thus we have respiratory and metabolic acidosis and alkalosis. One must remember that bicarbonate changes pH in same direction (increase in bicarbonate will increase pH and decrease in bicarbonate will decrease pH) and CO_2 changes pH in opposite direction. Lungs primarily control respiratory component in body and the metabolic component is controlled by kidneys. *Thus pH is a ratio between renal and pulmonary functions*. Carbon dioxide in the body behaves like an acid and thus when it accumulates causing acidic pH, it is respiratory acidosis and when CO_2 levels are down changing the pH to alkaline it is respiratory alkalosis.

Compensation: With primary alteration in respiratory system (hypo or hyperventilation) body compensates by altering the metabolic component. Modulating respiratory system compensates for primary change in metabolic factors (change in bicarbonates). Compensation will never bring the pH to normal (7.40) but will pull it towards normal. Renal compensation takes several days, respiratory compensation occurs in hours. There is nothing like overcompensation and this should suggest a mixed disturbance.

Anion gap: Anion gap measures the difference between the concentration of unmeasured anions (phosphates, lactate, ketones etc.) and cations. Anion gap = $[Na^+] - ([Cl^-] + [HCO_3^-])$.

Normal value is 8-12 mEq/L. It is useful in classifying acidosis.

PRACTICAL APPROACH TO ABG REPORT

One looks at the three values for rapid analysis of ABG (Table 14.1).

pH Normal 7.35 to 7.45
$PaCO_2$ Normal 35 to 45
HCO_3^- (Calculated parameter) Normal 22 to 26

Step 1: *Look at the pH.*
Normal 7.35 to 7.45
Below 7.35 is acidosis
Above 7.45 is alkalosis
Normal pH does not rule out an ABG disorder.

Step 2: *What is responsible for the change in pH?*
Look for bicarbonate. Is the value abnormal? If bicarbonate is responsible for the change in pH, then the pH will change in the direction of the change in bicarbonate. (Low bicarbonate should lower pH and high bicarbonate will increase pH).

Look for $PaCO_2$ value. Is the value abnormal? If carbon dioxide is responsible for the change in pH, then the pH will change in opposite direction of the change in CO_2.

At the end of this step one should be able to diagnose primary ABG disorder.

pH low ... acidosis
Low bicarbonate... Metabolic acidosis
High $PaCO_2$ ... Respiratory acidosis
pH high ... alkalosis
Low $PaCO_2$ ... Respiratory alkalosis
High bicarbonate ... Metabolic alkalosis.

Step 3: Look for Compensation (Table 14.2)
Metabolic acidosis: Expected $PaCO_2$ = Last two digits of pH (if pH is 7.20 expected $PaCO_2$ is 20).

Respiratory acidosis
Expected $PaCO_2$=Last two digits of pH (if pH is 7.20 expected $PaCO_2$ is 20) : $PaCO_2$ = rise of 6

Table 14.1: Classification of acid base disturbances and changes in $PaCO_2$ and HCO_3

Disorder	*pH*	*$PaCO_2$*	*HCO_3*	*Compensations*
Metabolic acidosis	Low	Low	Low	Fall in $PaCO_2$ Acidic urine
Metabolic alkalosis	High	High	High	Rise in $PaCO_2$ Alkaline urine
Respiratory acidosis	Low	High	High	Acidic urine
Respiratory alkalosis	High	Low	Low	Alkaline urine

Table 14.2: Expected compensatory changes for primary acid base disorders

Primary change	*Compensatory change and its rate*
HCO_3 ↓	↓ $PaCO_2$ by 1.0-1.5 mmHg per 1 mEq/l
HCO_3↑	↑ $PaCO_2$ by 0.5-1.5 mmHg per 1 mEq/l
Acute PCO_2↑	↑ HCO_3 by 1 mEq/l for each 10-mmHg increase
Chronic PCO_2 ↑	↑ HCO_3 by 4 mEq/l for each 10-mmHg increase
Acute PCO_2 ↓	↓ HCO_3 by 1-3 mEq/l for each 10-mmHg decrease
Chronic PCO_2 ↓	↓ HCO_3 by 2-5 mEq/l for each 10-mmHg decrease

mm per 10 mEq rise in bicarbonate.

Respiratory disorders

For acute change in $PaCO_2$ of 10 ... pH will change by .08, and $[HCO_3^-]$ by 1 mM.

For chronic change in $PaCO_2$ of 10 ... pH will change by .03 and $[HCO_3^-]$ by 3-5 mM.

Respiratory acidosis

Acute: For every increase of $PaCO_2$ of 10, pH will fall by 0.08

Chronic: For every increase of $PaCO_2$ by 10 the pH will fall by .03.

Respiratory alkalosis

Acute: For every decrease of $PaCO_2$ by 10 the pH will increase by .08.

Chronic: For every decrease of $PaCO_2$ by 10 the pH will increase by .03.

Metabolic Alkalosis: There is compensatory increase in $PaCO_2$, by 0.6 mmHg for each 1mM in $[HCO_3^-]$.

Step 4: Look for Mixed Disturbance (Table 14.3) When pH is normal and:

Bicarbonate is high—Metabolic alkalosis + respiratory acidosis.

Bicarbonate is low—Metabolic acidosis + respiratory alkalosis.

Bicarbonate is normal and anion gap is high—Metabolic Acidosis + Metabolic alkalosis.

When bicarbonate is normal and:

pH is in acidic range—Chronic respiratory acidosis + respiratory alkalosis.

pH is in alkalemic range—Metabolic alkalosis + respiratory alkalosis.

PCO_2 and bicarbonates are shifted from normal in opposing directions.

Anion gap is elevated and clinic and laboratory data suggest a diagnosis other than metabolic acidosis: Certain other rare conditions in patients with chronic renal and pulmonary diseases and patients on long-term diuretics.

Step 5: All the blood gas reports need to be seen in respect with the patient's age (Table 14.4), electrolytes, oxygenation status anion gap, clinical condition of the patient and the earlier reports of blood gases. Single report may fail to give the complete clinical picture of the patient and thus needs to be evaluated comprehensively.

Table 14.3: Recognition of type of disturbance in acid-base balance

$paCO_2$	*HCO_3 (mEq/L)* <21	21-26	>26
>45	Combined metabolic acidosis plus respiratory acidosis	Respiratory acidosis	Mixed *metabolic plus respiratory acidosis
35-45	Metabolic acidosis	Normal	Metabolic alkalosis
<35	Mixed* metabolic acidosis plus respiratory alkalosis	Respiratory alkalosis	Combined respiratory alkalosis plus metabolic alkalosis

* pH reflects which mixed disorder is primary and which is secondary because compensation is never complete.

Table 14.4: Normal blood gases in room air at different ages

Arterial blood	*pH*	*$PaCO_2$*	*PO_2*	*BE*	*HCO_3*
Newborn (Ist 24 hrs.)	7.30	33	68	- 6	20
Infants	7.40	34	90	- 3	20
Child	7.39	37	96	- 2	22
Adult	7.40	40	100	0	24

Metabolic Acidosis

Metabolic acidosis results from either excessive production or decreased excretion of H+ ions or excessive loss of bicarbonates from the body. The most important compensatory changes is hyperventilation to decrease PCO_2. Others include buffering by bicarbonate and proteins in plasma, hyperventilation to decrease PCO_2 and renal excretion of acid and regeneration of bicarbonate.

Anion Gap: Anion gap is defined as the difference between measured cations (Na+ and K+) and measured anions (Cl^- and HCO_3^-). Anion gap occurs due to the accumulation of anionic substances (acids); usually nonvolatile metabolic byproducts such as lactates, ketoacids etc. Which are not measured by routine laboratory techniques.

Anion gap = $(Na^+ + K^+) - (HCO_3 + Cl)$

The usual anion gap range is 15-20 mEq/1. It represents primarily phosphates, sulfates and organic acids. A high anion gap is associated with increased severity of illness and mortality.[6] Increased anion gap occurs due to increased unmeasured anions as seen in pateints with diabetic ketoacidosis (acetoacetic acid and beta hydroxybutyric acid), lactic acidosis (lactic acid), salicylate, isoniazid, iron and alcohol poisoning, and azotemia (sulfuric and organic acids). In metabolic alkalosis as compensation, plasma proteins release their H^+ ions leading to increase in their negative charge. The anionic value of protein increases, which is not measured. Therefore, a spurious decrease in measured anions occur resulting in increased anion gap. Decreased anion gap occurs in children with increased unmeasured cations (high Ca^{++}, Mg^{++}) or decreased unmeasured anion (hypoalbuminemia).

Causes: *Metabolic acidosis without an increase in anion gap:* Severe diarrhea (bicarbonate loss in stools), renal tubular acidosis, hyperalimentation and enteric fistula, and drugs (cholestyramine, amphotericin, acetazolamide).

Metabolic adidosis with increased anion gap: Diabetic ketoacidosis, poisonings (salicylates, methyl alcohol), shock, hypoxia (lactic acidosis), azotemia and inherited aminoacidurias.

Clinical Picture: Mild metabolic acidosis is asymptomatic. Non-specific symptoms may be present in the form of headache, nausea and vomiting, abdominal pain. At pH below 7.2, there is Kussmaul's breathing with signs of peripheral vasodilatation. A release of catecholamines occurs to counter balance some of the detrimental effects of acidosis. These are arteriolar dilation and hypotension. severe acidosis (pH <7.2) has several adverse effects on the body viz. myocardial depression, increased pulmonary vascular resistance, and depressed cerebral and cellular metabolism. Severe metabolic acidosis may also lead to hyperkalemia with additive cardio-toxic effects.

Treatment: Correction of acidosis is usually not recommended in mild and moderate cases. Treatment of the underlying condition improves acidosis. Severe acidosis (pH <7.2) or base excess more than-10 mMol/l requires urgent correction. Sodium bicarbonate is the safest and most effective alkalinising agent[22]. The dose is estimated for correcting only half of the deficit. The total body water is 60 percent of the body weight in which acid base imbalance is present. However, the correction is calculated for 30 percent of the body weight by the following formula:

mEq of bicarbonate = body weight (kg) x (bicarbonate desired-actual) x 0.3

One-half of the calculated bicarbonate may be given immediately and the rest over 12-24 hours as as slow infusion. In the state of severe cardio-respiratory instability of resuscitation the dose may be infused over 10-30 minutes[32]. Sodium bicarbonate (7.5% solution provides 0.9 mEq/ml) must be diluted with at least equal volume of distilled water or double volume of D5W before administration. Concurrent administration of potassium is essential to safeguard against development of hypokalemia due to shift of K+ from ECF into the cells. Following correction of acidosis, hypocalcemic tetany may occur due to fall in ionized calcium level. Calcium gluconate 10% (0.5-1.0 ml/kg) should be administered separately and not mixed in fluids containing sodium bicarbonate; otherwise it may get precipitated. *Sodium overload should be kept in mind while correcting acidosis with sodium bicarbonate.*

Other alkalinising agents such as THAM (tris-hydroxymethyl- aminomethane) rapidly increases pH of body fluids and tissues including CNS and transiently lowers PCO_2. It may be helpful in severe acidosis associated with severe hypernatremia (Na^+>155mEq/1) where $NaHCO_3$ administration is considered hazardous. Severe acidosis in the presence of renal failure or hyperosmolar state is best treated by peritoneal or hemodialysis.

Metabolic Alkalosis

Metabolic alkalosis results from either loss of H^+ ions or an excess of bicarbonate ions in the body. Loss of chloride and body fluids because of persistent vomiting (especially due to hypertrophic stenosis) or prologed gastric aspiration leads to alkalosis due to loss of H^+ ions. Hypokalemia causes alkalosis by shift of H^+ ions in order to conserve K^+ and due to urinary loss of H^+ ions in order to conserve K^+ in the renal tubules. Prolonged diuretic therapy (thiazide, furosemide, ethacrynic acid) and excessive intake of alkalies may also lead to metabolic alkalosis. Metabolic alkalosis without volume and chloride depletion (saline resistant alkalosis) is seen in children with primary hyperaldosteronism, cushing's syndrome and Bartter's syndrome. The saline responsive and saline resistant alkalosis can be differentiated on the basis of urinary chloride levels. In saline responsive variety, urinary chlorides are less than 10 mEq/l and in saline resistant it is usually more than 10 mEq/l and in saline resistant it is usually more than 10 mEq/l. An increase in pH by 0.1 causes on an average a fall of 0.5 mEq/l in serum potassium.

Clinical Picture: The patients have signs and symptoms of underlying disease and features of hypokalemia. At pH above 7.55 the patient may be confused, drowsy or comatose. The child may develop tetany, laryngospasm or convulsions due to decreased ionic calcium, and cardiac arrhythmia because of hypokalemia.

Treatment - Treatment is advised at pH value greater than 7.5 and is aimed at reducing blood pH value to 7.5. Saline responsive variety responds to administration of saline and potassium chloride. When intravascular volume is restored with saline, excessive secretion of aldosterone stops, excessive loss of potassium in the urine is arrested and excretion of bicarbonate takes place that corrects metabolic alkalosis. Acetazolamide 5 mg/kg/24 hr in 1-4 divided doses may be used if volume expansion is risky, such as in patients with congestive cardiac failure[32].

Saline resistant alkalosis - The mild cases respond to sodium chloride restriction, mineralocorticoid antagonist (spironolactone) and potassium chloride supplements. Severe cases should be treated with HCl (0.1 N solution i.e. 100 mEq of H^+ ions/l) or HCI producing substances such as ammonium chloride[7]. The HCl solution should be administered through central venous line. Ammonium chloride can be given through peripheral venous line in a dose of 3 mEq/l at a rate of about 0.5 mEq/min, or orally in a dose of 75 mg/kg/24 hours in four divided doses[32]. Cimetidine (20 mg-40 mg/kg/24 hours) IV or oral reduces acid excretion by stomach and thus reduces the pH of body fluids.

Respiratory Acidosis

In respiratory acidosis there is decreased elimination of carbon dioxide from the body due to poor ventilation, which leads to accumulation of carbon dioxide in the body and generation of carbonic acid.

Acute respiratory acidosis is characterized by a primary rise in PCO_2 above 45 mmHg, which remains at this high value for no longer than 6 to 12 hours[32]. Sustained elevation of PCO_2 beyond 12 hours is defined as chronic respiratory acidosis. During acute respiratory acidosis the rise in HCO_3 concentration rarely exceeds 4 mEq/l and renal compensation does not occur. However, chronic respiratory acidosis is accompanied by renal excretion of H^+ ions as NH_4 CI, and increased bicarbonate production. Hypochloremia is a common feature of chronic respiratory acidosis because of renal chloride excretion.

Acute respiratory acidosis may occur due to airway obstruction (severe bronchospasm, birth asphyxia, foreign body or laryngeal edema), hyaline membrane disease, extensive pneumonia, pneumothorax, pulmonary embolism and pulmonary edema, hypoventilation because of neuromuscular disease (poliomyelitis, Guillain-Barre syndrome) and overdose of opium and sedatives. Chronic respiratory acidosis is associated with chronic lung disease (interstitial fibrosis, bronchiectasis, chronic cor-pulmonale), kyphoscoliosis, asphyxiating thoracic dystrophy, paralysis or weakness of respiratory muscles.

Clinical Picture: Signs and symptoms are related to the degree of hypercapnia. Child develops headache with either irritability or depression due to increase in ICP. There is impairment of consciousness varying from drowsiness to deep coma. Muscular tremors can occur. Tachycardia, flushing of skin or perspiration may be present. Blood pressure may be low with signs of shock. Ventricular fibrillations may occur.

Treatment: The immediate dangers of respiratory acidosis are carbon dioxide narcosis and anoxic damage. Treatment is directed at the underlying cause and improvement of alveolar gas exchange by assisted ventilation. Oxygen administration with high flow rates may help to wash out carbon dioxide. However, in-breathing in a tight fitting mask or head box may cause a dangerous elevation of PCO_2. If hyperkalemia or ventricular fibrillation develops in a child with acute respiratory acidosis, sodium bicarbonate may be life saving. It should be administered after establishing ventilation. Metabolic alkalosis may develop because of previous chloride losses and will need replacement.

Respiratory Alkalosis

In this condition there is a fall in arterial PCO_2. It usually occurs due to hyperventilation (assisted ventilation), psychogenic or neurogenic hyperventilation. It may be one of the earliest signs of sepsis. Acute respiratory alkalosis last no longer than 6 to 12 hours. The compensatory response to this phase involves consumption of HCO_3 by body buffers without any renal involvement. In the chronic phase renal suppression of H+ ion excretion and chloride retention occurs to offset the falling HCO_3 Hyperchloremia is a common feature in chronic phase.

Clinical Picture: Usually there is hyperventilation with features of tetany as alkalosis decreases blood levels of ionized calcium.

Treatment: Breathing in a closed circuit would cause a accumulation of carbon dioxide. The underlying condition should be treated. Sodium bicarbonate therapy is not indicated.

Mixed Acid base Disorders

Mixed acid base disturbances are conditions where more than one primary acid disturbance occurs. The four commonly encountered mixed acid base disorders are: respiratory acidosis+ metabolic acidosis, respiratory + metabolic alkalosis, respiratory alkalosis+ metabolic acidosis and respiratory alkalosis+ metabolic alkalosis. The most serious acid base disorders are of mixed type when respiratory and metabolic disturbances result in a pH change in same direction.

In order to diagnose a mixed acid base disorder one needs to distinguish between combined primary changes in PCO_2 and HCO_3 and simple acid base disorder where one variable changes secondary to a primary change in the other. As a rule, if values of either PCO_2 are compatible with expected compensatory values to a simple acid base disorder, a mixed disturbance should be considered.

Chapter fifteen

Acute Renal Failure

Acute renal failure (ARF) is a common problem in pediatric intensive care units (PICUs) especially in a setting of predisposing conditions like dehydration, glomerulonephritis or nephrotic syndrome. Often sick children having respiratory problems, sepsis, intracranial pathology etc., are treated without attention to "renal protection" and ARF is discovered when raised levels of blood urea and creatinine are found. ARF needs to be anticipated and suspected early so that life-threatening complications can be avoided with proper management. Often, however, very sick children already in ARF are referred to PICUs. A PICU therefore should have services of a pediatric nephrologist available round the clock and preparedness to institute peritoneal dialysis at a short notice.

DEFINITIONS

Acute renal failure is defined as sudden decline in glomerular filtration rate, resulting in inability to excrete nitrogenous waste and maintain fluid and acid-base balance. In 95% patients it is potentially reversible. It is frequently associated with oliguria (urine output < 0.5 ml/kg/h, <1 ml/kg/h in neonates) but it may occur without oliguria.

Acute on chronic renal failure is suggested by poor growth, history of polyuria and polydipsia, and evidence of renal osteodystrophy and hypertensive retinopathy.

COMMON CAUSES OF ARF

Pre-renal failure accounts for 50-70% of all renal failure. It occurs because of a fall in renal perfusion pressure and consequent decrease in glomerular filtration. Reduced renal perfusion caused by hypovolemia, low cardiac output states, or profound shock leads to reductions in glomerular perfusion and urine output. Afferent vasodilation and efferent vasoconstriction of the glomerular vessels (mediated by dilating prostaglandins and angiotensin II, respectively) initially maintain glomerular perfusion pressure at the cost of compromising tubular perfusion. If renal hypoperfusion persists, acute tubular necrosis, and established renal failure inevitably develop. NSAIDs and ACE inhibitors exacerbate prerenal renal failure by interfering with these compensatory mechanisms.

Pre-renal failure may be caused by a true decrease in intravascular volume *(dehydration, GI losses, salt-wasting, third space losses—sepsis, nephrotic syndrome)*, septic shock (*vasodilation and volume redistribution*) and circulatory failure (*CCF, pericarditis, cardiac tamponade)*.

Intrinsic renal disease accounts for 25% of all renal failure. In most cases it is caused by acute tubular necrosis (caused by *ischemic-hypoxic injury, or drug and toxins)*. It may occur because of interstitial nephritis *(drug-induced, idiopathic)*, glomerulonephritis *(post-infectious, membrano-proliferative, Henoch schonlin purpura nephritis, nephritis of chronic infection, idiopathic rapidly progressive glomerulonephritis and other types)*, hemolytic uremic syndrome, vascular lesions (*renal artery/ vein thrombosis)*, acute hemolysis, rhabdomyolysis, tumour lysis syndrome, cortical necrosis, and infectious causes *(sepsis, pyelonephritis)*.

Obstructive uropathy accounts for 15-25% of all renal failure. It may occur because of obstruction in a solitary kidney or bilateral ureteric obstruction, urethral obstruction etc.

DIAGNOSTIC EVALUATION

Diagnostic evaluation should include obtaining the history of urinary output, fluid loss *(diarrhoea, vomiting)*, recent drugs , fever, previous UTIs, urinary symptoms, family history of renal problems. Commonly used drugs that can interstitial nephritis include aminoglycosides, amphotericin B, cephalosporins, penicillins, vancomycin, anti-epileptics, nonsteroidal analgesics, diuretics, ranitidine and acetazolamide. On examination after attention to airway and breathing (respiratory rate, work of breathing and color and oxygen saturation), circulation should be assessed carefully. This should include state of hydration (peripheral perfusion, edema), heart rate, blood pressure, signs of cardiac failure (gallop rhythm, palpable liver, raised JVP), rash, palpable kidneys or bladder. A low blood pressure implies shock. Remember to plot height and weight on growth chart.

Investigations

The important laboratory abnormalities that occur with acute renal failure include:

1. Raised urea and creatinine.
2. Hyperkalemia.
3. Metabolic acidosis.

All patients should have the following investigations:

- Urea, creatinine, electrolytes, Ca, PO_4, alkaline phosphatase, albumin, LFTs
- Urgent renal ultrasound scan (large bright kidneys suggest an acute process; small kidneys suggest CRF)
- Chest X-ray
- Urinalysis
- Complete blood count, blood culture and CRP
- Arterial blood gases
- Urate (disproportionably high urate suggests tumour lysis syndrome)

Other additional investigations are dictated by clinical presentation:

For suspected HUS:

- Peripheral blood smear, Platelet count, Stool culture

For acute nephritis:

- ESR, Complement (C_3, C_4, C_3 nephritic factor)
- Throat swab, ASOT, anti-DNAse B
- ANA, dsDNA, anti-GBM, ANCA.

Imaging: The role of imaging modalities is very limited.

Renal biopsy: A renal biopsy is indicated as soon as possible where renal function is deteriorating and the etiology is not certain.

Laboratory indices: Distinction between prerenal and intrinsic renal failure may be difficult (Table 15.1). Of various diagnostic indices proposed to distinguish pre-renal from established renal failure (acute tubular necrosis) measurement of fractional excretion of Na^+ (FE_{Na+}) is considered as most reliable discriminator, provided saline or furosemide has not already been administered. In pre-renal ARF values <1 are obtained whereas in acute tubular necrosis it is >1.

The fractional excretion of Na^+ (FE_{Na+}) is calculated as follows:

$$FE_{Na+} = (U_{Na}/Pl\ Cr_{Na}) + (U_{Cr}/Pl_{Cr}) \times 100$$

Where U_{Na} = urea sodium, Pl_{Na} = plasma sodium, U_{Cr} = urea creatinine, and Pl_{Cr} = plasma creatinine.

Table 15.1: Distinction between prerenal and intrinsic renal failure

Variable	*Prerenal*	*Intrinsic*
Specific gravity	>1.020	1.010
Urine [Na^+]	< 10mmol/L	>20 mmol/L
FE_{Na+}	< 1%	> 1%
Casts	Hyaline	Tubular epithelial cells and debris

A change in serum creatinine concentration and creatinine clearance has been used to classify patients with renal injury and renal failure. In renal injury creatinine is elevated 2 times above base line and creatinine clearance is decreased by 50%. In renal failure creatinine rises 3 times above base line (or acute rise of $\geq$ 0.5 mg/dL) and creatinine clearance is decreased $\geq$ 75%.

MANAGEMENT

The aim of treatment is to restore renal perfusion before intrinsic renal failure sets in by establishing adequate monitoring, aggressive fluid resuscitation, restoration of systolic blood pressure, avoidance of nephrotoxins and maintenance of adequate oxygenation.

Hypoxemia, hypotension and hypovolemia should be rapidly corrected. Under as well as overhydration must be avoided. Insensible losses are replaced with electrolyte-free dextrose solution and aspiration/drainage fluids and urine with 0.45% saline containing 1 mEq/kg of $NaHCO_3$. Appropriate modifications are made depending upon blood electrolyte values. The insensible losses are decreased with administration of humidified oxygen and increased with fever, tachypnea and use of overhead warmer. The child should be accurately weighed every 12 hours. Weight gain, appearance of edema and hyponatremia indicate fluid overload.

Correction of Hydration

Prerenal factors account for oliguria of short duration in most cases. Provided the child is not obviously over hydrated, he should be administered 20 ml/kg boluses of isotonic saline intravenously over a period of half an hour. That should restore renal perfusion and lead to increase in urine output (2-3 ml/kg/hour). If urine flow does not increase with correction of dehydration, IV infusion of furosemide 1-2 mg/kg/hour over 4 hours may be given. After carefully excluding congestive heart failure, the volume challenge can be repeated *once* using plasma or 5% albumin especially in children with nephrotic syndrome. If volume expansion fails, established ARF should be presumed and standard management of ARF instituted. Administration of "renal dose" of dopamine (1-2 μg/kg/min) that was widely used despite the fact that it did not influence the outcome of ARF, is no longer recommended

Intrinsic Renal Failure

Renal perfusion should be maintained to eliminate prerenal failure. Measures should be taken to exclude and treat obstructive renal failure. Once intrinsic renal failure is established, general measures include the following:

Fluid balance: Fluid intake should be restricted to 300 mL/m^2/day plus losses (nasogastric, drains, diarrhea, etc.) until renal replacement therapy has been instituted

Nutritional support: Adequate nutrition is of considerable importance and should be enteral if at all possible. Maintenance of nutrition becomes crucial if ARF extends beyond a week or so. Appropriate calories and proteins should be provided along with vitamins and micronutrients. Caloric requirements may be high in hypercatabolic patients (30-35 kcal/kg/day). Protein requirements are similarly high (1.5-2g/kg/day). Although protein intake should be restricted until renal replacement therapy is instituted. In an infected, hypercatabolic infant parenteral nutrition may be required.

Prevention of infection: All the infection control measures should be observed. All procedures must be done with strict aseptic precautions. Besides fever, tachycardia and rapid increase in blood urea levels suggest infection. Antibiotics should be judiciously used and their doses appropriately modified.

Treatment of Complications

Hyperkalemia: Treatment is required if ECG changes of hyperkalemia are present or K^+ is >6.5mmol/L. ECG changes include: peaked T waves, loss of P wave, broadened QRS complex, slurring of ST segment into T wave and sine wave leading to asystole.

Dangerous levels of raised serum K+ are urgently controlled with infusion of 10% calcium gluconate over 10 minutes with ECG monitoring. Calcium stabilizes membrane potential and antagonizes myocardial toxicity of potassium. IV infusion of sodium bicarbonate 2 mEq/kg over 10 minutes or insulin 0.1 unit/kg with dextrose 0.5 g/kg over 2 hours can subsequently be used. Both of these measures lead to a shift of K+ into cells, but the effect is short lived: peritoneal dialysis should be set up while these are being undertaken. Hyperkalemia is best controlled with dialysis.

Hyponatremia: Although hyponatremia is almost always dilutional reflecting excessive fluid administration, serum Na levels < 120 mEq/l may cause cerebral dysfunction and seizures. In such cases 3% hypertonic saline should be infused very slowly to raise the serum Na+ level to 125 mEq/l. The amount to be given is calculated as follows: 125 - actual serum level × 0.6 = mEq of Na to be administered. Divide that number by 2 (3% NaCl has 0.5 mEq Na/ml); it gives the amount of hypertonic saline *to be infused over 6-8 hours.*

Hypertension: Profound elevation of BP may be associated with nephritis and vasculitis. However, milder degrees of hypertension are due to hypervolemia. Hypertensive emergency may be treated with infusion of sodium nitroprusside with careful monitoring. Nifedipine 0.25-0.5 mg/kg or captopril 0.05- 0.2 mg/kg orally 3-4 times a day (often much smaller doses suffice) can be used to control hypertension.

Cause-specific Therapies

- Mannitol and $NaHCO_3$ in acute rhabdomyolysis.
- Imunosuppression in SLE.
- Plasmapheresis, fresh frozen plasma, and prostacyclin in the hemolytic uremic syndrome.
- Seroids in allergic interstitial nephritis.

Monitoring

Intake and urine output and body weight are accurately recorded. Blood electrolyte and acid base status are measured every 12-24 hours or more frequently if necessary. Careful physical examination should be done particularly to assess hydration and detect evidence of infection.

Dialysis

Indications for acute dialysis include:

- Fluid overload–leading to pulmonary edema, or severe hypertension
- Severe Acidosis (pH < 7.1)
- Hyperkalemia
- Uremia with signs of encephalopathy
- Toxins removable by dialysis

There is no absolute level of blood urea and creatinine at which therapy should be started, but it is often considered appropriate when blood urea reaches 300 mg/dL. Early dialysis might shorten the course of acute tubular necrosis; excessive dialysis might prolong the maintenance phase via complement activation and hypovolemia. Timely institution of peritoneal dialysis is essential to treat and prevent serious complications of ARF, particularly in oligo-anuric ARF. In non-oliguric ARF overhydration and hyperkalemia are relatively less problematic in the overall management.

Peritoneal dialysis in the child is not a difficult procedure. Appropriate sized dialysis catheters are available. Technical details of peritoneal dialysis can be found in the Procedure section.

With careful aseptic precautions and usual care the complication of peritonitis is rare. If prolonged dialysis is anticipated, a Tenckhoff catheter should be surgically placed. Besides the control of biochemical abnormalities, fluid removal by dialysis permits volume support needed for administration of the necessary medications and nutrition. Other modalities of renal replacement such as hemodialysis and hemofiltration require considerable expertise and equipment.

Drugs in renal failure: Dosage regimens of many drugs commonly used in the ICU need to be modified in renal failure to avoid accumulation and toxicity. For further information consult individual drug information sheet.

Continuous Arteriovenous Hemofiltration (CAVH)

CAVH with or without countercurrent dialysis (CAVH/D) involves diversion of blood flow through an extracorporeal circuit and filter cartridge, which produces a large volume of ultrafiltrate. Only a part of this ultrafiltrate is replaced with an electrolyte containing solution to achieve a negative fluid balance. The procedure is particularly useful in patients who are hemodynamically unstable to tolerate dialysis, and in those with pulmonary edema and multiple organ failure. It has been observed that children with pulmonary edema, remain hemodynamically stable at a ultrafiltration rate of 8-10 ml/kg/hour, tolerate net negative fluid balance of 1.9-5.4 ml/kg/hour, and show a dramatic improvement in oxygenation.

Chapter sixteen

Acute Liver Failure

Acute liver failure is characterized by severe injury to hepatocytes or massive necrosis. Loss of hepatocytes function sets in motion a multiorgan response, and death may occur even when the liver begun to recover.

DEFINITION

Clinically liver failure is defined as altered mental status (hepatic encephalopathy) and coagulopathy in the setting of an acute hepatic disease. It is called ***hyper acute*** if acute liver failure develops within 7 days of onset of illness, ***acute*** if within 8-28 days, and ***subacute*** if within 5-12 weeks. Patients with faster onset of encephalopathy tend to have a better prognosis.

Subfulminant or late onset hepatic failure implies development of hepatic encephalopathy after 26 weeks of onset of illness.

ETIOLOGY

A likely cause of acute liver failure can often be identified in infants with hepatic insufficiency whereas determinant tends to be elusive in the older child. Metabolic disorders like tyrosinemia, fructose intolerance, galactosemia and Zellweger syndrome must be considered when severe hepatic dysfunction appears in the late perinatal period. In most series, the foremost cause of acute liver failure in childhood and young adulthood is acute viral hepatitis with each of the five primary hepatotropic viruses (A through E) with the possible exception of Hepatitis C virus. Drugs are another common etiology for development of acute liver failure e.g. acetaminophen, isoniazid, sodium valproate, phenytoin, and halothane. Some commonly used drugs when used in combinations may cause synergistic toxicity by idiosyncrasy e.g. trimethoprim and sulfamethoxazole, rifampicin and isoniazid, amoxicillin and clauvalinic acid. Certain miscellaneous causes may also lead to acute liver failure in childhood and early adulthood like ischemia/hypotension, malignant infiltration by lymphoma or leukemia, Wilson disease, α-1 antitrypsin deficiency and Reye's syndrome. Chemical toxins like carbon tetrachloride, phosphorus and Amanita phalloides may also lead to acute liver failure.

PATHOGENESIS

Although the causative agent is frequently known a full understanding of the pathogenesis of acute liver failure eludes us. A shock like state and cerebral edema, shared by all forms of liver failure suggest a unified pathogenetic mechanism. Endotoxemia is common but it cannot explain these complex metabolic changes alone. Tumor necrosis factor $\alpha 1$, an endogenous mediator of septic shock is increased in some patients with acute liver failure whereas it is not so in others. Similarly prostaglandin metabolism is perturbed in some cases and PGE_2, thromboxane A_2 and prostacyclin have found to be increased in a mouse model of acute liver failure. A single pathogenetic mechanism is unlikely to explain all the abnormal events in this condition.

CLINICAL FEATURES AND LABORATORY FINDINGS

Usual presentation is with nonspecific symptoms such as malaise, anorexia and nausea, which is followed by appearance of jaundice and thereafter altered mental status and coma. Seizures may occur at any stage of encephalopathy. Agitated delirium is common in children and fetor hepaticus is often pronounced. Shrinkage of liver size is a distinctive clinical feature of viral hepatitis. Early development of ascites indicates a poor prognosis. Bleeding manifestations due to coagulopathy and altered mental status are the hallmarks of acute liver failure.

Laboratory abnormalities reveal hyperbilirubinemia, markedly raised aminotransferase (SGOT and SGPT) concentration, vitamin K resistant prolongation of prothrombin time, hypoglycemia, leukocytosis, thrombocytopenia and hyperammonemia. Low albumin and low blood urea nitrogen suggests underlying chronic liver pathology.

Coagulopathy

Severe changes in coagulation are typical of acute liver failure. Decreased levels of factors II, V, VII, IX and X are responsible for prolonged prothrombin and partial thromboplastin time. Factor VII has the shortest $T_{1/2}$ of -2 hrs. Hence it is the first factor to get depleted in severe hepatocellular dysfunction and also the first to recover with improved liver function. Measurements of prothrombin time and factor V levels are the most widely used tests to follow the patient's clinical condition. Disseminated intravascular coagulation with increased level of fibrin or fibrinogen degradation products and decreased levels of plasminogen activator, plasminogen and platelets may also occur. Thrombocytopenia with thrombaesthenia may both be a feature of acute liver failure.

Renal Functional Impairment

Acute liver failure may be complicated by prerenal azotemia, acute tubular necrosis and functional renal failure, also called hepatorenal syndrome. Prerenal azotemia occurs because of dehydration, hypovolemia and hypotension as well as increased intestinal nitrogen absorption when gastrointestinal bleeding occurs. Oliguric renal failure, which occurs in approximately half the patients with acute live failure, worsens the prognosis. Renal failure may also occur due to the direct toxic effect of etiological agents like acetaminophen or hydrocarbons.

Cardiovascular Changes

The circulatory changes, which occur in acute liver failure are hypotension, hypovolemia, decreased systemic vascular resistance with compensatory increase in cardiac output and increased interstitial edema.

Respiratory Dysfunction

Respiratory dysfunction may result from aspiration pneumonia/pneumonitis, CNS-driven hyperventilation, fluid overload (particularly if associated with acute renal failure), and acute lung injury resulting from sepsis or as part of the spectrum of systemic inflammation.

Metabolic Changes

Hypoglycemia occurs because of deficient hepatic gluconeogenesis and decreased metabolism of insulin by the liver causing increased peripheral insulin level. Pancreatic glucagon synthesis increases when hypoglycemia persists, resulting in a decrease of insulin/glucagon ratio, which accelerates muscle protein catabolism and release of amino acids, which the failing liver cannot utilize.

Hypokalemia results from respiratory alkalosis induced by raised intracranial pressure and resultant renal potassium excretion in place of hydrogen ions. This may further be aggravated by diuretic therapy.

Hyponatremia may result from hemodilution and impairment of sodium potassium pump. Hypophosphatemia may also be present.

Infections

Patients with acute liver failure are very prone to bacterial infections. Bacteremia is common in these patients as they are comatose, have numerous indwelling catheters, and receive H_2 receptor blockers, steroids or broad spectrum antibiotics. Most common organisms are *staphylococcus aureus,* gram negative bacilli and *streptococci*. In acute liver failure there is serum complement deficiency, multiple defects in neutrophils function and diminished serum opsonic activity. Disseminated fungemia in this condition is an ominous feature.

Encephalopathy and Cerebral Edema

Encephalopathy in acute liver failure is abrupt in onset and a prominent clinical feature of this condition. It progresses through 4 stages (Table 16.1). In stage I child is conscious but may have abnormal sleep pattern, confusion, altered mood or behavior. Asterix may be present and patient has difficulty in drawing line figures. EEG is normal at this stage. In stage II the child becomes disoriented and has abnormal behavior, fetor hepaticus may appear and EEG reveals generalized slowing. In stage III child becomes stuporous with brisk tendon reflexes, decrebrate posturing and has a markedly abnormal EEG. In stage IV patient becomes comatose and completely flaccid and areflexic and EEG may become isoelectric.

The pathophysiology of encephalopathy remains elusive. Currently it is thought that (1) it results from accumulation of toxic substances in brain because of impaired hepatic filtering e.g. ammonia, which is generated in the GI tract by the action of colonic bacteria and mucosal enzymes on endogenous and exogenous protein. (2) Impaired hepatic function alters the plasma aminoacid profile i.e. an increase in aromatic aminoacids and methionine and lowered branched chain aminoacid levels. This results in accumulation of false neurotransmitters and depletion of true neurotransmitters. (3) There are increased levels of neuroinhibitory substances such as gamma-aminobutyric acid or GABA in the brain tissue.

Table 16.1: Staging of hepatic encephalopathy

Grade 1:	Altered mood or behavior, sleep disturbances, irritability, normal EEG
Grade 2:	Drowsy, inappropriate behavior, minimal confusion, slowing on EEG
Grade 3:	Stuporous but speaking and obeying simple commands, inarticulate speech, marked confusion, marked abnormal EEG
Grade 4:	Coma, flaccid and areflexic.

Cerebral edema occurs in 75-80% of patients who progress to grade IV encephalopathy. The rapid increase in the water content of the brain results from a loss of cell membrane integrity and an alteration in the permeability of blood brain barrier. Patients with cerebral edema frequently have reflex systemic hypertension and bradycardia and increased muscle tones progressing to decerebrate rigidity and posturing with abnormal pupillary reflexes (usually dilation) and finally to brain stem respiratory patterns and apnea. The signs of raised intracranial pressure occur late and thus do not provide a reliable guide for therapeutic intervention.

MANAGEMENT

There is no specific therapy for AHF. Intensive care management of these patients is designed specifically to define and correct biochemical, cardiovascular, pulmonary, cerebral and renal complications of the condition. Cerebral edema is the most important cause of death in AHF, therefore major effort is directed at controlling the factors which affect intracranial pressure, and improve cerebral perfusion.

Immediate Care

- Establish peripheral IV lines
- Start maintenance fluids, Place Nasogastric tube for drainage/feeding, urinary catheter
- Establish central venous line (preferable)

- Initiate care of bowel, bladder, back, skin, eyes, input/output charting
- Transfer to ICU with frequent monitoring of vitals
- Identify cause if possible
- Look for potential complications and their management-look for and treat complications.

Respiratory Care

Respiratory dysfunction may result from aspiration pneumonia, pneumonitis, CNS driven hyperventilation, fluid overload, or acute lung injury secondary to SIRS or shock. Treatment consist of attention to airway, oxygen intubation and mechanical ventilation before protective airway reflexes are lost.

Fluid, Electrolytes and Metabolic Complications

Hypotension

N-saline or Ringer's lactate as per assessed losses should be given while avoiding overloading. Plasma or blood may be given depending on the need and availability. Vasopressors i.e. dopamine/noradrenaline are required to maintain blood pressure.

Child should be infused 60-80 ml/m^2/hr of intravenous fluids in the form of 10% dextrose for combating hypoglycemia.

Hyponatremia (Na+ < 125 mEq/L)

It may be due to SIADH and hemodilution. Fluid should be restricted to 65-75% of the maintenance and Na^+ infusion restricted to <2 mEq/kg body weight/day. Impaired free water excretion leading to hyponatremia should not be treated with excess sodium replacement as this may lead to ascites in the presence of renal sodium retention. Instead judicious fluid restriction according to central venous pressure monitoring should be achieved. Unfortunately colloids and blood products which are used frequently for combating hypotension and bleeding manifestations have a high sodium content.

Obvious cause of loss of sodium should be searched for before replacing sodium.

Hypernatremia (Na+> 150 mEq/L)

Hypernatremia may occur with lactulose administration, therefore reduce or stop lactulose, and give N/5 or N/6 fluids including correction fluids.

Hypokalemia

Hypokalemia occurs frequently. It should be prevented and potassium should be administered in the dose of 2-3 mEq/kg/day. Potassium can be supplemented as the phosphate salt in order to combat hypophosphatemia. Calcium and magnesium replacement may also be required.

Hypokalemia causing ECG changes should be treated with rapid KCI infusion 0.35-0.5 mEq/kg/hour till ECG is normal. It should be followed by maintenance KCl/100 ml IV fluid : 2 mEq if serum K^+ >3 mEq/L, 3 mEq if serum K^+ 2-3 mEq/L, 4 mEq if serum K^+ 1.5-2 mEq/L , 5 mEq if serum K^+ <1.5 mEq/L. (see Chapter 22).

Hyperkalemia

If there is hyperkalemia patient should be screened for possible causes viz. hepato-renal syndrome, hemolysis etc., intravenous potassium is stopped and other standard treatments given (for details see Chapter 22).

Metabolic Acidosis

It is most often due to hypovolemia. Correction of fluid deficit to ensure adequate intra-vascular volume is therefore, first step in the treatment. Albumin may be infused slowly to expand volume. $NaHCO_3$ infusion is advised only in presence of very severe acidosis i.e. blood pH < 7.00. The emphasis still remains on fluid replacement; $NaHCO_3$ may do more harm than good.

Metabolic Alkalosis

Increase KCl infusion till pH is <7.5, even if the serum potassium levels are within normal range.

Hypoglycemia (blood glucose< 60 mg/dl)

All IV fluids are prepared in 10% dextrose as a routine. If blood sugar goes below the hypoglycemia level, bolus of 25% dextrose solution (2 ml/kg body weight) is recommended.

Other Metabolic Complications

For Hypocalcaemia and Hypomagnesaemia (see Chapter 22).

Infections

High index of suspicion should be maintained. If fever, cough, etc. Common organism recovered are *Staphylococcus aureus, Esch.coli, Klebseilla sp.* Initial antibiotics therapy should therefore cover these organisms. The suggested empiric therapy should include Cloxacillin, and Amikacin. It may be modified according to microbiological reports and clinical response. If there is deterioration or no improvement in clinical condition antibiotics should be added/modified in a stepwise manner to cover for *Pseudomonas aeruginosa,* fungal sepsis, and anaerobic organism.

Coagulopathy/Bleeding

Upper and lower GI bleed

Objective should be to maintain the gastric pH> 5 by gastric wash with cold saline, H_2 receptor antagonist and antacids (0.5 ml/kg/dose after every gastric wash) (See Chapter 18).

Coagulation Defects

Objective should be to maintain prothrombin time < 18 seconds by using fresh frozen plasma, or fresh whole blood, and Vitamin K 5-10 mg/day for 3 days.

Disseminated Intravascular Coagulation and Platelet Disorders

Thrombocytopenia is treated with platelet concentrates, and fresh blood if there is bleeding.

Fresh frozen plasma or blood is used for DIC.

Cerebral Edema

Cerebral Edema is difficult to detect. Ideally ICP should be monitored. If raised ICP is suspected following measures should be instituted:

General Measures such as head in neutral position, head end raised to 30-45°, minimal handling of the patient should be strictly observed in all patients suspected of raised ICP. **Mannitol** (20%): 2-5 ml/kg body weight/dose: infused over 15 minutes at 4-6 hrly interval; maximum for 48 hours, should be used in patients with clear signs of raised ICP. There is no role for steroids. If ICP monitoring is possible cerebral perfusion pressure (CPP = MAP–ICP) should be maintained at about 60 mmHg.

Mechanical ventilation: Elective ventilation for short duration be undertaken after proper sedation and paralysis. $PaCO_2$ should be maintained between 30-35 mm Hg.

Encephalopathy

- Dietary protein intake is reduced to provide only 4-5% of total caloric need, preferably as vegetable proteins.
- *Bowel washes 6-8 hourly:* Acidify tap water with acetic acid or vinegar. (1 tsf/cup of water)
- *Lactulose:* Per oral/nasogastric/rectal catheter, 10-30 ml 4-6 hrly till > 2 loose stools per day (monitor hydration and watch for hypernatremia). There is no convincing proof of its efficacy though so far.

Avoid sedation especially benzodiazepines: if necessary, give short acting ones e.g. ketamine (1-2 mg/kg/dose).

- *Anticonvulsants:* Phenytoin 5-8 mg/kg/day may be given to all patients. Phenobarbitone may be used but no benzodiazepine.

Other Modalities

- Benzodiazepine antagonist e.g. flumezenil
- Extracorporeal liver support device
- Molecular Adsorbent Recirculating System (MARS)
- Charcoal perfusion
- Hemodialysis
- Liver transplantation.

Hepatorenal Syndrome

Definition: Oliguria which is unresponsive to fluid challenge, urinary $Na^+ < 10$ mEq/L in contrast to acute tubular necrosis with urinary Na+> 20 mEq/L, urinary creatinine: plasma creatinine ratio of> 30, urinary osmolality > 100 mosmols higher as compared to that of plasma.

In such patients water and Na+ intake should be restricted and be guided by the urine output. Hemodialysis/peritoneal dialysis may be needed. Role of low dose dopamine infusion (2-5 microgm/kg body weight/minute) is unproved.

Baseline Investigations

- Liver function tests: total and differential bilirubin levels, ALT/AST, alkaline PO_4ase, total protein, albumin: globulin ratio, prothrombin time
- Viral markers
- Blood counts, platelet counts, cultures (blood, urine), X-ray chest
- Serum electrolytes, sugar, urea, creatinine, blood gases, calcium and PO_4.

Monitoring the Progress of the Patient

A. Clinical Monitoring

- BP, pulse, respiration (hourly)
- Coma grade: once in a day
- Clinical indicators of cerebral edema: pupillary reaction, deep tendon reflexes, plantar reflex, abnormal posturing, neurogenic hyperventilation, bradycardia
- Clinical indicators of sepsis e.g. fever, leukocytosis, DIC.

B. Biochemical and Laboratory Monitoring

- Serum electrolytes: 4-12 hourly; reduce frequency after condition stabilizes
- Blood sugar: 2 hourly if hypoglycemia, thereafter with electrolytes
- Blood gases and acid base status (if available): with serum electrolytes
- Blood urea once daily; creatinine twice weekly; urinary electrolytes and creatinine if suspected to have hepato-renal syndrome
- Prothrombin time: monitor daily till it reaches < 18 seconds, Coagulation profile as required
- Liver function tests once in two days
- Serum calcium: baseline and thereafter if convulsions occur
- Repeat counts and cultures at every change of antibiotics
- Central venous pressure should be monitored and intra-arterial line should be inserted for blood pressure monitoring as well as sampling.

Outcome of Acute Liver Failure

Despite best efforts, the mortality of these children remains high. Mortality is particularly significant (> 70%) if following poor prognostic features are present: Prothrombin time > 40 seconds at admission, total bilirubin levels >10 mg/dl at admission, presence of sepsis, and infection due to hepatitis viruses other than HAV and HEV.

As there is no specific therapy for acute liver failure (except for toxin antidotes) *intensive supportive care is the key to management of such cases. Patients should be isolated unless it is absolutely known that the cause of the liver failure is non-infectious.*

Chapter seventeen

Severe Infections: Diagnosis and Antibiotics

A Pediatric Intensivist deals with diseases of infectious nature that may be cause or consequence of critical illness. All such patients with severe sepsis require admission to a critical care unit. For most part these disorders carry a high risk of mortality if unrecognized and untreated. These illnesses also tend to result in an unfavourable outcome even when specific antimicrobial therapy is appropriately administered.

DIAGNOSIS

The diagnosis of life-threatening infection is based on the suspicion of infection and the presence of characteristic clinical manifestations.

A. Predisposing Conditions

The presence of predisposing conditions should alert the physician to patients at higher risk of developing life threatening infections. These are neonates, immunocompromised patients, patients with malignancies, multiple trauma, sickle cell disease, splenectomy, or burns; patients receiving chemotherapy or corticosteroids, hepatic failure or malnutrition and patients with AIDS, and those undergoing invasive procedures.

B. Clinical Manifestations

The clinical manifestations may be subtle or flagrant and systemic or site-specific.

1. Systemic Signs and Symptoms

Fever is the most frequent systemic manifestation of infection. Hypothermia occasionally occurs, particularly in neonates. Other systemic manifestations include chills, rash (patechial or other kind) tachypnea, dyspnea, and nausea and vomiting. Hypotension may be initially present or develops, and results in signs of septic shock. Altered mental status is common and ranges from lethargy/ irritability to coma. Inactivity, poor cry, excessive sleepiness and lack of responsiveness could be only manifestation in very young babies.

2. Site-Specific Signs and Symptoms

- Infections of the central nervous system (CNS) may be associated with irritability bulging AF, altered mental status, headache, seizures, meningismus, or focal neurologic findings.
- Respiratory tract infections may result in dyspnea, tachypnea, cough, crepitations, rhonchi, or altered breath sounds.
- Intra-abdominal infection may cause abdominal pain, distension, nausea and/or vomiting, diarrhea and anorexia.
- Urinary tract infection may produce abdominal pain, tenderness, dysuria, hematuria, and oliguria.
- Life-threatening cutaneous infections may produce erythema, edema, abscess.

C. Laboratory Manifestations

Routine laboratory tests are not specific for making the diagnosis. WBC count is usually elevated with a shift to left. Malnourished children and young infants may have a normal WBC count or neutropenia. Toxic granulation of neutrophils may be noted. Thrombocytopenia is an early clue to the presence of infection.

At this stage it is worthwhile to know some definitions pertaining to sepsis and shock. A consensus committee of ACCP and SCCM in 1992 proposed more precise definitions using specific clinical characteristics and thresholds to define sepsis. Since then these definitions have been refined further and adapted for use in children. These are given in Table 17.1.

Table 17.1: Definition of terminology for sepsis and septic shock

Term	*Definition*
Infection	Infection is defined as invasion of normally sterile body sites by microbes or an inflammatory response to presence of microorganism in body
Bacteremia	Positive blood culture
Septicemia	Old term, no longer used
Systemic inflammatory response syndrome (SIRS)	**SIRS** is a response to variety of clinical insults including infection and is characterized by two or more of the following: • Tachypnea (respiration > age appropriate breaths/min or $PaCO_2$ <32 torr) • Tachycardia (heart rate > age appropriate beats/min.) • Hyperthermia or hypothermia: core or rectal temperature > 101°F (>38°C) or < 96.1°F (<35.5°C). • WBC > 12,000 cells/mm³ or <4000 cells/ mm³ or 10% band cells.
Sepsis	Clinical evidence of infection with • Tachypnea (respiration >age appropriate breaths/min) • Tachycardia (heart rate >age appropriate beats/min) • Hyperthermia or hypothermia (core or rectal) Temperature >101° F (>38°C) or <96.1 °F (<35.5°C)
Severe sepsis syndrome	Sepsis, plus evidence of altered organ perfusion (including one or more of the following): • Acute changes in mental status • $PaO_2/FiO_2 \leq 280$ (without other pulmonary or cardio-vascular disease as the cause) • Increased lactate (more than upper limits of normal for the laboratory) • Oliguria (documented urine output <0.5 mL/kg body weight for at least 1hr (in patients with bladder catheter in place)
Presence of the following in a child with sepsis	Hypotension OR Need for vasoactive drug to maintain BP above 5th centile range (dopamine >5 mcg/kg/min or dobutamine, epinephrine, or norepinephrine at any dose) OR Signs of hypoperfusion- any three of the following: decreased pulse volume (weak or absent dorsalis pedis pulse), capillary refilling time >3 sec, tachycardia (heart rate as defined in table -1), core (rectal/oral) to peripheral (Skin-toe) temperature gap >3°C, and urine output <1 mL/kg/hr (<20 mL/hr in >20 kg child). OR Sepsis and cardiovascular organ dysfunction as defined in Table 2.
Refractory or nonresponsive septic shock	Sepsis syndrome with hypotension that lasts for >1hr. that is not responsive to IV fluids (20 ml/kg of normal saline over 30 mins) or pharmacologic intervention (requiring vasopresors: e.g., dopamine >10 µg/kg/min).

SIRS can be caused due to tissue injury e.g. surgery, trauma etc., acute adrenal insufficiency, malignancy, or infection.

Septic Shock

Shock is a clinical syndrome that results from an acute circulatory dysfunction and consequent failure to deliver sufficient oxygen and other nutrients to meet the metabolic demands of tissue beds. Septic shock is defined as sepsis associated with hypotension [Systolic BP < 70 mmHg + (age × 2) or fall in mean arterial pressure by >10 mmHg from base line] and perfusion abnormalities (such as oliguria, altered mental status, lactic acidosis and increased CFT).

Refractory or Non-responsive Septic Shock

Sepsis with hypotension that lasts for >1 hour, not responsive to fluids (20 ml./hour or N.Saline over 30 min.) or pharmacologic intervention (requiring vasopressors: e.g., dopamine> 10 µg/kg/minute).

SIRS, Sepsis, severe sepsis and septic shock represent a continuum of clinical and pathological severity. The process begins with infection with or without SIRS, may progress to systemic response with severe sepsis or septic shock. There is a stepwise increase in mortality from SIRS to septic shock.

Management:

Approach to Life Threatening infections

Treatment of a life threatening process of the disease must take precedence over specific therapy aimed at the underlying illness. Although early administration of disease directed therapy (antibiotics) may prevent development of shock or respiratory failure, but the job of early recognition of shock and respiratory failure and initial intervention is one of the first priority.

Once airway breathing and circulation has been established a quick examination must be performed and highlights of patient history should be obtained. This would enable the physician to make a presumptive diagnosis and choose reasonable antimicrobial agent if an infection is suspected.

Based on the information gathered in this limited fashion, broad categories of infection can be considered and a wide spectrum antimicrobial coverage should be provided (Table 17.2 and 17.5). Over next several hours, further history is elucidated and the efforts are made to identify the pathogen by various techniques. The objectives of antibiotic therapy are shown in Table 17.3.

Choice of Antibiotics (Criteria)

1. *Age of the patient*
   The particular susceptibilities of a neonate differ from that of an older infant, child and adolescent, a pediatric intensivist must be familiar with each group and their idiosyncrasies, for example:
   a. A neonate has immature B cell system, which results in inadequate levels of specific IgG to protect against gram negative organisms or to provide opsonization of group B *streptococcus*.
   b. Organisms that require production of specific subclasses of immunoglobulins may be encountered repeatedly by the infants and young children until the ability to produce specific immunoglobulin has been developed. This is true for *Haemophilus influenza type b*, which is the most frequent cause of bacterial meningitis in this age group.
2. Coexistence of any premorbid condition leading to impaired immune response. For example leukemia, burns, cystic fibrosis (*pseudomonas and staphylococcus*), Diabetes (anaerobes and *staphylococcus*), HIV (*Pneumocystis carinii,* Candida).
3. Whether infection is community acquired or hospital acquired. For example surgical patient shifted to PICU after surgery going into septic shock may have a hospital acquired infection, which is caused by pathogens with complex anti-microbial resistance and requires different

Table 17.2: Important characteristics of antibiotics commonly used in critically ill patients

Aminoglycosides (Gentamicin, Netilemicin, Amikacin, Isepamicin)
- Drug of choice for gram negative infection
- Do not cross blood-brain barrier; excreted unchanged by kidney.
- Toxic: nephrotoxic-5-20% after 1 week, needs drug level monitoring and dose adjustment if renal failure
- After empiric use-review after 2-3 days, stop if culture negative or other drugs as effective
- Maintain good vascular volume, limit diuretic use
- Peak concentration dependent bactericidal effect: good in single daily dose.

Quinolones (Ciprofloxacin, ofloxacin, Levofloxacin, Gatiflox, Trovoflox)
- Activity against gram negatives including *P. aeruginosa*
- Oral use- 100% bioavailability, very good concentration in respiratory tract
- Long half life, does not cross BBB
- Useful in gram negatives nosocomial infections incldluing *P. aeruginosa*, resistant *S. typhi, S. paratyphi, shigella, V. cholera*
- Newer generation also active against M. pneumoniae and C. pneumoniae

The B-Lactams (Pencillins, Cephalosporins, Carbapenems and Monobactams).
All have B-lactam ring with variable rings and side chains are one bactericidal.

Third generation Cephalosporins (Cefotaxime, Ceftriaxone, Ceftazoxime, Ceftazidime for IV use and Cefixime, Cefrodoxime for oral use)
- Superior gram negative coverage; also gram positive cover including *staphylococcus (but less than first generation)*
- Ceftriaxone-prolonged half life, may be used in once a day regimen
- Oral Cefixime-once a day, 50% bioavailability, best gram positive cover
- Cefrodoxime-also active against *staphylococcus aureus*
- Useful: in suspected/proven serious gram positive infections if aminoglycoside ineffective/resistance e.g. in CNS infections.
- Best reserved for LRTI

Fourth generation Cephalosporins (Cefepime and Cefpirome)
- Broad coverage-*Enterobacteriacae*, other gram negatives *H. influenzae, N. meningitidis, N. gonorrhoeae, Pseudomonas*, Acinetobacter (better than Ceftazidime)
- Cefpirome-active against gram positive, *S. aureus; against pneumococcus* comparable to cefotaxime
- Diffuses more rapidly into bacteria, low inducer of beta-lactamases
- Reserve for hospital acquired infections, immuno-compromised host and highly resistant gram negative infections

Carbapenems (Imipenem, Meropenem Ertapenam)
- Broadest spectrum among all available antibiotics: against gram positive, including vancomycin resistant *Enterococcus* and *S. aureus;* against gram negative, including anaerobes, *Pseudomonas* aeruginosa
- Resistant to B-lactamases; emergence of carbopenemase producing bacteria is reported.
- Imipenem—neurotoxic, may cause seizures in children
- Meropenem—distributed in most tissues and fluids

Glycopeptides: (Vancomycin, Daptomycin)
- Activity against all Gram positive cocci: MRSA, *CONS, Cl.difficle*
- Crosses inflamed meninges, excreted unchanged through kidney
- Useful in compromised host, nosocomial infections, methicillin resistant *Staph. aureus* (MRSA), and high penicillin resistant pneumococci
- Useful as a single agent in all infections resistant to standard antibiotics, nosocomial pneumonia, UTI, sepsis, polymicrobial infections etc.
- Ototoxic in 2% nephrotoxic in 5%, phlebitis and sclerosis occur in 10-15%, with purified preparation; can cause Red man Syndrome

Contd.

Contd.

- Daptomycin works on vancomycin resistant enterococci.
- Drug level monitoring essential if renal failure
- Simultaneous use of aminoglycoside is to be avoided

Teicoplanin

- A glycopeptide, active against both aerobic and anaerobic gram positive bacteria
- Therapeutic indications are – severe enterococcal infections, neutropenic sepsis, infective endocarditis, severe LRI with presumed gram positive bacteria.
- Dosage : Children – 10 mg/kg 12 hrly for first 3 doses then 10 mg/kg once daily, neonates – 16 mg/kg Ist day then 8 mg/kg once daily.

Oxazolidinone (Linezolid)

- Acts against gram positive bacteria – *S. aureus, other staph, streptococci, entercocci*, as effective as Vancomycin against MRSA, MRCONS.
- May need fewer days of IV therapy, oral preparation available
- Indications are – clinically significant infections due to vancomycin-resistant *Enterococcus faecium* nosocomial and MRSA skin and soft tissue infections.
- Dosage: 7.5 mg/kg 8 hr × 10-14 days

Monobactams (Atreonam)

- Active against most aerobic gram negative bacilli including *P. aeruginosa*. Primarily used as alternative to aminoglycoside, as a combination therapy for mixed aerobic and anaerobic infections —UTI, lower resp infections.
- Can be given IV, IM, 8 hourly
- No nephrotoxicity, coagulopathy.

Table 17.3: Objectives of antibiotic therapy in ICU

- Eradication of bacteria
- Clinical cure
- Prevention of relapse
- Prevention of early and late complications, sequelae and mortality
- Minimizing risks of super infection
- Minimizing emergence of resistant organisms

set of anti-microbials.

4. *What is the site of primary infection*
   For example meninges (*S. pneumoniae, N.meningitides and H. influenza*), endocardium (aerobic gram positive cocci, *S. aureus, S.viridans*) urinary tract and biliary tree (enteric aerobic gram negative bacilli).
5. Local patterns of antibiotics resistance by common infecting organism.
6. *Understanding of pharmacology of the antimicrobials.*

Bactericidal drugs are required for meningitis because the complement levels are decreased and there is lack of surface phagocytosis. In Endocarditis vegetations are impermeable to white cells so a bactericidal drug should be used for such infections. Bacteriostatic drugs are usually adequate if host defenses are intact. General principles of antibiotic threapy in PICU are shown in Table 17.4.

Table 17.4: General principles of antibiotic therapy in ICU

- *Dose:* depends on intensity of infection, patient's weight, renal functions
- *Route:* initially always IV, but IV seldom needed for > 14 days
- *Duration:* must be long enough to eradicate the infection but not too long
- *Culture:* must always be obtained from site of infection, and blood
- *Reassess:* 48-72 hours later, for clinical improvement and culture
  If no improvement–think of possibilities that antibiotic is not reaching the site of infection, is not appropriate for infection, or it is not a bacterial infection
- After culture report/stabilization-Streamline

Table17.5: Antiviral Agents and Antifungal Agents commonly used in PICU

Antiviral Agents

- **Acyclovir**
  - Active against herpes simplex types 1 and 2, varicella zoster and, in high doses, Epstein-Barr virus.
  - Drug of choice in treatment of herpes encephalitis, and disseminated herpes and zoster infections in the immunocompromised patient.
  - Parenteral dose: 5-10 mg/kg every 8 hours.
- **Ganciclovir**
  - Used in treatment of live-threatening cytomegalovirus infections
  - Causes anemia and neutropenia
  - Parenteral dose: 5mg/kg every 12 hours

Antifungal Agents

- **Amphotericin-B**
  - Drug of choice in systemic fungal infections, but high risk of hypersensitivity and nephrotoxicity
  - Lipid preparations (lipid complex) - less toxic, but expensive; improves the therapeutic index of amphotericin by facilitating the ability to administer higher doses of the drug. useful in patients with renal insufficiency,or who are intolerant or refractory to conventional amphotericin B, manifested by development of renal dysfunction (serum creatinine >2.5mg/dL) during antifungal therapy; or severe or persistent infusion-related adverse events.
  - Dose- 1 mg test dose, followed by 250mcg/kg daily, gradually increasing to a maximum of 1.5 mg/kg per day in severe infections.
- **Azoles**
  - **Fluconazole** is less toxic alternative to amphotericin in treatment of Aspergillus and some Candida infections. Dose: 12mg/kg initially, followed by 6-12 mg/kg daily.
  - **Itraconazole** is an oral agent with a broad spectrum of activity against several fungal strains, including *Candida, Histoplasma, Blastomyces,* and *Aspergillus.*
  - **Voriconazole** is treatment of choice for invasive aspergillosis; has broad spectrum of activity against *Candida spp., Cryptococcus neoformans, Aspergillus* spp., *Blastomyces,* and *histoplasma.* Voriconazole's anticandidal activity includes fluconazole-resistant strains of *C. krusei* and *C. glabrata.* The drug has a high oral bioavailability and is extensive distributed throughout the body including the CNS
- **Flucytosine**
  - Active in systemic Candida and cryptococcal infections, used in combination with amphotericin to prevent resistance.
  - Parenteral dose: 50mg/kg every 6 hours.
- **Echinocandins (Caspofungin)**
  - Rapidly fungicidal against Candida spp. including species resistant to the azoles. Approved and used for the treatment of invasive aspergillosis
  - Not active against *C. neoformans.*
  - $T^{1/2}$ of 10 to 12 hours, allowing once-daily dosing,
  - Must be administered parenterally.

- Broad spectrum empiric regimen to narrow spectrum, single antibiotic
- Intravenous to oral

Empiric Initial Antimicrobials

Following is a broad guideline for initial antibiotic therapy, individual situation may vary:

1. *Sepsis in neonate < 7 days:* Focus is not relevant

   Common organisms are *Klebsiella sp., E. coli, Staph. aureus, Staph epidermidis,* less commonly *Pseudomonas* and *Candida sp.* Gentamicin–5 mg/kg/dose at 24 hours interval, Or Amikacin–15 mg/kg daily *plus* or Cefotaxime–100 mg/kg/day divided 12 hourly.

2. *Sepsis in neonate who are > 7 days:*

   A. No focus, respiratory infection or CNS focus:

Table17.6: Choice of empirical antibiotic in patients with shock with respect to clinical settings

Clinical Setting	Usual Pathogens	Preferred Therapy	Alternate Therapy
Unknown source, community acquired	*Salmonella typhi/paratyphi* *S. pneumoniae* *H. influenzae* ***Enterobacteriaceae*** ***B. fragilis*** ***E. fecalis*** **Think of malaria & dengue**	Ceftriaxone plus Metronidazole OR Meropenem OR Imipenem	Quinolone (Cipro/Levo) *plus* either Metronidazole OR Clindamycin
Lung source	*S. pneumoniae* *H. influenzae* *Staphylococcus aureus* *M pneumoniae*	Ceftriaxone/ cefotaxime/ amox-clav and azithro/ clarithro	Substitute new fluoroquinolone (levo/gati/moxi) for macrolide
IV line sepsis	*S.epidermidis* *S. aureus (MSSA)* *Klebsiella* **Enterobacter** *Serratia*	Vancomycin PLUS Meropenem OR Imipenam OR Cefepime OR Piperacillin-Tazobactum	May substitute linezolid for vancomycin Add antifungals if fungus suspected
Urosepsis	*Enterobacteriacae*	Ceftriaxone OR Cefotaxime OR Quinolone	Aztreonam OR Ampicillin + Amikacin
Meningitis	*S. pneumoniae* *H. influenzae* meningococci	Ceftriaxone	Add vancomycin if drug resistant pneumococci suspected
Intrabdominal source	*Enterobacteriacae* ***B fragilis*** *Enterococci*	Ceftriaxone plus Metronidazole OR Piperacillin+ tazobactum OR Meropenem OR Imipenem	Quinolone (Cipro/Levo) *plus* either Metroindazole OR Clindamycin

Ampicillin–200 mg/kg/day divided 8-12 hourly and

Gentamicin–2.5 mg/kg/dose given 8-18 hourly

Or

Ceftriaxone–100 mg/kg as loading dose then 100 mg/kg/day divided 12 hrly or Cefotaxime 100 mg/kg/day divided 12 hrly.

B. No focus, CNS or respiratory infection in a baby with central line

Add Vancomycin to above, 10-15 mg/kg dose at 8-12 hrs. interval

C. Neonate as above and with an endotracheal tube and suspected NNEC Consider Ticarcillin/clavulanate–300 mg/kg/day, 8 hourly and

Metronidazole–15 mg/kg loading dose then 7.5 mg/kg/dose at 8 hourly interval

Or

Clindamycin–15 – 20 mg/kg/day, divided, at 6-8 hourly interval.

3. *Community aquired severe sepsis in previously healthy children > 2 months, H. influenza, Streptococcus pneumoniae, N. meningitides and Staph aureus, β hemolytic streptococcus* are the commonest organisms in this age group as cause of sepsis without focus, pneumonia, meningitis, CNS infection, and skin and soft tissue infections.

A. No focus or respiratory infection. Ampicillin and Gentamicin 5-7.5 mg/kg/day or Ceftriaxone: 100 mg/kg. loading, then 100 mg/kg/day in 12 hourly divided doses.

B. *Focus CNS—Meningitis:* Ceftriaxone. Start immediately without waiting for lumber puncture result, continue further after confirmation.

C. *Gastrointestinal Focus:* Add metronidazole to above regime–15 mg/kg load then 7.5 mg/kg/dose at 6 hourly interval. If resistant organisms are suspected imipenam or piperacillin/tazobactam plus aminoglycoside.

D. *UTI:* Cefotaxime, ceftriaxone or quinolones.

E. *Cellulitis:* Cloxacillin + penicillin G. If MRSA suspected–Vancomycin.

4. *Sepsis in previously ill children:*

A. No focus, in an immuno-compromised host: Ceftazidime–150 mg/kg/day–at 8 hourly interval and amikacin–15 mg/kg/day.

B. No focus in immuno compromised child with central line:

Above regime + add cloxacillin or vancomycin.

Encephalitis: Many viral agents can cause encephalitis, but only herpes simplex encephalitis is amenable to therapy. If herpes encephalitis is suspected, a 14 to 21-day course or acyclovir should be promptly initiated.

Brain Abscess: Brain abscesses are rare but should be suspected in patients with chronic suppurative otitis or congenital cyanotic heart disease and in patients with suppressed immune systems such as in AIDS. Infections are often polymicrobial and etiologic organisms include aerobic and anaerobic *streptococci*, Gram-negative bacteria and *staphylococci*. A recommended initial choice of antibiotics includes cloxacillin, amikacin and penicillin or metronidazole, cephalosporins. Vancomycin can be substituted for cloxacillin.

Pneumonia–Immunocompromised patients: Besides the usual antibiotics recommended for community acquired pneumonia, immunocompromised patients, especially patients with AIDS, with radiographic evidence of interstitial pneumonia or a normal chest radiograph should receive trimethoprim/sulfamethoxazole in appropriate doses or pentamidine for possible *Pneumocystis carinii* infection. Consider the addition of steroids in *P. carinii* pneumonia associated with significant hypoxemia. If fungal organisms are considered, amphotericin B should be initiated. Tuberculosis should also be considered.

Nosocomial Infections and Ventilator–Associated Pneumonia: Gram-negative organisms (*Klebsiella pneumonia, E. coli, P. aeruginosa, enterobactor species*) are frequent causes of nosocomial infections and pneumonia. *Staphylococcus* is also common, enterococci is getting frequent. An aminoglycoside plus a third-generation cephalosporin with beta lactamase inhibitor or imipenam should be used.

If *pseudomonas* is strongly suspected in those with neutropenia or cystic fibrosis, two anti-pseudomonal antibiotics (Ceftazidime, aminoglycoside, fluoroquinolones, piperacillin-tazobactam imipenem/meropenem) should be instituted. Vancomycin should be considered if a sputum gram stain suggests gram-positive *staphylococci.*

Intravascular Catheters

In patients with known or suspected intravascular infection and systemic infections complications related to indwelling catheters, the catheter should be promptly removed. Vancomycin is recommended in the immunocompromised patient with coagulase-negative *Staphylococcus* line infection or the patient with systemic manifestations. If *S.aureus* is the infecting organism, then cloxacillin or equivalent is recommended unless there is a high rate of methicillin-resistant *S. aureus* (MRSA) in the hospital or MRSA is confirmed, in which case vancomycin should be used.

Immunocompromised or Neutropenic Patient

If no focus–combination therapy is recommended in severely ill patients.

- Third-or fourth-generation cephalosporins or Ceftazidime 150 mg/kg/day or cefoperazone + aminoglycoside (Amikacin or Gentamicin)
- Imipenam or
- Ticarcillin-clavulanate, (300 mg/kg at 4-6 hourly interval)
- Piperacillin-tazobactam
- Add Vancomycin if central line Gram positive organisms are likely.

If fungal infection is suspected: Fluconazole in less severely ill and Amphotericin B in severely ill.

Patient with Renal Failure

Avoid/modify—aminoglycoside, vancomycin. Relatively safe—Quinolones, ceftriaxone, cefoperazone.

Patient with Liver Failure

- Avoid—Cefalosporins
- Realtively safe—Quinolones and aminoglycoside.

Chapter eighteen

Gastrointestinal Mucosal Damage and Upper GI Bleed

A majority of critically ill patients having respiratory failure, coagulopathy, hypotension, sepsis, hepatic failure, renal failure and glucocorticoid therapy may develop stress-related mucosal damage. Clinically-relevant bleeding causing hemetemesis and/or malena, hypotension, tachycardia, or anemia may occur. Patients who develop stress-related mucosal damage, endoscopic signs of bleeding or clinically important bleeding have a higher risk of death. Upper GI bleed (stomach, esophagus or small intestine) is more frequently seen then lower GI haemorrhage. The incidence of upper GI bleed in PICUs has been estimated at 25%.

MECHANISMS

Decreased blood flow, mucosal ischemia, hypoperfusion and reperfusion injury all lead to splanchnic ischemia. As a consequence the mucous layer that protects the mucosal surface epithelium from hydrogen ions may be compromised. Acid-pepsin attacks the mucosa of the upper GI tract, leading to peptic erosions or ulcerations and the risk of hemorrhage.

In the lower GI tract through disrupted intestinal mucosa gut bacteria or their toxins cross into the portal circulation and then systemically. Such leakage, called as 'bacterial translocation' fuels the inflammatory processes of systemic inflammation and multiple organ dysfunction syndrome.

PREDISPOSING FACTORS

1. Previous history of ulcer or liver disease
2. Use of Nonsteroidal anti-inflammatory drugs, Anticoagulants
3. Multiple trauma, Burns > 30%
4. Head injury, Spinal cord injury CNS infections
5. Hypotension
6. Severe Sepsis
7. Adult respiratory distress syndrome (ARDS).
8. Mechanical ventilation > 48 hours.

ENDOSCOPY

Endoscopy may be used to reveal the site of upper GI bleeding, the degree of ulceration, and the amount of tissue injury, or to control bleeding, sigmoidoscopy or colonoscopy may reveal the site of lower GI bleeding.

LABORATORY STUDIES

1. Decreased hematocrit (Hct) may reflect blood loss.
2. Hypovolemia and hyponatremia may be present because of nasogastric suction.
3. WBC count may be elevated, usually return to normal 24 to 48 hours after bleed stops.
4. Blood urea may be elevated related to the absorption of blood from the GI tract or hyporolemia.
5. Prolonged clotting times may be related to coagulation disorder.

MANAGEMENT

1. General Approach

In any patient with GI bleed first step is assessment of vital signs: airway, breathing, circulation (heart rate), and documentation of blood loss, Quantitation of the amount of blood lost is needed to assess the severity of bleed. Next step is to determine site of bleed i.e. Gastrointestinal vs extragastrointestnal. A bloody NG aspirate confirms an upper GI source. If bile is present in a non bloody NG lavage, an upper GI bleed is unlikely on acute surgical conditions should be ruled out, as also trauma, drugs, toxins, and foreign body, Signs of systemic disease such as fever, splenomegaly, vascular malformation should be looked for. Patients should be investigated for coagulopathy or bleeding diathesis, particularly if petechiae, ecchymosis and bleeding from puncture sites are seen.

2. Acid suppression

Acid suppression may be achieved by various means. These include direct acid neutralization such as antacids, blockade of stimulation of parietal cell along the cascade by histamine and gastrin, blockade of cholinergic pathways and blockade of the acid-producing proton pump at the parietal cell.

There are two major forms for acid suppression

a. *H_2 blockers* (e.g., ranitidine) block the pathways mediated by histamine. They may reduce the risk of stress-related mucosal ulceration, but they do not treat clinically-important bleeding. H_2 receptor antagonists are able to elevate pH > 4.0 only. This level of acid suppression appears to be insufficient to control or prevent rebleeding episodes. A pH > 6.0 may be necessary to maintain clotting in patients at risk of rebleeding. Furthermore, tachyphylaxis appears to develop to continuous IV infusion within 72 hours.

   Continuous infusion of H_2 blockers is the most effective method of maintaining gastric acid inhibition, intermittent dosing is currently the favored regimen for stress ulcer prophylaxis.

b. *Proton pump inhibitors (PPIs)* block histamine-2, gastrin and cholinergic mediated sources and are currently the agents of first choice. This class of drugs are weak bases that, when activated, bind to the proton pump and inhibit its ability to produce gastric acid. For intravenous use, omeprazole and pantoprazole are available. The ease of use, reliability of elevation of gastric pH, and absence of clinically significant drug interaction make pantoprazole an attractive therapy in settings, such as acute upper gastrointestinal hemorrhage, high risk stress ulcer patients, and patients who cannot tolerate an oral PPI. Oral preparation of pantoprazole appears to carry the same level of suppression.

   Alkalinization of gastric pH, may lead to increased bacterial colonization of gastric mucosa, and has been linked with increased risk of nosocomial pneumonia in ventilated patients.

Table 18.1: Commonly used drugs for gastric acid suppression/mucosal protection

H_2 Blockers	
Cimetidine	PGE analogue
Ranitidine (1-2 mg/kg/dose)	Misoprostol
Proton Pump Inhibitors	Sucralfate
Omeprazole	
Pantoprazole	

3. Sucralfate

A complex of aluminium hydroxide and sulfated sucrose, is thought to act by protecting the gastric mucosa from acid-pepsin attack. *It requires an acid environment to act, and should not therefore be combined with H_2 blockade or PPIs.* Gastric acidity is maintained, which may help to protect against nosocomial pneumonia. It is given in dose of 1-2 g, (40-80 mg/kg/ 24 hours) by nasogastric tube 4-6 hourly.

Sucrafate is effective in reducing overt bleeding from gastric erosions in critically ill patients.

Sucralfate can bind to a number of drugs and reduce their absorption; drugs relevant to pediatric patients are as follows.

1. Diagoxin
2. Fluoroquinolones
3. Phenytoin
4. Ranitidine
5. Theophylline
6. Warfarin

These drugs should be given at least 2 hours before surcralfate.

It has an added advantage of decreasing the risk of nosocomial pneumonia. Rantidine is superior to sucralfate for the prevention of bleeding from gastric erosions, while sucralfate is superior to ranitidine for the prevention of pneumonia.

Given the effectiveness of other prophylactic measures, the use of PPIs for stress ulcer prophylaxis seems unnecessary. Furthermore, the potency of PPIs in raising gastric pH will create greater risks from bacterial overgrowth in the bowel than the H_2 blockers.

4. Enteral Nutrition

Enteral nutrition combats stress ulceration and helps maintain intestinal mucosal integrity. A daily rest period allows gastric acidity to be restored. Many believe that patients on full enternal feeding regimens require no other prophylaxis.

5. Maintenance of Splanchnic Oxygenation

a. **Standard support to circulation and respiration** is believed to contribute to the preservation of mucosal perfusion.
b. Splanchnic vasodilators such as dopamine (2-5 μg/kg/min) may improve splanchnic perfusion and so help preserve mucosal integrity; however, dopamine may interfere with enteral nutrition by slowing gastric emptying

6. Other Measures

Other measures include antacids (Aluminium or Magnesium salts, 0.5 ml/kg/dose 6 hourly), and prostaglandin E_1 analogues. Generally, these are less effective than the therapies above.

Choosing Whom to Treat

In the setting of the ICU two groups of patients warrant acid suppression, those with high risk of GI bleeding and those having upper GI bleed to prevent rebleed. Patients at high risk of gastrointestinal bleeding–stress ulcers are those with raised intracranial pressure, coagulopathy, shock, burns, and those who require mechanical ventilation. The risk increases 16-fold in patients undergoing mechanical ventilation and 4 fold with coagulopathy.

Chapter nineteen

The Metabolic and Nutritional Response to Critical Illness and Nutritional Management

The nutritional support is an important issue in the management of critically ill patients. Integrity and functioning of most of the cells of the body depend on continuous delivery of the nutrients. Early nutritional depletion is common in ICU patients. This has a deleterious effect on immunocompetence, wound healing, and recovery from infections. In addition, malnutrition decreases muscle-mass and strength of respiratory muscles especially diaphragm, which impairs the ability to wean from a ventilator.

Nutritional needs of critically ill children are higher than normal because of catabolic stress (resulting from infections, trauma and other disease states), and metabolic needs of reparative processes and growth. The goal of nutrition supplementation therefore is to minimize nitrogen (protein) wasting and provide adequate nonprotein substrate.

All nutritional intervention must be based on a thorough understanding of metabolic and nutritional alteration in critically ill. Sepsis causes much the same metabolic disturbance as trauma or injury but the response seems to be exacerbated, is more variable and more difficult to counteract.

THE METABOLIC AND NUTRITIONAL RESPONSE TO CRITICAL ILLNESS

Changes that occur may be driven by any/all of the following:

- Lack of nutrient intake (starvation)
- Physiologic insult to the gastrointestinal tract
- The endocrine/mediator response to the "stress" of critical illness.

Metabolic Effects of Starvation and Hypercatabolic Response to Critical Illness

The initial response to starvation is glycogenolysis. Glycogen stores, become exhausted within 2-3 days and structural body proteins are broken down for gluconeogenesis. Process is slowed by:

1. An adaptive process and tissues metabolize ketones.
2. A significant reduction in basal metabolic rate.
3. Energy production by oxidation of lipid stores. When the lipid stores are almost depleted protein breakdown and gluconeogenesis again become significant.

The hypercatabolic response that accompanies critical illness is characterized by increased basal metabolic rate, caloric requirements, increased secretion of 'stress' hormones (catecholamines, cortisol etc.) and impaired capacity to use carbohydrate and fat as energy source, resulting in an increased protein breakdown as alternative energy source, and massive nitrogen losses from the breakdown of muscle protein. The catabolic state does not get reversed by resumption of adequate nutrition.

Physiologic Insult to the Gastrointestinal Tract

Decreased gut perfusion and oxygenation occur frequently with critical illness and may persist. Even short period of circulatory compromise may result in prolonged gut ischemia/hypoxia, causing cell injury, necrosis and loss of mucosal integrity and barrier function especially if this is combined with a prolonged lack of nutrients in the gut lumen. Translocation of bacteria/endotoxin may increase with resultant endotoxinemia and increased intestinal permeability.

Endocrine Responses

The early response is stimulation of the hypothalamic-pituitary-adrenal (HPA) axis, increased prolactin and growth hormone (GH) levels and often a reduction in thyroid hormone secretion in protracted critical illness. In protracted critical illness there is suppression of anterior pituitary hormone secretion. Pulsatile release of GH, prolactin and TSH is markedly reduced, predominantly in amplitude, whereas the frequency of secretory pulses is maintained. Cortisol levels however, remain high.

Adrenal Glucocorticoids

In critical illness, plasma cortisol levels are usually increased but exhibit loss of the normal circadian rhythm. However, adrenal insufficiency during critical illness is being described, with increasing frequency, particularly in association with systemic sepsis with shock. This probability should be considered in patients with sepsis/septic shock with increasing inotropic requirements despite adequate antimicrobial therapy and the absence of convincing evidence of ongoing or worsening infection. Important of adequate cortisol levels in critical illness is clear.

Growth Hormone

Growth hormone increases plasma glucose levels and facilitates protein sparing, lipolysis, immunocompetence and sodium and water retention. During stress or illness, baseline GH is often elevated and diurnal variation reduced. However, continuing stress, as typified by critical illness, may be associated with reduced GH and IGF-I and therefore an attenuation of anabolic processes. Administration of high dose GH (5-10 times standard replacement dosage) has been shown to improve nitrogen balance in patients with burns after trauma early sepsis and in postoperative surgical patients, but worsen the mortality.

Leptins

Leptin stimulates energy release from fat by oxidation of fatty acids and can be considered as stress-related hormone. It suppresses adrenal synthetic activity and may be responsible, in part, for the functional adrenocortical insufficiency sometimes seen in sepsis.

MEETING NUTRITIONAL NEEDS

Energy

Estimates of resting energy expenditure (REE) by standard formulas are difficult to extrapolate to intensive care setting in which metabolic rates fluctuate according to patient's condition. Total energy expenditure is generally 1.2-1.5 times higher than REE in most critically ill patients. Thus, energy requirements are increased. Hypocaloric, hyperproteic regimens are superior to those that provide excess calories. Hypercaloric nutritional support can not prevent the intense protein catabolism associate with sepsis and results in a number of complications. These include increased energy expenditure, increased carbon dioxide production, hyperglycemia and when nutrition is parenteral, complications of lipid emulsions. The goal should be to provide appropriate calories with adequate proportion of carbohydrates, proteins and lipids. In practice, an energy supply of 25-30 kcal/kg/d is adequate in 90% of cases. During recovery phase this amount may be increased to avoid risk of malnutrition, to achieve energy balance and to avoid endogenous fat oxidation.

How Much Glucose?

The literature on this topic is controversial. During frankly hyperglycemic phase, a minimum glucose supply is necessary to suppress glucose supply dependent tissues particularly as peripheral amino acid utilization is inadequate. It is a common practice to increase glucose infusion to maximal tolerance apparently to optimize protein metabolism. In sepsis deficient glucose oxidation is not a problem. The maximum rate of glucose oxidation is of the order of 5-6 mg/kg/min and recommended glucose supply for septic patients is therefore about 3-5 g/kg/day. Doses higher than 6 g/kg/d do not fully suppress gluconeogenesis and markedly exacerbate acute stress. Glucose intake is best guided by blood sugar levels. Blood sugar levels should be maintained <150 mg/dl. Addition of insulin (0.1 units/kg) is justified to keep blood glucose < 150 mg/dl. Hyperglycemia can predispose to infection and has been associated with poor outcome. Aggressive treatment of hyperglycemia appears to lower the risk of infection.

Lipids

Fatty acid oxidative capacity is not altered during sepsis. Long chain triglycerides (LCT) emulsions therefore, appear to be the most logical choice when higher caloric input is required. In severe sepsis, however, when glucose and insulin are high, clearance of lipid from blood falls rapidly suggesting that not much is utilized as energy substrate. Increasing the proportions of calories given as fat may however, be useful in controlling hyperglycemia and hypercapnia. There continue to be concerns about the immunosuppressive and other complications of intravenous fat emulsions.

It is not known whether formulations containing long and medium chain triglycerides (MCTs) are superior to those containing long chain triglycerides only. MCTs may have a potential advantage such as rapid clearance from plasma and rapid oxidation. 50:50 blend of medium chain triglycerides and long chain triglycerides also result in even balance of ω-3 and ω-6 fatty acids and increased amounts of antioxidants such as α-tocopherol. There is some evidence that the medium chain/long chain triglycerides mixture may have some advantages in critically ill patients with sepsis—for example, improved pulmonary hemodynamic and gas exchange parameters—but no evidence that the infection risk is reduced.

In practice it seems best to limit lipid supply to 20-35% of non-protein caloric input and even less in patients who are very seriously septic.

Protein

Main goal of protein supply in critically ill is to attenuate muscle catabolism while maintaining adequate nutrient supply to liver for synthesis of certain proteins especially those involved in immune defenses. Severe sepsis increases muscle catabolism, an increase in hepatic protein synthesis (acute phase reactants) and a decrease in total body protein synthesis. Overall, nitrogen balance is negative. In practice amino acid supply shown to meet the demands of protein synthesis and to achieve nitrogen equilibrium is approximately 1.5 gm protein per kg body weight per day. The ideal non-protein caloric to nitrogen ratio in critically ill septic patients is approx. 100:1.

The branched chain amino acids (leucine, isoleucine, and valine) can be oxidized peripherally by skeletal muscle and have been proposed to be a preferred substrate in sepsis.

Micronutrients—Electrolytes, vitamins and trace elements—the antioxidant concept

As part of the acute phase response to injury and sepsis there are altered dynamics of many trace elements, particularly zinc, iron and copper. Characteristically, plasma zinc and iron concentrations fall and plasma copper concentration rises probably as result of activation of neuroendocrine and cytokine pathways. They are thought to be beneficial aspects of the early acute phase response and require no specific treatment unless the illness is prolonged.

In severe infections, phosphorus requirements may be upto 10 times higher than normal in patients with respiratory distress, and also when glucose input is high. Some authors believe that iron deficiency is a normal defensive response to infection or trauma. In the opinion of other authors, iron deficiency, if sufficiently severe, impairs resistance to infection and should be corrected. Deficiency of zinc can lead to the persistence, and even the onset of sepsis due to immuno-deficiency. Selnium levels fall rapidly in sepsis and septic shock. (A minimal daily amount of about 200 μg could be required to normalize the serum concentration).

Immunonutrition

Some substances have metabolic benefits beyond their nutritional value. These have potential to alter cellular responses to inflammatory mediators. To obtain this effect, these nutrients are required in doses higher than those required for general nutritional support. Use of these nutrients is called immunonutrition. Various nutrients known to enhance immune function are dietary peptides, arginine, glutamine, Vitamin C, Vitamin A, Vitamin E and nucleic acids.

Glutamine: is an important nutrient for enterocytes and prevents mucosal atrophy in experimental models of starvation. Glutamine increases neutrophil phagocytic activity, enhances the production of reactive oxygen species by neutrophils *in vitro,* and thus increases protection against cellular injury in ischemia/reperfusion.

Arginine: is another conditionally essential amino acid involved in process of protein synthesis, and production of nitric oxide. It stimulates immune function in general and has been associated with improved bactericidal activity and wound healing. Arginine enhances T-lymphocyte activation, which increases the mean CD4 phenotype of patients with impaired cellular immunity. Supplementation with arginine upregulates immune function and reduces the incidence of postoperative infections.

Taurine: Its immunoregulatory effects are based on modulation of key proinflammatory cells, particularly the neutrophil and T lymphocyte. In neutrophils, taurine maintains phagocytic and microbicidal function in aged cells and prevents apoptosis. It has a role in membrane stabilization, bile salt formation, antioxidation, calcium homeostasis growth modulation, and osmoregulation. Its potential role in immunonutrition requires further study.

Omega-3 fatty acids: The ω-3 series family of long chain fatty acids cannot be synthesized in humans and therefore are essential components of the diet. They are incorporated into cell membranes and influence membrane stability and fluidity, cell mobility and the formation of binding of receptors. They are also involved in activation of intracellular signaling pathways. In clinical studies, consumption of ω-3 fatty acids has resulted in reduction of cardiovascular diseases, including arrhythmias and protection from renal disease, improvement in reduced episodes of rejection and protection from infection.

Phospholipids, incorporated into the structure of cell membranes, represent a reservoir of potential metabolic mediators. Under enzymatic action, the phospholipid membranes release fatty acid molecules.

Nucleotides are the structural subunits for DNA and RNA synthesis. Dietary nucleotides are broken down in the small bowel lumen into nucleosides and purine/pyrimidine bases. These may be absorbed by the enterocytes.

Immune-enhancing diets, parenteral or enteral in critically ill patients after trauma, sepsis, or major surgery reduce the incidence of infection, number of ventilator days, the length of hospital stay, but had no effect on intensive care stay. Apart from the extra cost involved, no detrimental effect of immunonutrition was identified. Taken together, all these studies suggest strongly that immunonutrition has a place in the treatment of critically ill patients.

ENTERAL NUTRITION

Who is Eligible for Enteral Nutrition?

Any patient with intact gastrointestinal tract, is a candidate for receiving enteral nutrition. In contrast to the usual belief, presence of bowel sounds is not a prerequisite for starting enteral feeds.It has been shown that 90% of critically ill adult patients tolerate feeds irrespective of presence of bowel sounds.

Intensivists are reluctant to start EN in the early stages of sepsis because of the risk of exacerbating intestinal ischemia and of favoring the ischemia-reperfusion phenomenon. Minimal EN may be implemented early and gradually increased at the expense of IV intake. Enteral feeding can be administered in the presence of gastrointestinal hemorrhage. A protective role of enteral feeding in gastrointestinal hemorrhage (GIH) in critically ill patients on mechanical ventilation has been shown.

Minor gastrointestinal problems e.g. bloating, vomiting and diarrhea should not be taken as absolute contraindications to enteral feeds. These are potentially manageable by changing the feeding volume and rate, using gastric motility agents and change in fiber content of the feed.

There are only a few contraindications to early enteral feeding. These are acute pancreatitis, distal bowel anastomosis and small bowel pathology. With the aid of jejunal feeding tubes and prokinetic agents, the majority of critically ill patients can be fed enterally.

Any patient who is not able to eat is a candidate to receive enteral feeds. The earlier EN is established the greater the benefit.

Available Feeding Mixtures

Following are the various categories of feeding mixtures from which selection should be made for a given patient:

1. Elemental Diets

These are monomeric formulas of low molecular weight and require minimal digestive effort, are easily absorbed without leaving much residue. Carbohydrates are present in these diets as oligosaccharides, sucrose and glucose. Proteins are present in form of short chain peptides and fat is usually in the form of medium chain triglycerides along with small amounts of essential fatty acids. As these diets are predigested, they are easily absorbed and are ideal for patients with pancreatic insufficiency or short bowel.

2. Polymeric Formulas

These diets consist of intact proteins, complex carbohydrates, fat and residue. Following are the various types of polymeric formulas:

a. Milk based diets.

b. Lactose free diets are preferred in critically ill patients and of course in lactose-intolerant patients.

Polymeric diets are of high molecular weight and are of relatively low osmolality. Therefore, they are preferred for duodenal and jejunal administration.

3. Modular Diets

These formulas are available as individual nutrients. Various nutrients can be mixed according to need of the patient.

Various enteral formula used at our center are shown in Table 19.1.

Selection of Diet Formula in Specific Conditions

1. Sepsis, Trauma and Burns

Stress caused by sepsis, burns and trauma, results in release of various hormones in the body. These hormones cause skeletal muscle proteolysis and hydrolysis of branched chain amino acids (BCAA). Therefore in such stress conditions, formulas rich in BCAAs are preferred.

In sepsis it must be emphasized that infectious and non-infectious complications are more frequent. As long as the situation remains unstable, it is probably harmful to start complex nutritional support.

It is best to begin nutrition as soon as patient is stable to help avoid the onset of severe metabolic disorders and/or nosocomial infections that can lead to irreversible multiple organs failure (MOF). Nutritional (metabolic) support is aimed at preventing or limiting malnutrition and its consequences (particularly for the immune system), and at correcting immediate metabolic deficiencies, which can be cofactors in the morbidity and mortality associated with sepsis states. Nutrient supply should consist simply of sufficient glucose to meet the requirements of glucose

Table 19.1: Enteral formulas used at PGIMER, Chandigarh (Prepared by our Dietetic Department)

Type of Formula	*Contents*		*Nutritional*	*Value/100ml*
Elemental	Protinex	50gm	Calories	110
	Glucose	100gm	Proteins	2.6gm
	Refined oil	30gm	CHO	19.5gm
	Water	to make 1000 cc	Fats	3 gm
Polymeric (Milk based) (Suji kheer)	Milk	500gm	Calories	150
	Sugar	50 gm	Proteins	4gm
	Suji	20 gm	CHO	4gm
	Oil	20gm	Fats	7.5gm
Polymeric (Lactose free)	Rice	50gm	Calories	66
	Sugar	45gm	Proteins	3gm
	Oil	30gm	CHO	8.4gm
	Water	to make 1000cc	Fats	3.7gm
Special formulas (Renal formula)	Skimmed milk powder	25gm	Calories	344
	Fats	125gm	Proteins	3gm
	Sugar	150cc	CHO	33gm
	Tonned milk	250cc	Fats	22gm
Special formulas (Hepatic formula)	Milk	250cc	Calories	100
	Sugar	50gm	CHO	20gm
	Rice	150gm	Proteins	2gm
	Cornflour	25gm	Fats	1.5gm
	Oil	5gm		
	Water	to make 1000cc		

dependent tissues, plus electrolytes and vitamins (e.g. Phosphorus and folinic acid).

Table 19.2: Specific metabolic support for sepsis, systemic inflammatory response syndrome, and septic shock

Energy requirements
1.3–1.5 times the average estimated resting energy expenditure (REE)
Carbohydrate <6 g/kg/d
Lipid (LCT or MCT/LCT) 0.5-1 g/kg/d
Proteins—1.2 g/kg/day protein
Conventional crystalline amino acid solution or polymeric diets (EN)
Vitamins—Standard balanced formula, vitamin K, B_1, B_6, A, C & E.
Trace-elements—Standard balanced formula with + Zn, + Se.
Electrolytes—Based on day to day plasma concentrations Na+, K+, Ca++, P, Mg.

2. Pulmonary Compromise

Increase intake of carbohydrates can lead to increase in CO_2 production and oxygen consumption, which can complicate and delay weaning in artificially ventilated patients. Therefore, in patients with pulmonary compromise, a formula containing decreased carbohydrate calories should be selected.

3. Hepatic Failure

High concentration of BCAA and low concentration of aromatic amino acids may help in normalizing the altered amino acid profile in patients with hepatic encephalopathy. Deliberate restriction of proteins is unjustified.

4. Renal Failure

Diets for patients with renal failure should contain high concentrations of essential amino acids combined with a large calorie to nitrogen ratio.

Routes for Enteral Feeds

Naso-enteric Feeds (Nasogastric, Nasoduodenal or Nasojejunal Tubes)

If enteric nutrition is needed for a short period, nasoenteric feed is preferred because of its temporary nature, ease of administration and simple technique of insertion. Among all naso-enteric routes, nasogastric is the preferred site. If there is increased risk of aspiration, feeding can be administered into distal duodenum or jejunum (post pyloric feeding). Tubes can be passed beyond the pylorus i.e. nasoduodenal or naso-jejunal along with the peristaltic movements. If peristalsis is not successful, tubes can be passed through pylorus endoscopically under fluoroscopic guidance.

Alternative Routes (Gastrostomy and Jejunostomy)

If requirement for enteral nutrition is expected for more than 4 weeks, these routes are chosen. In the past, these tubes were being inserted at the time of surgery. However, now-a-days percutaneous insertion techniques are available using local anesthesia. Overall there is no evidence in favour of either small bowel or gastric feeding.

Methods of Enteral Feeding

1. Bolus feeding
2. Intermittent feeding
3. Continuous drip feeding.

Bolus feeding: It has advantages of requiring less amount of time and equipment and reduced risk of contamination. However, there are more chances of aspiration after a bolus feed. Patients with short bowel or malabsorption who run the risk of physiologic intolerance to the bolus of carbohydrate/protein or fat do not tolerate this type of feeding.

Intermittent feeding: This is given as 2 ml/kg every 4-6 hourly, each time for 20-45 minutes. This type of feed is usually well tolerated.

Continuous drip feeding: This type of feeding has advantage of leaving smallest residual volume, has least potential for aspiration, bloating and diarrhea. However, it requires close monitoring and has danger of causing bacterial overgrowth. In small bowel, continuous drip-feeding is preferred, whereas jejunal feed may be given by smaller but more frequent feeding increment than given into the stomach.

Feed should be started with small volumes, 1 ml/kg/hr of half strength formula. If tolerated for 24 hrs, it can be increased by 0.5 ml/kg/hr until the desired volume is delivered. Once the required volume is achieved, concentration can be increased to full strength.

Initiation of Enteral Feeds

Initiation and success of enteral feeding requires help of clinical nutritionist, gastroenterologist and dietician. A specific, yet flexible plan should be made for each patient before starting enteral feeds. There should be a written estimation of fluid, caloric and electrolyte requirements for that particular patient. Protocol for patient's monitoring should be clearly defined before initiating enteral feeds.

The selected formula should initially be used at one quarter to half strength; at a volume approximately half of the required 24 hrs volume and further increments in volume and strength should be made gradually.

Monitoring of Patients on Enteral Feeds

Frequency of monitoring of patients on enteral feeds depends on nutritional and clinical condition of the patient. The suggested monitoring schedule is shown in Table 19.3.

Table 19.3: Monitoring protocol for patient on enteral nutrition

Tolerance	Nausea Vomiting Diarrhea Constipation Abdominal distension
Nutrition and metabolic	Body weight Serum Na^+, K^+, osmolality Acid base balance Blood glucose, urea, nitrogen. Serum Mg^{++}, Ca^{++}, PO_4^{++} Urine examination Liver function tests
Mechanical	Confirm tube patency and location before each use. Irrigate feeding tube after intermittent feeds, crushed medication administration.

Complications of Enteral Feeds

The two major risks of EN are aspiration pneumonia due to functional ileus and the onset of diarrhea. Diarrhea can usually be controlled by reducing the flow rate of the mixtures and by providing sufficient intraluminal sodium.

1. *Pulmonary aspiration of gastric contents:* This complication is usually due to prolongation of gastric emptying time, which may lead to vomiting resulting in aspiration. Use of cisapride or domeperidone, gastrointestinal prokinetic drugs has been shown to increase gastric emptying. Other methods, which help to decrease the risk of vomiting are elevation of the patient's head to approximately 30 degrees and administration of enteral feeds beyond the pylorus.
2. *Diarrhea:* It is a frequent problem in patients on enteral formula. The causes of diarrhea include use of hyperosomolar formula, rapid feeding of large volumes, contamination of the feed, low serum albumin, concurrent antibiotic therapy or administration of lactose containing formulas to lactose deficient patients. If these

factors can be taken care of, diarrhea does not remain an absolute contraindication for enteral feeds.

3. Other adverse gastrointestinal effects of specialized enteral formulae include nausea, vomiting, cramping and abdominal pain. These can be caused by rapid administration of hypertonic feeds or by use of inappropriate formula. Therefore, increment in formula strength, volume and rate of administration must be made gradually.
4. *Nutrient deficiencies:* There is risk of development of excess or deficiencies of various nutrients and electrolytes. To overcome this, there should be a strict and accurate recording of all the sources of fluids, electrolytes and nutrients.
5. *Mechanical problems*: Occlusion, displacement of feeding tubes can be avoided by taking proper monitoring precautions as mentioned earlier.

PARENTERAL NUTRITION (PN)

Total PN (TPN) is indicated when enteral administration is inappropriate or has failed, the value of brief periods (< 1 week) of PN is uncertain.

Feeding Regimens

Daily energy and nitrogen requirements remain as stated above but modified as follows:

1. Nitrogen is given as amino acids, at least 25% of which should be essential amino acids. Glutamine supplements may help preserve muscle mass and support immunocompetence.
2. Energy is delivered as a combination of glucose and fat, the latter making up approximately one-third of the total calorie intake.
3. Fat is delivered as a proprietary 10 or 20% emulsion of soyabean oil in glycerol and egg phosphatides. This has a higher calorific value than glucose, and therefore has a particular advantage when fluid overload is a problem. Excessive lipemia may be a problem in some very ill patients (severe sepsis, liver failure, pancreatitis), although the clinical consequences of this are unclear. Increasing the glucose concentration of TPN solutions to avoid the adverse effects of fat emulsions is not advised, it can result in hyperglycemia.
4. Appropriate water and fat soluble vitamin supplements should be added to the solutions.
5. Although the various components of a TPN regimen can be given independently, this requires parallel administration of amino acid and glucose/fat solutions, which complicates administration and increases the risk of infection. As a result, many centers now use composite TPN solutions, in which all the requirements for a 24-hour period (glucose, fat, amino acids, vitamins, and trace elements, etc.) are mixed aseptically in the hospital pharmacy into a single bag. Drugs such as ranitidine and insulin can also be added as required.

Parenteral alimentation is difficult to organize with limited facilities. However, it should be possible with ready commercial availability of lipid solution (Intralipid), and amino acid (AA) mixtures. Plasma is not a good substitute to amino acid mixture, but may be given for a short period of time. Parenteral solution, bulk of which is made of 10% glucose, should contain all essential electrolytes and vitamins (Table 19.4). It may be given through a peripheral vein, but central vein is preferable. Intralipid, dextrose and amino acids should all be infused through separate IV sets attached through 3-way stop cocks to IV cannula, just before it enters the vein. Parenteral nutrition should be introduced gradually, reaching full volume by 5th day.

Administration

Standard solutions are an irritant to small veins due to their high osmolarity, and therefore need

Table 19.4: Typical requirement for parenteral nutrition in children and suggested parenteral solution

Solution	*Volume (kg/day)*	*Amount (kg/day)*
Aminoacid solution (10%)	25 ml	2.5 g
Intralipid (10%)	10-30 ml	0.5-3 g
Glucose (50%)	10 ml	
KCl (15%)	1 ml (2mEq)	K 2-3 mEq
$MgSO_4$ (10%)	0.2 ml	Mg 0.25 mEq*
Calcium gluconate (50%)	3.5 ml	Ca 1.5 mEq
Sodium chloride (25%)	6 ml (3Eq)	Na 3 mEq
Trace metals (mix)	1 ml	Zinc, Chromium magnesium
Multivitamin	1 ml	
Glucose 10% to make	120 ml	

Note: Supplement Vit K-1 mg, Vit B_{12} – 50 μg, Folic acid 1 mg (weekly).
* Potassium phosphate equal to 1 mEq of K^+/kg should used to provide phosphate, if available.

to be given centrally. In the long-term convalescent patients, TPN should be via a single-lumen tunneled central line (usually an infraclavicular approach to the subclavian vein that has been sited under strict asepsis) that is not used for any other purpose, so as to minimize the risk of line infection. In the acute critically ill patient this is often inappropriate, but at the very least TPN solutions should be delivered via a dedicated lumen of an aseptically sited multi-lumen catheter. Solutions can be given peripherally providing osmolarity is restricted to 900 mOsm, with most of the calories given in the form of lipid.

Complications

1. *Catheter-related:*
   a. complications of insertion and residence
   b. sepsis (entry site, bacteremia).
2. *Metabolic:*
   a. hyperglycemia; insulin often required
   b. lipemia
   c. hypophosphatemia, leading to muscle weakness, reduced tissue oxygen delivery (lack of 2,3-diphosphoglycerate, shifting oxyhemoglobin dissociation curve to the left)
   d. Metabolic acidosis.
3. *Vitamin and trace element deficiencies.*
4. *Intestinal mucosal atrophy:* Intestinal mucosa derives most of its nutritional requirements from the lumen of the gut. Failure to deliver nutrition enterally may lead to atrophy of the intestinal mucosa and result in translocation of gut bacteria.

Route of Administration—Enteral or Parenteral?

Nutritional support in critically ill patients can be given via the enteral or parenteral route. Over the past decade or so it has become increasingly apparent that enteral nutrition is superior if it can be established. Most of the complications associated with TPN can be avoided by using the enteral route for nutritional support in the critically ill. Therefore, enteral nutrition (EN), if available, is the route of choice for nutrition in all patients. Only EN can preserve gut integrity and function, maintain bile secretion, maintain secretory immunoglobulin A and gut associated lymphoid tissue and enhances splanchnic blood flow and mesenteric oxygen utilization in sepsis. Enteral feeding is also preferred because of ease of administration, decreased cost, decreased prevalence of infection, no need for central venous access and improved gastrointestinal function. EN is also as effective as antacids in the prophylaxis of stress ulceration in ICU patients.

CONCLUSION

Nutrition management is an essential component of critical care. There is no cook-book formulae available; management should be more flexible, tailored to metabolism and goal oriented. Enteral nutrition is as good as parenteral nutrition with added advantages of being less costly and easier to administer. Successful enteral nutrition requires an intelligent selection of enteral formula and careful monitoring of patients on enteral feeding. Most of the complications associated with enteral feeding are potentially avoidable and manageable. Intestinal obstruction and intestinal fistulae are the only contraindications for enteral feeds.

Chapter twenty

Sedation and Analgesia

The correct management of sedation is one of the most important aspects of Intensive Care management. Unfortunately it is also one of the most difficult, mainly because patients cannot communicate easily how they feel and what they need to feel better.

Indications

Some degree of sedation (i.e. analgesia ± hypnosis) is often required to allow patient co-operation with organ system support and the associated nursing care. An agitated patient has a higher basal metabolic rate and may reduce the efficiency of supportive care. *Most important indication of sedation and analgesia is any situation requiring anxiolysis and analgesia to comfort the child.* Sedation is a mandatory prerequisite prior to, and during administration of neuromuscular blockers. The patient should never be subjected to paralysis without sedation. An additional benefit of sedatives is amnesia.

Most common procedures requiring sedation in PICU are endotracheal intubation and mechanical ventilation. In addition to mechanical ventilation, many other procedures require sedation such as CT or radiation therapy. Oxygen, suction, and resuscitation and monitoring equipment should be available and only trained and experienced personnel should administer sedation to ensure safety of the pediatric patient. As much as possible, PICU procedures should be planned ahead of time, so that adequate preparation can be made in PICU (e.g. liver or bone biopsy and high risk endoscopy).

Aims

1. *All patients must be comfortable and pain free.*
2. Anxiety should be minimized. The most important way of achieving this is to provide compassionate and considerate care.
3. *Patients should be calm, co-operative and able to sleep when undisturbed.* This does not mean that they must be asleep at all times.
4. Patients must be able to tolerate appropriate organ system support.
5. Patients must not be paralysed and awake.

COMMON SEDATIVE DRUGS

Characterstics of commonly used sedatives are given in Table 20.1.

Benzodiazepines

The primary pharmacological action of benzodiazepines is sedation. They also provide for anxiolysis, muscle relaxation, and anticonvulsant activity and induce anterograde amnesia. Benzodiazepines have no analgesic benefits. Diazepam and Midazolam have greater lipophilicity, enabling them to cross the blood brain barrier quickly. They have a much more rapid onset of action and are the appropriate choices when immediate sedation is required. Their long-term use causes dependency and abrupt discontinuation causes a withdrawal syndrome resulting in rebound agitation, and even seizures in some patients.

Flumazenil, a benzodiazepine antagonist can be used to reverse benzodiazepine induced sedation, if available.

Table 20.1: Commonly used sedatives and analgesics

Benzodiazepines

	Midazolam	*Lorazepam*	*Diazepam*
Onset	0.5-2 minutes	5 minutes	1-3 minutes
Duration	2 hours	6-10 hours	1-6 hours
Metabolism	Hepatic	Hepatic (less influenced by age and liver disease)	Hepatic
Elimination	Renal (Active metabolite)	Renal (no active metabolite)	Renal (Active metabolite)
Anxiolysis	++++	++++	++++
Analgesia	±	±	±
Hypnosis	++++	++++	++++
Amnesia	++++	+++	++++
Seizure threshold	+++	++++	+++
Dyspnea	+	+	+
CV effects	Venodilation, ↓BP	Venodilation, ↓BP	Venodilate, ↓BP
Respiratory effects	Shift CO_2 response curve to right	Shift CO_2 response curve to right	Shift CO_2 response curve to right
Side effects	Occasionally paradoxical agitation	Occasionally Paradoxical agitation	Occasionally paradoxical agitation

Opioid analgesics

	Morphine	*Pethidine*	*Fentanyl*
Onset	10 minutes	3-5 minutes	0.5-1 minutes
Duration	4 hours	1-4 hours	0.5-1 hours
Metabolism	Hepatic	Hepatic	Hepatic
Elimination	Renal	Renal	Renal
Anxiolysis	+	+	+
Analgesia	++++	++++	++++
Hypnosis	±	±	±
Amnesia	No	No	No
Seizure threshold	No effect	May ↓	No effect
Dyspnea	++++	++++	++++
CV effects	Venodilation, ↓BP	Venodilation, ↓BP	Venodilation, ↓BP
Respiratory effects	Shift CO_2 response curve to right	Shift CO_2 response curve to right	Shift CO_2 response curve to right
Side effects	Nausea, ileus, itching, histamine release	Seizures (norpethidine) nausea, ileus, itching	Nausea, ileus, itching

Pharmacologic properties based on single dose

Diazepam: is rapidly distributed to brain following an IV injection. The concentration in plasma declines rapidly owing to redistribution with an initial half-life of 10 to 15 minutes. However, drowsiness often returns with an increased concentration of diazepam in plasma after 6-8 hours. This effect is due to absorption from the gastrointestinal tract after excretion in the bile.

Lorazepam: has an intermediate duration of action. It has no active metabolite, so it is a more steady agent for long-term maintenance of sedation. Half life of redistribution of this drug is more than twice that of diazepam, therefore onset of drowsiness is less rapid. It is useful when anterograde amnesia is particularly desirable.

Midazolam (Versed) is the benzodiazepine of choice for short-term sedation because it has the highest lipid solubility, the fastest onset, and the shortest duration of action of all the intravenous benzodiazepines. Infusions of midazolam lasting more than a few hours can produce prolonged sedation after the drug infusion is stopped. Accumulation in the central nervous system, accumulation of an active metabolite, especially in renal failure and hepatic insufficiency, may lead to over sedation.

Opiates

Commonly used opiates are morphine, fentanyl and pethidine. The primary pharmacological action of opiates is to relieve pain or the sensitivity to noxious stimuli via opioid receptors. Opiates do not provide appreciable amnesia. A very significant secondary action of opiates is sedation and anxiolysis. Other effects include emesis, urinary retention, ileus, respiratory depression and hypotension. Hypotension occurs due to a combination of venodilatation, sympatholysis, vagal mediated bradycardia and histamine release.

Morphine should be given in smallest effective dose and as infrequently as possible to minimize the development of tolerance and physical dependence. Single pediatric dose should not exceed 10 mg. The active metabolite morphine-6-glucuronide accumulates in renal failure and extend the duration of action.

Fentanyl is a synthetic opiate with 100 times the potency of morphine. It has a more rapid onset of action due to greater lipophilicity. Fentanyl induces less hemodynamic instability because it does not induce histamine release like morphine. Fentanyl may therefore be preferred in patients with circulatory shock. Like morphine, it should be given in the smallest effective dose and as infrequently as possible to minimize the development of tolerance and physical dependence. As a word of caution, in neonates and younger infants, fentanyl can induce chest wall rigidity following rapid IV injection leading to severe respiratory depression, compounding the effect of centrally induced depression of the respiratory centre.

To provide general anesthesia without additional anesthetic agents, fentanyl doses of 50-100 µg/kg may be administered IV in conjunction with oxygen and skeletal muscle relaxant.

The standard reversal agent in the setting of opiate overdose is Naloxone, a competitive antagonist. Dose of naloxone is 0.01 mg/kg IV slowly. Rapid infusion can result in withdrawal seizures in patients receiving morphine on a chronic basis.

Ketamine

Ketamine hydrochloride is *phenycyclidine derivative.* It induces a state of sedation, immobility, amnesia and marked analgesia. It induces dissociative anaesthesia i.e. strong feeling of dissociation from the environment. It has been extensively used in pediatric patients for procedural analgesia.

Ketamine is ideal sedative in a relatively hypovolemic patient, with bronchospasm and shock. It causes release of catecholamines resulting hypertension and bronchodilatation. It should be avoided in patients with hypertension and raised intracranial pressure.

IV dose is given over a period of about one minute. The sensation of dissociation is noticed within 15 seconds and unconsciousness becomes apparent within 30 seconds. Intense analgesia and amnesia are established rapidly. Following a single dose, unconsciousness lasts 10-15 minutes and analgesia persists for 40 minutes, amnesia may be evident for 1-2 hours following the initial injection. If anaesthesia of longer duration is required repeat dose equal to half of the initial dose may be administered.

Muscle tone may be increased, purposeless movements may sometimes occur and violent and irrational responses to stimuli occur. Pharyngeal and Laryngeal reflexes are retained and although cough reflex is depressed, airway obstruction does not normally occur. Airway resistance is decreased and bronchospasm may be abolished. Ketamine, it acts on receptors in the cortex and limbic system. Awakening may be characterized by disagreeable dreams and even hallucinations. Some of these may occur days or weeks later.

Propofol

Propofol (2,6-diisopropyl) is an IV anaesthetic that is given to critically ill children for titrable sedation and hypnosis. Propofol has a wide array of benefits, including anxiolysis, anticonvulsant activity, anti-emesis, and the ability to reduce intracranial hypertension. Similar to the benzodiazepines, propofol has no analgesic activity. The most important advantage of propofol is its rapid onset and offset of action. This behavior of a "rapid on, rapid off" feature, accounts for the increasing popularity of propofol. Because the onset of action after a single dose is rapid, and its effect brief (10-15 minutes) due to high lipophilicity and central nervous system penetration, propofol is given only by continuous infusion when used for sedation.

Given in conjunction with midazolam, propofol provides satisfactory anaesthesia for emergency surgical procedures, radiological procedures etc.

The most significant adverse effect of propofol is hemodynamic destabilization. ***Propofol can substantially reduce cardiac output*** because it is both a negative inotrope and negative chronotrope. Additionally, it is a vasodilator. These effects ***can cause significant hypotension.*** It is also potent respiratory depressant.

Dexmetomidine: Dexmetomidine was introduced as an intravenous sedative that does not produce respiratory depression. Dexmetomidine is a highly selective α_2 – adrenergic agonist that produces sedation, anxiolysis, mild analgesia, and sympatholysis. With a bolus dose of the drug, sedation is evident in a few minutes, effect lasts less than 10 minutes. Because of the short duration of action, dexmetomidine is usually given by continuous infusion.

Dexmetomidine is given as a loading dose of 1 mg/Kg (infused over 10 minutes), followed by a continuous infusion of 0.2 to 0.7 mg/Kg/hour. Mild hypertension in response to the loading dose is observed in 15% of patients. Drug infusions should not be continued for longer and the dose should be reduced in patients with severe liver dysfunction. Adverse effects during dexmetomidine infusion include hypotension (30%) and bradycardia (8%)

Haloperidol: Haloperidol has little or no risk of cardio-respiratory depression. It produces its sedative and antipsychotic effects by blocking dopamine receptors in the central nervous system. Following an intravenous dose sedation is evident in 10 to 20 minutes; the effect lasts for hours. The prolonged duration of action makes haloperidol poorly suited for continuous infusion. Due to its delayed onset of action, haloperidol is not indicated for immediate control of anxiety. A benzodiazepine can be added to achieve more rapid sedation. Drug can be used to sedate ventilator-dependent patients, and to facilitate weaning from mechanical ventilation. Dopamine antagonism in the basal ganglia can cause extrapyramidal reactions; these are uncommon when haloperidol is given intravenously in combination with a benzodiazepine.

Dose for acute agitation: 3-12 years: initial 0.025-0.05 mg/kg/day divided 2-3 times; maintenance 0.01-0.03 mg/kg/day. Above 12 years: 0.1-0.2 mg/kg, IM or 1-15 mg/dose oral.

Chloral Hydrate (Trichlophos)

Chloral hydrate is used principally as an oral/rectal

hypnotic. It may be used as a routine oral sedative agent. The drug is used pre-operatively to allay anxiety and produce sedation and as adjunct to opiates and analgesics. It is also used for non-stimulating procedures requiring sedation only e.g. prior to EEG.

Toxicity can manifest as gastritis, skin eruptions or parenchymal renal damage may develop following prolonged administration of chloral hydrate. Prolonged use may also produce tolerance and physical dependence. Chloral hydrate over dosage produces symptoms that are similar to those of barbiturate over dosage like coma, hypotension, hypothermia, respiratory depression and cardiac arrhythmias. Treatment of chloral hydrate intoxication consists of general supportive therapy including maintenance of adequate airway, assisted respiration, oxygen administration and maintaining body temperature and circulation. Gastric lavage may be performed following over dosage if an endotracheal tube with cuff inflated is in place to prevent aspiration of gastric contents.

PRACTICAL APPROACH TO SEDATION IN PICU

Sedation in children is usually performed with one or combination of benzodiazepines, opiates, neuroleptic agents and anaesthetic agents such propofol and Ketamine. Each of these groups of medications has their particular benefits: benzodiazepines provide the greatest analgesia and propofol is the most easily titrable and has a more rapid reversal of sedation other than providing amnesia. For short non-stimulating procedures requiring sedation only, chloral hydrate alone may be used. Doses of commonly used sedatives are given in Table 20.2.

Ketamine or narcotic supplementation should be given before painful procedures such as central line, arterial line insertions and chest tube placement. Older children require muscle relaxants in addition to sedation, especially in cases of acute respiratory distress syndrome or other low compliance lung disease.

Table 20.2: Doses of various sedatives used in PICU

Drug	*Dose*
Diazepam	0.2-0.5 mg/kg IV; may be repeated 4-8 hourly
Midazolam	0.1-0.3 mg/kg IV; effect lasts 1-2 hour Alternatively 0.15-0.2 mg/kg IV loading; 1-3 mcg/kg/min
Morphine	0.1-0.2 mg/kg IV bolus; repeat 4-6 min
Chloral hydrate	50 mg/kg oral (hypnotic), 20 mg/kg oral (sedation)
Thiopental	2-8 mg/kg stat IV, 2-5 mg/kg/hour, IV infusion
Ketamine	2-3 mg/kg IM, 1-2 mg/kg bolus; 10-15 µg/kg/min (0.5 mg/kg/hour) by IV infusion (minimal risk of cardiorespiratory depression)
Fentanyl	1-2 mcg/kg/dose, IV; IV infusion 1 mcg/kg/hour

Sedation for Short Procedures

Midazolam and other benzodiazepines are useful as sole agents for procedures that do not require analgesia. For sedation before short diagnostic or endoscopic procedures, midazolam may be used alone or in combination with Ketamine or opiate agonist). For per oral procedures e.g. (upper Gastrointestinal endoscopy, bronchoscopy), use of a topical anesthetic is recommended and for bronchoscopy, use of an opiate analgesic for pre-medication is also recommended. When used concomitantly with opiates, midazolam dosage should be decreased by 30% to adjust for sedative effect of opiates as well as to reduce chances of respiratory depression. For maintenance of sedation midazolam may be administered in incremental IV doses of approximately 25% of the initial dose when lightening of sedation is evident.

Table 20.3: Sedation scoring systems: Cambridge sedation scale

Level	*Clinical characteristic*	*Sedation*
1. Agitated	Show anxiety or pain	Inadequate
2. Awake	Alert, not distressed	Adequate
3. Roused by voice	Lightly asleep, easily aroused	Ideal level
4. Roused by tracheal suction	–	Higher than necessary level
5. Unaroused by tracheal suction	–	Deep coma
6. Asleep	Normal sleep	

Sedation scoring systems: Ramsay sedation scale

1. Anxious, agitated, or restless
2. Co-operative, orientated, and tranquil
3. Responds to commands only
4. Asleep, but brisk response to glabellar tap or loud auditory stimulus
5. Asleep, sluggish response to glabellar tap or loud auditory stimulus
6. No response

Sedation scoring systems: Sedation agitation scale

Level	*Clinical characteristic*
7. Dangerous agitation	Pulling ETT, striking at staff, thrashing
6. Very agitated	Doesn't calm, bites ETT, needs restraints
5. Agitated	Anxious, tries to sit up, calms to verbal instruction
4. Calm and cooperative	Awakens easily, follows commands
3. Sedated	Awake to verbal stimulus or gentle shaking, follows commands
2. Very sedated	Arouses to physical stimulus, doesn't follow commands
1. Unarousable	Minimal response to noxious stimulation

Sedation in Ventilated Patients

All patients require sedation of some degree during mechanical ventilation. The most important goal in the sedation of these patients is to achieve patient comfort and patient-synchrony to avoid any mishaps during ventilation such as accidental extubation, circuit disconnection or kinking of circuits. It is important to remember that most common condition causing agitation in a child on ventilator is hypoxia due to mechanical reasons such as secretions, endotracheal tube misplacement, kink or pneumothorax. This must be addressed with adequate oxygen delivery, clearance of secretions, delivery of adequate tidal volume, ensuring proper placement of endotracheal tube and treating pneumothorax as the case may be, before sedating the child for anxiolysis and comfort.

In ventilated patients one should start with an infusion of an opioid, usually morphine or fentanyl. Fentanyl has the advantage of avoiding hypotension from histamine release. Once proper analgesia has been established, an infusion of a sedative benzodiazepines: midazolam,or diazepam should be added. If no painful procedures are contemplated, midazolam infusion alone is sufficient.

Midazolam is initiated with an IV loading dose administered over at least 2-3 minutes, followed by continuous IV infusion to maintain the clinical effect. Continuous IV infusion of midazolam should be initiated at the rate of 1-2 µg/kg per minute; i.e. 60-120 µg/kg/hour. The infusion rate may be increased or decreased generally by 25% of the initial or subsequent infusion rate to achieve the desired effect.

The response to sedative agents, particularly to benzadiazepines may show marked variation between patients. Hence it is desirable to monitor the level of sedation. Simple and clinically oriented sedation scores such as those developed at Cambridge or Ramsay scale may be used for this purpose (Table 20.3). Cerebral function monitor or cerebral function analyzing monitor may be used to evaluate neurological function.

Complications of Sedation in the ICU

While it is clear that leaving a patient agitated and distressed is detrimental to their care this is equally true of over sedation. All sedative agents share the following problems:

1. Cardiovascular instability—detrimental effects on the circulation leading to increased inotrope requirements.
2. Detrimental effects on the pulmonary vasculature—increasing VQ mismatch leading to increased ventilatory support with the consequent increase in complications.
3. Gastric stasis and impaired enteral nutritional support.
4. Reduced mobilization and muscle wasting.
5. Drug accumulation and consequent prolonged duration of action, delaying weaning from mechanical ventilation increasing complications and consequently morbidity and mortality.
6. Nosocomial pneumonia.
7. Tolerance during sedation and withdrawal syndromes (typically seen in patients receiving continuous infusion for several days without interruption).

It is therefore vital that sedation is managed as precisely as possible and given the priority attention that it deserves.

Reduction of Sedative Requirements in ICU

All sedatives can accumulate in critically ill patients leading to prolonged effect. This may increase duration of mechanical ventilation, ICU length of stay, hospital length of stay, and complications of critical illness (e.g., ventilator-associated pneumonia). A strategy to reduce drug accumulation such as daily interruption of sedative infusions until the patient awakens or a nursing-directed administration protocol based on a targeted level of sedation should be implemented.

In summary, one must follow a practice of judicious use of sedatives in PICU to try to make stressful and traumatic experience smoother for the child as well as for the parents. One must not forget to use analgesia where painful procedure is anticipated in a child. Availability of proper resuscitative equipment as well as trained personnel is extremely important to ensure safety of the child during all procedures, specially those performed in radiology or endoscopy rooms. Routine use of muscle relaxants can be avoided, these should to be reserved for mechanically ventilated patients with severe acute respiratory syndrome or raised intracranial tension.

Chapter twenty-one

Neuromuscular Blockade (Muscle Relaxants)

Drug-induced neuromuscular blockade is a common practice in ICUs. It is needed in children on mechanical ventilation for managing ventilator-dependent patients who are agitated and difficult to ventilate. These are also needed sometimes during procedures such as endotracheal tube placement.

Indications

Indications for prolonged neuromuscular blockade include:

1. Refractory hypoxemia in patients with acute hypoxemic respiratory failure (particularly acute respiratory distress syndrome [ARDS])
   - to facilitate ventilation (particularly inverse ratio ventilation and permissive hypercapnia)
   - to reduce skeletal muscle oxygen consumption.
2. Patients with critical intracranial hypertension in whom unwanted motor activity cannot be prevented by sedation alone.
3. Tetanus (improves chest wall compliance).

Neuromuscular blocking agents (muscle relaxants) act by binding to acetylcholine receptors on the postsynaptic side of the neuromuscular junction. The depolarizing agents act like acetylcholine produce a sustained depolarization of the postsynaptic membrane, which blocks the propagation of electrical impulses along the muscle. The nondepolarizing agent act by blocking acetylcholine-induced activation of the post-synaptic membrane.

Avoidable Agents

Succinylcholine is a depolarizing agent and is used infrequently. This agent is ultra-short acting and is, most often used to facilitate tracheal intubation. An intravenous dose of 1 to 2 mg/kg produces paralysis within 2 minutes, and the effect disappears within 10 minutes. The prolonged use may cause life-threatening increase in serum potassium.

Pancuronium (Pavulon) is a relatively long-acting neuromuscular blocker (duration of action is 1 to 2 hours). It can accumulate with repeated use and has vagolytic effect, which can produce tachycardia and hypertension. Pancuronium can be given by continuous infusion, but it is usually given as intermittent bolus doses because of the risk of drug accumulation. Pancuronium is excreted by the kidneys, and dosage reductions are often necessary in renal failure.

Vecuronium (Norcuron) is an analog of pancuronium but is shorter acting and has no vagolytic effects. Because of its short duration of action (30 minutes), it is often given by continuous infusion.

Atracurium is also shorter acting (duration of action 25-30 mins) and can be given by continuous infusion. This can release histamine from mast cells and produce hypotension when given too rapidly.

Infusions of short-acting non-depolarizing relaxants such as vecuronium, atracurium, or cisatracurium are generally used, and should be titrated against response using a monitor of neuromuscular blockade. The metabolism of atracurium and cis-atracurium is independent of hepatic metabolism and renal excretion, although the excitatory metabolite laudanosine may accumulate in patients with renal failure who are given atracurium—cis-atracurium also has more hemodynamic stability than atracurium. Vecuronium may accumulate in patients with hepatic impairment and is not considered a first line drug in critically ill patients.

Commonly used muscle relaxants and their doses are given in Table 21.1.

Table 21.1: Muscle relaxants used in PICU

Drug	*Dose*
1. Pancuronium	0.01 mg/kg for priming or defasciculating 0.1 mg/kg/hour (loading dose 0.1 mg/kg) full dose
2. Vecuronium	0.01 mg/kg for priming 0.05-0.1 mg/kg/hour (loading dose 0.1 mg/kg)
3. Atracurium	5-10 µg/kg/min (loading dose 0.5 mg/kg)
4. Cis-atracurium	1-5 µg/kg/min (loading dose 0.1-0.2 mg/kg)
5. Succinylcholine	2 mg/kg IV in infants 1.5 mg/kg in children (need defasciculation dose)

Disadvantages

Inadequate Sedation: It is impossible to determine whether sedation is adequate in a patient who is paralyzed. Generous sedation is therefore mandatory. Opiates may be preferred to achieve sedation with analgesia.

Prolonged Paralysis: Routine use of muscle relaxants to facilitate ventilation is associated with accelerated muscle atrophy, and weaning difficulties. Prolonged neuromuscular paralysis after discontinuing therapy with neuromuscular blocking agents may occur after prolonged neuromuscular blockade (longer than 1 week). It can also occur after just a few doses of neuromuscular blockers. There is no evidence that this problem is related to the drug that is used. Shorter periods and intermittent cessation of neuromuscular blockade have been recommended to limit the risk of prolonged paralysis.

Hypostatic/Nosocomial Pneumonia: Clearance of respiratory secretions is inadequate during neuromuscular paralysis resulting in pooling of secretions in dependent lung regions. This can lead to hypostatic/nosocomial pneumonia.

Venous thromboembolism because of loss of the milking action of muscle contraction on the venous return from the legs.

Prolonged administration of nondepolarizing muscle relaxants without objective monitoring of physiologic responses may result in relative or absolute overdoses. Concurrent administration of other drugs and/or certain disease states may enhance effects of nondepolarising muscle relaxants. With prolonged administration, pharmacologically relevant concentration may accumulate and thus prolong the duration of blockade.

In summary, the risks of neuromuscular paralysis are considerable enough to consider avoiding the use of neuromuscular blocking agents.

Practical Points

Adequate analgesia and amnesia should be provided before administration of muscle relaxants and continued throughout their administration. This will often obviate or at least diminish the need for muscle relaxant. Neuromuscular blockers should be avoided as far as possible. If these must be used, the period of use should be kept to minimum. If these are needed for a period longer than 2-3 hours continuous infusion should be preferred. An objective method must be used to assess development of neuromuscular blockade (Train of four method, post-tetanic count etc.). Application of peripheral nerve stimulators is mandatory to ensure such objectivity. If indicated, muscle relaxation should be reversed.

Chapter twenty-two

General Care of a Patient in an ICU

BASIC CARE

Basic care includes care of eyes, mouth, general hygiene, bowel, posture and prevention of bed sores specially in those who are unconscious or paralysed.

Care of Eyes

Eyes must be cleaned with normal saline every day, and an antibiotic cream or moisol drops should be applied. In comatose patients lids should be kept closed with a sterile cotton pad dressing. Exposure keratitis leading to blindness has been reported off and on from ICUs. It is a very high price to pay for intensive therapy.

Bowel Care

Most children develop changed bowel habit and constipation due to changes in the diet. A N-saline or glycerine enema may be required to keep the bowels clean. Changeover to special oral feeds invariably leads to loose motions and, therefore, should be done slowly over 2-3 days.

Care of Bladder

An indwelling bladder catheter is very useful to measure urinary output particularly in smaller children. However, catheterisation can lead to complications (infection, stricture of urethra) and should therefore be done only when specifically indicated. Urine bag or condom drainage should be preferred whenever feasible.

Skin Care

All skin areas should be frequently observed in patients bed ridden for more than a few days. Younger children and adolescents are at risk of developing pressure necrosis. Frequent rotation or use of air mattress will keep pressure off from any one area.

Maceration of intertriginous area of the neck, and diaper region are common, specially in ventilated, heavily sedated patients. Often they are secondarily infected. The area should be kept clean and dry. Child's bed sheets should always be kept dry so as to avoid skin infection and ulceration. Skin lesions occur as a result of intravenous (IV) infiltration or extravasation of infusions and drugs (such as hypertonic fluids, calcium, potassium, bicarbonate, sodium pentothal etc.). Careful maintenance of IV site and close observation of infusion may prevent the complication. It should be treated with warm compresses and elevation of the part. If the skin ulcerates, it should be treated as a burn.

PHYSIOTHERAPY

All unconscious patients and those with tracheal tubes need frequent respiratory physiotherapy. Postural drainage, vibration and percussion are needed to dislodge thick viscid secretions to prevent chest complications. Each patient should receive at least two or three sessions of chest physiotherapy daily. The frequency may be increased in those with a tendency to retain secretions. Simulated cough is used with physiotherapy to help clear secretions particularly in older children. A number of complications can arise during physiotherapy particularly in hypoxic patients. These include hypoxemia, fall in cardiac output, cardiac arrhythmias and pneumothorax.

Dysrhythmias seen during tracheobronchial suction are mainly due to hypoxia and vagal stimulation. It is thus imperative that the physician and nurse are available when chest physiotherapy is given.

Ventilated children may suffer a rapid loss of muscle mass in ICU due to lack of activity and inadequate nutrition in the presence of high catabolism. It may be severe enough to prevent weaning off a respirator even when the lung condition improves. Physiotherapists can prevent this by specific exercises. They can also chart muscle power and prepare special splints to prevent contractures and deformities in children requiring prolonged stay in PICU (also see Chapter 12).

FLUID AND ELECTROLYTE BALANCE

Fluid and electrolyte balance is crucial to the maintenance of the overall physiologic stability. A comprehensive knowledge of fluid, electrolyte and acid-base therapy is therefore, essential for care of critically ill children. The readers may refer to a recent text on this subject for management of common fluid and electrolyte problems in sick children.

The daily fluid and electrolyte requirement should include – maintenance plus ongoing losses and correction of deficit. The goals of fluid therapy are shown in Table 22.1.

Table 22.1: Goals of fluid-electrolyte therapy

The goals of fluid-electrolyte therapy are to:

1. MAINTAIN	–	normal daily fluid needs
2. REPAIR	–	pre-existing deficits
3. REPLACE	–	continuing abnormal losses
4. CORRECT/MONITOR	–	potential complications

The Replacement should give attention to abnormal GIT losses from diarrhea, vomiting, gastric aspirate, 3rd space loss, and ongoing losses particularly in septic and hypovolemic shock.

The Maintenance fluid should include allowance for urine output and insensible water loss from skin and lungs.

The Repair fluid should address acid base and electrolyte imbalances.

Normal requirement in a healthy child is best calculated based on caloric need or weight. The usual calculation is based on the simplified formula –100 ml/kg for first 10 kg, 50 ml/kg for next 10 kg and 25 ml/kg for the rest of the weight. In critically ill children this needs modification because of lower insensible loss in ICU's thermo neutral environment, humidification in ventilated patients, low or high metabolic rate, fever, sweating and abnormal urine output (Table 22.2).

Table 22.2: Modification in normal water requirement

Increased respiratory loss	Hyperventilation	Increase 5-20 ml/kg
Increased skin loss	Sweating-excessive	Increase 5-25 ml/kg
Increased metabolic rate	Fever	Increase 12% per°C
Decreased urine loss	Oliguria, Anuria	

Note: Fluid requirement is increased in fever, restlessness / delirium, warm ambient temperature. Fluid requirement is decreased in hypothermia, high humidity, oliguria/anuria, reduced consciousness, retention/edema, increased intracranial pressure.

Fluids that are available can be described as being from three categories:

- ***Isotonic-Fluids*** have the same osmolarity as plasma.
  Examples: Normal Saline (NS or 0.9% NaCl), Ringer's Acetate (RA), Ringer's Lactate (RL) These are used to increase ECF, replace acute/abnormal losses.
- ***Hypotonic-Fluids*** have fewer solutes than plasma.
  Examples: Dextrose water, half NS (0.45% NaCl), and D5W (5% dextrose in water) after the sugar is used up.

These fluids increase ICF > ECF, and are used for replacement of normal loss (IWL + urine).

- ***Hypertonic-Fluids*** have more solutes than plasma.
  Examples: 5% Dextrose in Normal Saline (D5 NS), 3% saline solution, D5 in RL. These are used in specific situations as repair solutions or as osmotic agents.

Hypovolemia during intensive care must be corrected with restoration of volume. Maintenance of microvascular blood flow by correction of hypovolemia is essential in improving tissue oxygenation. Crystalloids or colloids can be used to restore the volume as initial fluid. More volume of crystalloid is necessary to maintain intravascular volume because 75% of the administered solution gets distributed to extravascular compartment. If hypovolemia persists after initial fluid bolus, colloids must be used. Only relative contraindication to use of colloids is ARDS or noncardiac pulmonary edema.

Normal saline (0.9%) or Ringer's lactate 20 ml/kg over 5-10 minutes should be under BP and CVP monitoring. Repeated infusions at a rate of 10-20 ml/kg are given as many times as necessary to correct hypovolemia, till CVP is > 10 mmHg or BP is corrected.

Polyuria in ICU

It may be caused by:

1. Central diabetes insipidus—Deficient ADH secretion (idiopathic, trauma, pituitary surgery, hypoxic ischemic encephalopathy).
2. Nephrogenic diabetes insipidus—Renal resistance to ADH (hereditary, hypercalcemia), *cerebral salt wasting* (See Table 22.4).
3. Solute diuresis: Diuretics (furosemide, mannitol), glucosuria, high protein diets, post-obstructive uropathy, resolving ATN.
4. Primary polydipsia–occasional hypothalamic lesion affecting thirst center.

Central Diabetes Insipidus

Diagnosis: is made when there is polyuria, and inappropriately dilute urine (urine osmolality < serum osmolality). It frequently occurs in patients with acute brain injury.

Treatment: Treat hypovolemi shock with saline and start vasopressin infusion—beginning with 0.5 milli units/kg/hour, doubled every 15-30 minutes until urine flow is controlled.

DDAVP (desmopressin) may also be used.

Fluid replacement equal to urine volume should be given.

All patients should be closely monitored for development of hyponatremia/ hypernatremia.

Hypokalemia

Hypokalemia, serum potassium concentration below 3.5 mEq/L, is the most frequent electrolyte disorder seen in a PICU. The possible causes of hypokalemia that are likely to be encountered in the PICU are as follows:

1. Transcellular shift -Potassium movement into cells is facilitated by stimulation of β_2 adrenergic receptors by inhaled ß agonist (bronchodilators), alkalosis (respiratory or metabolic), hypothermia (accidental or induced), and insulin infusion.
2. Potassium depletion/loss- Renal potassium loss is one of the most common causes in PICU-The leading cause of renal potassium wasting is diuretic therapy. Other causes include nasogastric drainage, alkalosis and magnesium depletion. The urinary chloride is low (less than 15 mEq/L) when nasogastric drainage or alkalosis is involved and is high (greater than 25mEq/L) when magnesium depletion or diuretics are responsible. Magnesium depletion impairs potassium reabsorption across the renal tubules and may play a very important role in promoting and sustaining potassium depletion in critically ill patients. The major cause of extra-renal potassium loss is diarrhea.

Table 22.3: Hypokalemia: Signs and symptoms

Non-specific:	Anorexia, nausea, vomiting, polyuria
Neuromuscular:	Paralytic ileus, muscle weakness, respiratory muscle weakness, hypotonia, areflexia
Cardiac:	ECG changes – prominent U – waves, flattening and inversion of T waves, prolongation of QT interval and arrhythmias

Clinical Manifestations: Clinical features of hypokalemia are shown in Table 22.3. Severe hypokalemia, serum K below 2.5 mEq/L, can be accompanied by diffuse muscle weakness; milder degrees of hypokalemia (serum K 2.5 to 3.5 mEq/L) are often asymptomatic. Abnormalities in the ECG including prominent U waves, flattening and inversion of T waves and prolongation of the QT interval can be present in more than half of the cases. QT prolongation can be seen with hypocalcemia and hypomagnesemia as well.

Hypokalemia is often combined with other conditions that can promote arrhythmias (e.g magnesium depletion, digitalis, myocardial ischemia) and thus hypokalemia may enhance the proarrhythmic effects of these other conditions.

Patients with ECG changes, give intravenous potassium 0.25-0.5 mEq/kg/hour, in a solution containing 200 mEq/100 ml of normal saline, under continuous ECG and heart rate monitoring. Serum potassium is checked every hourly, and infusion is discontinued when ECG is normal or serum potassium is 3.0 mEq/L or more.

Hyperkalemia

Hyperkalemia (Serum K-greater than 5.5 mEq/L) can be a serious life –threatening condition.

Pseudohyperkalemia: Potassium released from traumatic hemolysis during the venipuncture can produce a spurious elevation in serum potassium. This is more common than suspected. An unexpected finding of hyperkalemia in an asymptomatic patient should always prompt a repeat measurement before any.diagnostic or therapeutic measures are initiated. Potassium release from cells during clot formation in the specimen tube can also produce pseudohyperkalemia when severe leukocytois (white blood cell count greater than 50,000/mm^3) is present.

Causes: Hyperkalemia can be caused by potassium release from cells or by impaired renal potassium excretion. If the source of the hyperkalemia is unclear, the urinary potassium concentration can be helpful. A high urine potassium (greater than 30mEq/L) suggests a transcellular shift and low urine potassium (less than 30 mEq/L) indicates impaired renal excretion.

A. Transcellular shift can be caused by acidosis, drugs etc. Drugs that can promote hyperkalemia include beta-receptor antagonists and digitalis. Rhabdomyolysis can release large amounts of potassium into extracellular fluid but if renal function is normal the extra potassium is promptly cleared by the kidneys.

B. Impaired renal excretion - Renal insufficiency can produce hyperkalemia when the glomerular filtration rate falls below 10ml/minute or the urine output falls below 1ml/kg/hr.

Adrenal insufficiency is a well known cause of hyperkalemia because of impaired renal potassium excretion. Drugs that impair renal potassium excretion include angiotensin – converting enzyme inhibitors, angiotensin receptor blockers, potassium sparing diuretics and nonsteroidal anti-inflammatory drugs, heparin, cotrimoxazole and pentamidine. All of these agents promote hyperkalemia by inhibiting or blocking the reniin – angiotensin aldosterone system.

Massive blood transfusions can promote hyperkalemia in patients with circulatory shock. The potassium load in blood transfusions normally is cleared by the kidneys and thus sustained rise in plasma potassium occurs because of poor renal perfusion.

Table 22.4: Clinical features and treatment of disorders of serum sodium

Parameter	*SIADH*	*Cerebral salt wasting*	*Diabetes insipidus*
Blood pressure	Normal	Low/postural hypotension	Low/normal
Heart rate	Low/normal	Resting/postural tachycardia	Normal/increased
Body weight (total body water)	Normal/increased	Low	Low/normal
Urea, creatinine	Low/normal	Normal/high	Normal/high
Blood			
Volume (CVP)	Increased	Low	Low
Hematocrit	Low	High	High
[Na+] mEq/L	<135	<135	> 145
Osmolality	<280 mOsm	< 280 mOsm	> 295 mOsm
Urine			
Volume	Low/normal	Normal	Increased
Specific gravity	> 1.010	> 1.010	< 1.004
$[Na^+]$ mEq/L	> 25	> 25	< 25
24-hour secretion of Na+	> 30 mmol	> 30 mmol	< 30 mmol
Osmolality	> serum osmolality	> serum osmolality	< serum osmolality
Treatment Na+	Supplement with 3% NaCl avoid rises in serum $[Na^+]$ > 10 mEq/day	Supplement with 0.9-3% NaCl, depending upon urgency of need to correct	Restrict
Water	Restrict 2/3 of normal	Supplement	Supplement
Others	Furosemide if overloaded	Fludrocortisone 50-100 µg/day	DDAVP 1-4 mg IV, Vasopressin infusion

Clinical manifestations: The clinical features of hypokalemia are shown in Table 22.3. The most serious consequence of hyperkalemia is the slowing of electrical conduction in the heart. The ECG can begin to change when the serum potassium reach 6.0 mEq/L and is always abnormal when the serum potassium reaches 8.0mEq/L. The earliest change in the ECG is a tall, tapering T wave that is most evident in precordial leads V_2 and V_3, as the hyperkalemia progresses , the P wave amplitude decreases and the PR interval lengthens. The P waves eventually disappear and the QRS duration becomes prolonged. The final event is ventricular asystole.

Management: See chapter 14 Acute renal failure

Hyponatremia

The usual signs and symptoms of hyponatremia such as apathy, nausea, vomiting, ataxia etc. are not easily identifiable in sick children. However, severe hyponatremia may manifest with seizures, coma and hypotension. The most common cause of hyponatremia in PICU is syndrome of inappropriate antidiuretic hormone secretions (SIADH) and sodium loss (Table 22.5).

Table 22.5: Causes of hyponatremia in critically ill children

1. ***Impaired water excretion***:
   a. *Elevated vasopressin—SIADH*, because of trauma, infection, malignancy, various medications, CNS disorders, positive pressure ventilation, "Stress".
   b. *Water retention*—in CCF, Acute renal failure, Nephrotic Syndrome, Hepatic failure, etc.
2. ***Salt and Water loss:***
   a. *Renal losses*—diuretic therapy, osmotic diuresis, *D. insipidus*

b. *GI losses*—diarrhea, tube drainage
c. Third space losses
d. Excessive Sweating

3. ***Redistribution (Translocation):***
a. Shift of water from cell–e.g. hyperglycemia, sick cell syndrome
b. Shift of sodium into cell

4. ***Fictitious (Pseudohyponatremia)***: diabetic ketoacidosis, hyperlipidemia

The following questions need to be answered to find the cause of hyponatremia and treat it:

1. Is it true hyponatremia or pseudohyponatremia because of lab. errors (Anion gap <9 mEq), hyperglycemia, hyperlipidemia, hyperproteinemia?
2. Is ECF depleted (Signs of dehydration present, no edema) or is there edema?
3. If no dehydration, no edema–what is urinary specific gravity or sodium excretion?

Hyponatremia with

	Signs of dehydration	*With edema*
Physiology	Due to Na^+ and water losses	Na^+ + water retention Total body Na - increased, Se Na low
Settings	GIT loss, diuresis, Adreno-cortical insufficiency, Cerebral salt wasting (CSW)	Congestive heart failure Nephrotic syndrome, cirrhosis
Treatment	Replace Na & water	Water restriction

If there is no edema and no dehydration SIADH is most likely. The criteria for diagnosis of SIADH are given in Table 22.6.

Table 22.6: Criteria for diagnosis SIADH

By definition, "inappropriate" implies having excluded normal physiologic reasons for release of ADH:
1. In response to hypertonicity.
2. In response to life threatening hypotension

Diagnosis requires demonstration of inappropriately concentrated urine in face of hyponatremia, and exclusion of normal physiologic release of ADH .

- Hyponatremia (Serum Na < 135 mEq/L)
- Low serum osmolality (< 280 mOsm/L)
- High Urinary Na+ (>20 mEq/L)
- Urine Osmolality > Serum osmolality
- Normal adrenal and renal function
- Absence of peripheral edema or dehydration

Principles of Correction of Hyponatremia

1. Ascertain whether hyponatremia is acute or chronic.
2. Is it asymptomatic vs symptomatic.
3. ***If acute symptomatic hyponatremia*** give correction with 3% saline, 5 ml/kg, (range) 1-2 ml/kg, maximum 12 ml/kg [rate 1 ml/min]. *If symptomatic with seizures*, immediately increase serum sodium by 5 mEq/L. Next, correct sodium to 125-130 mEq/L, the deficit is equal to (0.6) (weight[kg]) (125-measured sodium).
Rate of correction of serum Na^+-must not exceed an increase in serum Na^+ by 0.5 mEq/hr or 10 mEq in 24 hrs and 20 mEq per 48 hours.
4. ***Treatment of CSW***—Water and salt supplementation, and Fludrocortisone 0.05– 0.2 mg per day to minimise salt wasting.

Specific aspects of clinical features and treatment of some hyponatremic disorders is given in Table 22.4.

In PICU, two particularly critical electrolytes are calcium (Ca) and magnesium (Mg). Abnormalities of either occur frequently in critically ill children and can precipitate serious and potentially life threatening problems. Hypocalcemia and hypo- and hypermagnesemia are both associated with increased mortality and prolonged hospital stay.

Magnesium

Magnesium is essential in maintenance of several cellular functions through its role in activation of adenosine triphosphate (ATP). ***Hypomagnesemia*** is associated with prolonged PR interval, widened QRS-ocomplex, ST segment depression and low amplitude T-wave on ECG. It may potentiate dysrhythmia from hypocalcemia and digitalis toxicity. ***Hypermagnesemia*** produces tall peaked T-waves and narrow QRS complexes. Normal serum Mg concentration range between 1.5-1.9 mEq/L. Mg deficiency frequently develops in a wide variety of clinical conditions such as protein energy malnutrition, malabsorption, hypo-albuminemia, sepsis, following prolonged gastrointestinal suctioning, diarrhea, blood transfusion, catecholamine excess, aminoglycoside therapy, osmotic diuresis, use of diuretics etc. which are operative in ICU patients. We found that 60% PICU patients had serum Mg <1.4 mEq/L and PICU stay is significantly longer in hyper- and hypomagnesemic patients as compared to those with normal Mg. Refractory hypokalemia is a prominent feature of hypomagnesemia. Intractable arrhythmias, muscle weakness–including respiratory muscle weakness, neuromuscular excitability, seizures, and ECG changes such as prolonged QT interval on ECG are other features.

Daily intravenous administration of 0.25-0.3 mEq/kg can prevent Mg^{++} deficiency. Most patients with symptomatic magnesium depletion and normal renal function have an estimated deficit of 1 to 2 mEq/kg. About twice the estimated magnesium deficit is replaced at a rate of 1 mEq/kg for the first 24 hours and 0.5 mEq/kg/day for the next 3 to 5 days. Magnesium sulfate 50% solution provides 4 mEq/ml of elemental magnesium.

Hypermagnesemia is treated with diuretics, calcium gluconate 0.5-1 ml/kg infusion and if needed dialysis.

Calcium

Calcium in the ionized from is essential for myocardial contractility. It is also involved in control of vascular tone, mediation of action of several drugs and hormones, and function of skeletal muscles.

Normal range of serum total calcium concentration is 8.5 to 10.2 mg/dL Or 2.1 to 2.5 mM/L and ionized calcium 4.8 to 7.2 mg/dl Or 1.1 to 1.8 mM/L. It is difficult to predict ionized Ca levels from total serum Ca, even after corrections for proteins, albumin or pH.

Sepsis is often associated with hypocalcemia, ***Hypocalcemia*** may occur when calcium is chelated e.g. after blood transfusion. Changes in acid-base status may also alter total and ionized calcium values. Hypocalcemia was seen in 35% of our PICU patients at admission and another 13% developed it during PICU stay. The incidence of ionized hypocalcemia in our patients was 32.2 episodes /100 patient days. Hypocalcemia is often a laboratory diagnosis because the clinical manifestations are minimal or absent (Table 22.7). The manifestations that do surface are caused by neuromuscular excitability and decreased cardiac contractility. There is little evidence that hyperreflexia, tetany, and seizures as consequences of hypocalcemia, actually occur in the clinical setting of ICU. Mild degree of hypocalcemia (ionized calcium upto 0.8 mM or 3.2 mg/dL) are usually asymptomatic in the critically ill patient. One should treat hypocalcemia if symptomatic or if the ionized calcium concentration decreases to <0.8 mM. Hypocalcemia

Table 22.7: Signs and symptoms of hypocalcemia

Nervous system: Parasthesia, fasciculations, muscle spasm, Chvostek's and Trousseau's signs, tetany; irritability, movement disorders, seizures, organic brain syndrome, psychosis

Pulmonary: Bronchospasm

Cardiovascular: Arrhythmias, hypertension or hypotension (*Hypotension refractory to fluids and inotropes – think of hypocalcemia*), congestive heart failure.

Gastrointestinal: Dysphagia, abdominal pain, biliary colic

Symptomatic ionised hypocalcemia presents with neurological and cardiovascular features. All signs and symptoms may not be evident in a given clinical setting.

should be considered and treated in patients with hypotension refractory to fluids and pressor agents. The dose is 0.5-1.0 ml/kg of calcium-gluconate over 5-10 minutes followed by a continuous infusion 0.1-0.2 ml/kg/hour (equal to 0.5 to 2 mg/hr/kg).

Bolus dose of calcium increases the serum-ionized calcium concentration for a short period of time (1 to 2 hrs). One should monitor ionized calcium concentrations every 1 to 4 hrs. Concentration usually normalizes over 2 to 4 hrs with this regimen. Thereafter, maintenance rate of elemental calcium should be given at rate of 0.3 to 0.5 mg/kg/hr. Calcium chloride–10% soln, contains 1.36 mEq/ml or 27 mg/ml and calcium gluconate-10% soln, 0.45 mEq/ml or 9 mg/ml.

Ionised Ca and Mg should be routinely monitored together with Na, K, Cl in all ICU admissions, and abnormal levels must be corrected.

Hypophosphatemia

Hypophosphatemia (Serum phosphate less than 2.5 mg/dl) is uncommon. The usual causes are hyperglycemic hyperosmolar state, diabetic ketoacidosis, sepsis, stimulation of beta adrenergic receptors and respiratory alkalosis.

Clinical Features

Muscle: Muscle weakness, rhabdomyolysis, cardiomyopathy

CNS : Lethargy, seizures

Hematological: Decreased RBC ATP, hemolysis.

Treatment

Hypophosphatemia should be treated when serum $PO_4 < 1$ mg/dL or if it is symptomatic.

Parenteral: Sodium or potassium phosphate infusion (each of these provide 93 mg/mL) in a dose of 0.6 mg/kg body weight per hour. In mild hypophosphatemia with symptoms (serum $PO_4 < 2$ mg/dL) the dose is 0.9 mg/kg/hour.

Serum phosphate should be monitored in such patients 6 hourly. Once the patient is asymptomatic or serum $PO_4 > 2$ mg/dL oral replacement or phosphate retention enemas may be used.

BLOOD RED CELL AND PLATELET TRANSFUSION

Anemia is very common in critically ill patients; almost 95% of patients admitted to the intensive care unit (ICU) have a hemoglobin level below normal by ICU day 3. As a result, critically ill patients receive a significant number of RBC transfusions during their ICU stay.

More than 50% of all patients admitted to the ICU are transfused during their ICU stay. In the patients with a prolonged ICU length of stay, 85% received a transfusion.

A major factor contributing to anemia and the need for blood transfusion in the critically ill patient is phlebotomy.

Red blood cell production in critically ill patients is often abnormal, and a decreased RBC production factors into the development and maintenance of anemia observed in the critically ill. There is a growing literature suggesting that the anemia observed in the critically ill is an under-production anemia consistent with what is commonly referred to as the anemia of chronic inflammatory disease.

The expected benefit from RBC transfusion is to improve oxygen delivery, and thus prevent cellular injury. However, it has been difficult to demonstrate this benefit in clinical practice. Studies that compared a liberal transfusion strategy (hemoglobin 10 to 12 grams per deciliter with a transfusion trigger of 10.0 g/dL) to a restrictive transfusion strategy (hemoglobin 7.0 to 9.0 grams per deciliter with a transfusion trigger of 7.0 g/dL) found that restrictive strategy was at least equivalent and possibly superior in some patients (patients who were less ill) to a more liberal transfusion strategy.

Blood transfusion is currently indicated in those with active blood loss or if hemoglobin is below 10 g/dl. Active blood loss must be replaced volume for volume with whole blood. When clotting deficiency is suspected reconstituted blood (packed red cells + fresh frozen plasma) is preferable. Increasing patient's blood volume acutely by infusion of whole blood by an amount within 5% of estimated total blood volume per single transfusion is unlikely to produce circulatory over-load. However, CVP monitoring should be done.

RBC Transfusions are indicated in normovolemic patients who require an increase in oxygen carrying capacity, and oxygen delivery to tissues, particularly if excessive volume would be poorly tolerated. Studies have demonstrated that in septic shock patients, maximizing oxygen delivery to supranormal level by using fluid boluses, packed red cells and inotropes, have significant impact on ICU mortality. Pack cell transfusions (8-10 ml/kg over 1-2 hours) have been shown to improve oxygen delivery to tissues in children with septic shock whose mean hemoglobin was < 10 gm/dl.

If the patient needs RBC or blood transfusion, normal saline is the only fluid that should be used concurrently. Dextrose is hypotonic and may cause hemolysis; Ringer's lactate contains calcium which may cause clotting.

Indications for platelet transfusions

Active bleeding: In the presence of active bleeding other than ecchymoses or petechiae, platelet transfusion is indicated when:

- The platelet count is below 50,000 µ/L and there is no contraindication to platelet transfusion
- The platelet count is below 100,000/ µ/L and the bleeding is intracranial or there is a condition that impairs platelet adhesion (e.g. renal failure)

Prophylactic platelet transfusion: When there is no evidence of active bleeding other than ecchymotic, petechial hemorrhages and there is thrombocytopenia from bone marrow suppression prophylactic transfusion is indicated when

- The platelet count is < 10,000 µ/L
- The platelet count is <20,000 µ/L and there is a risk of hemorrhage
- The platelet count is <50,000 µ/L and invasive procedures such endoscopic biopsy, lumbar puncture, liver biopsy and major surgery is to be performed.

Central venous cannulation can be done safely in patient with platelet with counts down up to 10,000/ µL. More important is the expertise of the person doing the procedure.

Contraindication to platelet transfusion

Patients with thrombotic thrombocytopenic purpura, and heparin-induced thrombocytopenia because transfused platelets can aggravate the tendency for thrombosis in these conditions.

INFECTION CONTROL

Infection control is the most important concern of all those involved in delivery of intensive care especially more so in our set-up. Presence of serious underlying disease, invasive diagnostic and therapeutic procedures, and indwelling vascular catheters make patients in ICU at high risk of hospital acquired infection. Tracheal intubation also provides a conduit which bypasses normal defence mechanisms of upper airway, interferes with ciliary function and permits passage of organisms from supraglottic/oral flora directly to the lungs.

Respiratory and catheter related infections constitute the major portion of nosocomial infections observed in PICU. The most common infections observed by us are lower respiratory infections (pneumonia), bacteremia, urinary tract infections, and wound infections. The organisms commonly involved are *Klebsiella pneumoniae*, *Pseudomonas*, *Acinetobactor* and *Staphyloco-*

ccus aureus. Candida infections either as fungemia or disseminated infection are also common. CNS infections occur in about one fourth of the patients on intracranial monitoring devices. UTI occur in up to one third of all catheterized patients.

To prevent infections, strict anti-infection protocol must be developed. These should address to hand washing, using of clean linen and changing of soiled linen, strict asepsis before invasive procedures, catheterization and tracheal or oropharyngeal suction, care of IV sites, periodic change of indwelling cannula, catheters, IV infusion equipment, sterilization of ventilation accessories, patient circuits, humidifiers etc. We routinely cover all IV and cannula connections and ports with sterile dressing.

Routine microbiological surveillance of PICU and of individual patients for oropharyngeal and tracheal secretions, and urine and blood may be practiced to keep a check on infections. Colonization of buccal mucosa appears to be the crucial antecedent to endotracheal colonization in children.

Of all the methods of prevention of nosocomial infection, none is as important as single hand washing between patient contacts. All aseptic precautions (including gowning, mask) must be observed in insertion of intravascular catheters and other invasive procedures (Please also see Chapter 12 and the Appendix). Some measures may help specifically in prevention of pneumonia in ventilated patients. In patients who are receiving enteral feeding, use of intermittent rather than continuous nasogastric feeding, and the use of a prophylactic regime designed to prevent endogenous colonization of oral mucosa with Gram negative bacteria have been shown to be very effective in decreasing lower airway infections and resultant mortality. The regimen consists of oral application of non absorbable antibiotics (i.e. polymixin-2%, tobramycin, and amphotericin B-2%), administration of the same antibiotics through gastric tube four times a day and intravenous Cefotaxime 50-100 mg/kg daily during first 3 days.

PSYCHOLOGICAL SUPPORT

The goal of PICU team should be directed toward prompt and painless recovery with minimum disruption of the family structure. Treatment of children in various stages of social, emotional and physical development is unique to pediatric intensive care. An assessment of pain, anxiety and fear suffered by the child, based on previous experience must be made, and steps taken to reduce each of these stresses. Pain control is one area, which is often over looked in young children.

Support to child's environment should become an integral part of the child's care. Interaction between family and care givers regarding child's treatment and progress is also important in critical care. This helps parents to accept decisions better. Presence of one of the parents all the time with a critically ill child should be encouraged. The familiar face and voice of parents to a child who responds to stimuli, is very reassuring and promotes feeling of familiarity. It helps the child to adjust to the new surroundings and takes away anxiety and fear of the unknown. Parents are also valuable observers, and can greatly help in nursing care such as changing the wet sheets and clothes, and changing the posture. The active participation by parents in their child's care also helps the parents understand the situation better and cope with the emotional stress. During the process of recovery, presence of parents and their interaction with the child may simulate a home environment, which may greatly accelerate a child's recovery from trauma and stress of hospitalization.

Chapter twenty-three

Fever in the ICU

Practice guideline from the Society of Critical Care Medicine proposes that a body temperature above 38.3°C (101°F) represents a fever and deserves further evaluation to search for an infection. The appearance of hospital acquired fever in PICU patient requires attention.

Fever vs. Hyperthermia

Hyperthermia is the result of abnormal temperature regulation in the body while fever is a condition where the thermo-regulatory system is intact but is operating at a higher set point. Fever is the result of inflammatory cytokines and is an adaptive response.

Fever is a sign of inflammation, not infection. The distinction is important not only for the evaluation of fever, but also for curtailing the use of antibiotics to treat a fever. The severity of the fever is not an indication of the presence or severity of infection. High fevers can be associated with noninfectious process (e.g. drug fever), while fever can be mild or absent in patients with life-threatening infections.

Where to Measure Temperature

Rectal temperatures in infants and children provide an accurate reflection of core body temperature. Oral temperatures measured in intubated patients can also be a close approximation of core body temperature when electronic probes are placed in the right or left sublingual pockets. Axillary temperatures are on an average 1-2°C below oral temperatures.

Causes of Fever in a PICU

Any condition capable of triggering systemic inflammatory/immune response is capable of causing a fever. The common conditions associated with hospital-acquired fever in medical-surgical PICUs are - pneumonia, catheter associated sepsis, drug fever, urosepsis, translocation, sinusitis, wound infection in post-operative patients, etc. and less commonly pulmonary embolism, deep vein thrombosis, meningitis, bowel infarction, acalculous cholecystitis, endocarditis, pericarditis, etc.

Common Nosocomial Infections

Four infections account for over three-quarters of the nosocomial infections in PICU patients: pneumonia, urinary tract infections, bloodstream infections, and surgical site infections. Three of these infections are primarily related to indwelling devices. The pathogenic organisms isolated in three of the common nosocomial infections are: *Kleb. pneumoniae, Acinetobactor, Staphylococcus aureus* and *Pseudomonas aeruginosa Candida albicans,* are the most common isolates in our setup. E.coli and *Candida albicans* are the most common isolates in urinary tract infections.

Catheter Sepsis: Infections caused by indwelling vascular catheters should be suspected in any case of unexplained fever when a catheter has been in place for more than 48 hours, or when purulence is found at the catheter insertion site. If the patient appears toxic, or there is purulence the catheter should be removed and a distal segment of catheter should be sent for cultures. If the patient is not seriously ill and there is no purulence at the catheter insertion site catheter can be left in place. The decision to initiate empiric antibiotic therapy depends on the clinical condition of the patient. If there are no signs of severe sepsis antibiotics can be withheld. If empiric antibiotic therapy is needed, coverage for staphylococci is mandatory.

Pneumonia: Nosocomial pneumonia in the PICU is mainly a disease of patients on ventilator. Pneumonia should be suspected when there is a new infiltrate on chest x-ray and two of the following conditions are present: fever, leukocytosis, and purulent tracheal secretions. For more details please see chapter- Pneumonia in ICU.

Urinary Tract Infections: Urinary tract infection should be suspected as a cause of nosocomial fever in any patient with an indwelling bladder catheter for more than a few days. The demonstration of pyuria by gram stain or leukocyte esterase dipstick test can help in early identification of such.

Pseudomembranous Enterocolitis(antibiotic Associated Colitis): Enterocolitis from *Clostridium difficile* should be suspected for cases of nosocomial fever accompanied by diarrhea in patients who have received antibiotics within 2 weeks prior to the onset of the fever. Documentation of *C. difficile* toxin in stool samples or evidence of pseudomembranes on proctosigmoidoscopy is diagnostic. Empiric antibiotic (oral or intravenous metronidazole or oral vancomycin) is necessary if diarrhea is severe or the patient appears toxic.

Wound Infections: Wound infections typically appear at 5 to 7 days after surgery. Antimicrobial therapy should be reserved for cases of persistent erythema or for evidence of deep tissue involvement. Necrotizing wound infections that are produced by Clostridia or β-*hemolytic Streptococci* are evident in the first few postoperative days. Skin may have crepitance and fluid –filled bullae. Spread to deeper structures is rapid and produces progressive rhabdomyolysis. Treatment involves extensive debridement and intravenous penicillin. The mortality is high when treatment is delayed.

Postoperative abdominal abscesses typically become symptomatic at one to two weeks after laparotomy. Computed tomography will reveal the localized collection in more than 95% of cases. Initial antimicrobial therapy should be directed at gram-negative enteric pathogens, including anaerobes *Bacteroides fragilis*. Definitive treatment requires surgical or percutaneous drainage.

Other Infections: Endocarditis in patients with prosthetic valves, meningitis in neurosurgical patients and those with human immunodeficiency virus infection and spontaneous bacterial peritonitis in patients with ascites.

Noninfectious Causes

Systemic Inflammatory response Syndrome (SIRS): Possible sources of sign of systemic inflammation (e.g.,fever, leukocytosis) without evidence of infection include trauma, ischemia, or toxic insults, and translocation of endotoxins and bacterial antigens from the lumen of the gastrointestinal tract.

Drug Fever: Drug-induced fever can be the result of a hypersensitivity reaction, an idiosyncratic reaction, or an infusion-related phlebitis. Drug fever is a recognized entity in the PICU, but the significance and prevalence of this entity in the PICU is not known.

Drugs that are commonly associated with fever in a PICU are: cephalosporins, penicillins, amphotericin, phenytoin, and less commonly, vancomycin, cimetidine, carbamazepine, and rifampin.

Blood Transfusions

Postoperative Fever: Fever on the first day following major surgery is reported in about one-fourth of patients. In most of these cases there is no associated infection. It usually resolves within 24 to 48 hours. *Malignant Hyperthermia* is an inherited disorder characterized by intense muscle rigidity and hyperthermia in response to halogenated inhalational anesthetics and depolarizing neuromuscular blockers succinylcholine. It is seen in the immediate postoperative period.

Hemodialysis: Febrile reactions during hemodialysis are attributed to endotoxins contamination of the dialysis equipment, but bacteremia occurs on some occassions. Blood cultures are recommended for all. Empiric antibiotics are recommended only for patients who appear septic. Vancomycin plus ceftazidime should suffice pending culture results.

Bronchoscopy: Fiberoptic bronchoscopy is followed by fever in 5% of cases Fever usually appears 8 to 10 hours after the procedure, and it subsides spontaneously in 24 hours. The fever is often associated with leukocytosis but pneumonia and bacteremia are rare. Blood cultures or empiric antimicrobial therapy is needed only if the fever does not subside.

Venous Thromboembolism: Acute pulmonary embolism can produce a fever that lasts up to 1 week. Most cases of hospital-acquired deep vein thrombosis are asymptomatic.

Acalculous Cholecystitis: Acalculous cholecystitis is an uncommon but serious disorder reported in up to 1.5% of critically ill adults. This condition is believed to be the result of ischemia and stasis within the gallbladder, eventually leading to edema of the cystic duct that blocks drainage of the gallbladder. The clinical manifestations include fever and right upper quadrant tenderness. Diagnosis is possible with right upper quadrant ultrasound examination. The treatment of choice is cholecystostomy, or percutaneous cholecystostomy in patients who are too ill for surgery.

Endocrine Disorder known to produce fever in a PICU is adrenal crisis, which is a recognized complication of severe sepsis, disseminated intravascular coagulation (DIC) and anticoagulant therapy.

Infarction: Ischemic injury in any organ will trigger a local inflammatory response. Common ones are distal infarcts of extremities because of severe sepsis and vasculitis, and bowel infarction with abdominal sepsis. Myocardial and cerebrovascular infarctions are usually heralded by other symptoms, but can be clinically silent in patients with depressed consciousness.

Management Decisions

Blood Cultures

Blood cultures should be obtained whenever an infection is suspected. No more than one set of blood cultures is needed from each venipuncture site.

Empiric Antimicrobial Therapy

Empiric antibiotic therapy is indicated in the following situations:

When the likelihood of infection is high.

When there is evidence of severe sepsis or severe organ dysfunction (e.g. depressed consciousness, progressive hypoxemia, hypotension, metabolic acidosis, or decreasing urine output).

When the patient is immunocompromised

Empiric antibiotic therapy should be selected on the basis of antibiotic susceptibility patterns in each ICU. Empire coverage for gram-negative infections can include either a carbapenem; imipenem or meropenem, an anti-pseudomonal cephalosporin: ceftazidime or cefipime, ticarcillin-clavulnate, or piperacillin-tazobactam. In immunocompromised patients an aminoglycoside can be added for gram-negative coverage. *(For more details see chapter "Severe infections: diagnosis and antibiotics").*

Antipyretic Therapy

Prostaglandin E is believed to mediate the febrile response to endogenous. Drugs that interfere with prostaglandin E synthesis are effective in reducing fever. These drugs include paracetamol, aspirin and the nonsteroidal anti-inflammatory agents (NSAIDS). The usual dose of paracetamol for fever suppression is 15mg/kg every 4-6 hourly orally, by rectal suppository, or intravenous route. Ibuprofen may be used 10mg/kg every 6 hours.

In brief, in a child with new onset fever in PICU use a stepwise approach that begins by examining the patient to assess the severity of the condition. Next evaluate if anything has been done to the patient in the past 24 to 48 hours (e.g. a procedure, a change in drug therapy). If this does not give a clue, then use the patient's clinical condition to identify possible sources of the fever. Start antibiotics only if an infection is apparent or highly suspected or the patient is immuno compromised.

Chapter twenty-four

Acute Lung Injury and Acute Respiratory Distress Syndrome

ARDS was first described as adult respiratory distress syndrome in 1967 by Ashbaugh, as a syndrome of severe respiratory failure associated with pulmonary infiltrates similar to that seen in infantile respiratory distress syndrome (hyaline membrane disease).

ARDS is now recognized as a severe form of acute lung injury caused by a large number of systemic or pulmonary illness, and is defined in terms of severity of gas exchange defect.

Characteristically patients with ARDS have bilateral pulmonary infiltrates on chest X-ray (CXR), impaired oxygenation resulting in a ratio of PaO_2 to FiO_2 less than 200 and the absence of elevated pulmonary arterial occlusion pressure (PAOP) or left atrial pressure. Patients with acute lung injury (ALI) have a PaO_2/FiO_2 ratio <300, other features being similar to ARDS. In other words, ALI and ARDS is presence of pulmonary edema in the absence of volume overload or depressed left ventricular function.

Pathology and Pathophysiology

The basic pathology is widespread damage and loss of the integrity of the alveolocapillary membrane (diffuse alveolar damage), increased permeability of the membrane to plasma and resultant fluid accumulation within the airspaces of the lung (Exudative phase, noncardiogenic pulmonary edema). Fluid in alveolar space disrupts the function of pulmonary surfactant resulting in microatelectasis and impaired gas exchange. The lung becomes stiff and compliance decreases. Ultimately, regional variations in pulmonary perfusion, V/Q mismatch, shunting of blood through underventilated alveoli and an increased alveolar-arterial oxygen gradient occur resulting in hypoxemia resistant to oxygen therapy (Fig. 24.1). Initial inflammation, edema, and atelectasis rapidly progress to fibrosis in many patients. (Proliferative and fibrotic stages).

Causes

A number of clinical conditions have been associated with the development of ARDS (Table 24.1). These causes act by different mechanisms, such as: direct endothelial damage, decrease and alteration of surfactant, cellular damage by mediators of inflammation (cytokines, complement, products of coagulation, metabolites of arachidonic acid, proteases, and free oxygen radicals), and the activation of platelets and leucocytes. Direct damage to alveolocapillary membrane occurs becuase of diffuse injury to alveolar epithelium in pneumonia, aspiration pneumonia, pulmonary contusion, near-drowning and smoke inhalation injury, while in conditions like severe sepsis, severe trauma, fractures, multiple transfusions, tricyclic antidepressants and sedatives overdosage the damage is mainly due to a widespread systemic response causing endothelial damage.

Table 24.1: Causes of ALI and ARDS

Causes of acute lung injury

Direct	*Indirect*
Smoke/toxin inhalation	Severe Sepsis
Aspiration of gastric contents	Systemic Inflammation and multiple organ dysfunction syndrome
Near drowning	Anaphylaxis
Thoracic trauma	Cardiopulmonary bypass
Diffuse pulmonary infections, pneumonia	Neurogenic pulmonary edema
	Non-thoracic trauma
	Pancreatitis
	Massive transfusion
	Air embolism, Fat embolism

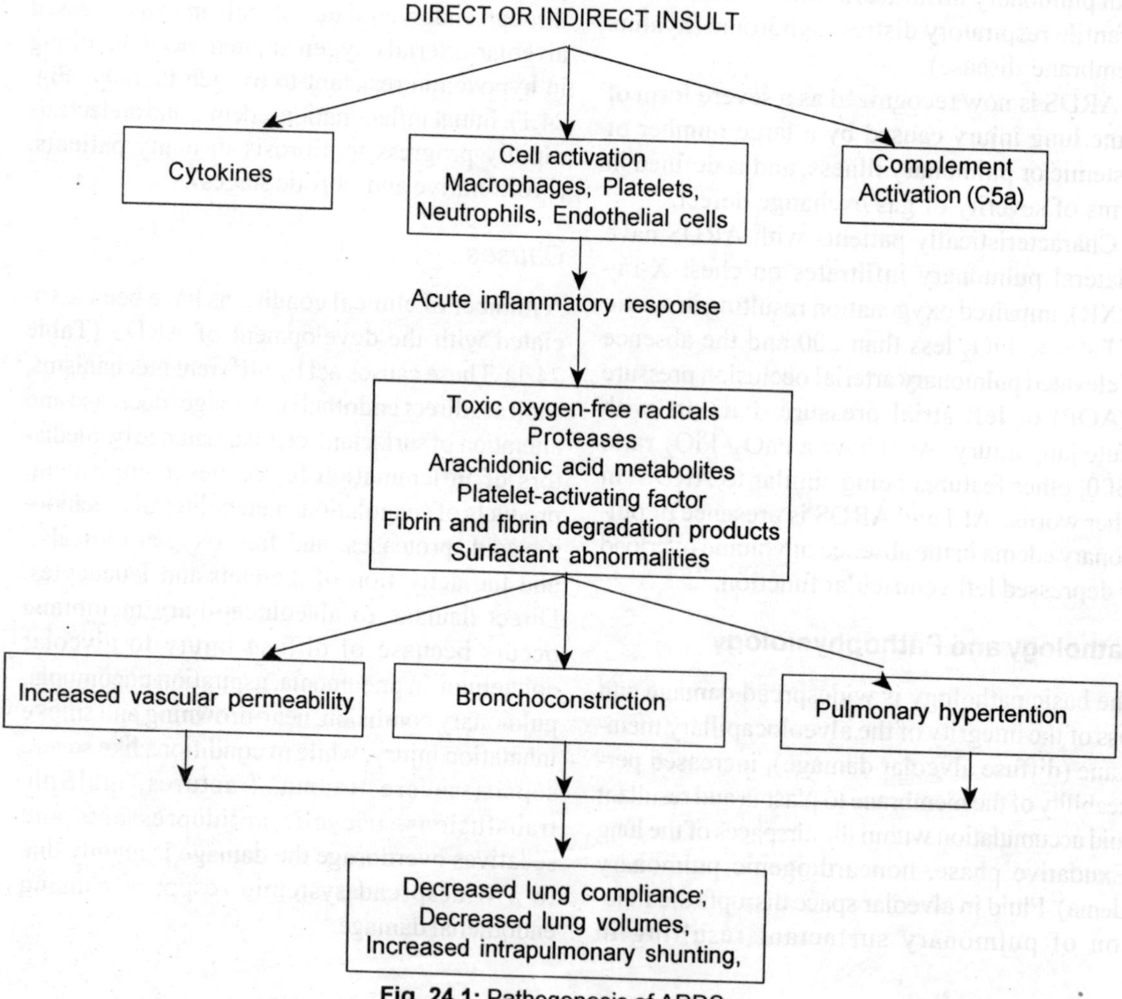

Fig. 24.1: Pathogenesis of ARDS

Severe sepsis and the systemic inflammatory response syndrome (SIRS) are the most common predisposing conditions. These are thought to result from systemic neutrophil-derived inflammatory mediators and the mediators in the lung . Severe trauma, especially multiple fractures, also causes ARDS through SIRS. Long bone fractures may result in ARDS through fat embolism. ARDS in association with head injury is thought to result from sudden discharge of the sympathetic nervous system, resulting in both acute pulmonary hypertension and injury to the pulmonary capillary bed. Multiple transfusions are another important risk factor, independent of the reason for transfusion or coexistence of trauma. The incidence of ARDS increases with the number of units transfused. Pre-existing liver disease or coagulation abnormalities further contribute to this risk.

Near-drowning victims can develop ARDS. Infiltrates and hypoxia develop in 12-24 hours after the initial accident. Aspiration of water leads to an osmotic gradient favoring the movement of water into the airspaces of the lung. Pulmonary contusions result in ARDS through direct trauma to the lung as also the infectious pneumonia and aspiration of gastric contents. Damage to lung tissue by smoke inhalation results from direct thermal damage to the lungs, toxic damage from chemicals and the effect of particulate matter carried into the lower lung. Narcotics overdose, salicylates, tricyclic antidepressants and other sedatives, and several toxins and drugs have been associated with the development of ARDS. This risk is independent of the risk from concurrent aspiration.

Clinical Features

Patients may present early in the course of the disease without symptoms or signs. Mild tachypnea may be the only manifestation. With time, severe respiratory distress ensues. On physical examination crepitations are often heard on both the lung fields; however, physical findings are usually minimal in early stage. Signs of volume overload, including an S3 on auscultation of the heart or jugular venous distention, are noticeably absent. In the later stages patient may show increased work of breathing and signs of hypoxemia—restlessness, agitation, pallor or cyanosis; diminished breath sounds and/or bronchial breathing.

Patients with smoke inhalation may initially be asymptomatic and should be monitored closely for the development of ARDS. In early stages ARDS may be confused with infectious pneumonia in a patient with sepsis and septic shock, aspiration syndromes, congestive cardiac failure, irritant inhalation pneumonia.

An ABG will usually reveal early in the course of the disease low $PaCO_2$ (<35 mmHg) and a respiratory alkalosis may be present. As the disease progresses, hypercarbia and respiratory acidosis develop. Hypoxemia, gradually getting refractory to oxygen therapy sets in because of V/Q mismatch, shunting and diffusion abnormality. A complete blood count (CBC), serum electrolytes, blood urea nitrogen and creatinine should be obtained. In cases of severe ARDS without a discernable cause, appropriate cultures should be obtained, as sepsis is the most common cause.

Imaging Studies

Early in the course of the disease the chest x-ray may be normal. Chest radiography most often shows bilateral diffuse parenchymal infiltrates, a normal sized cardiac silhouette and the absence of vascular redistribution. The chest X-ray rapidly progresses to complete white-out of both lung fields (Fig. 24.2).

Management

The syndrome has been frustratingly resistant to treatment, and no specific therapy has proved beneficial. Although recent case series suggest

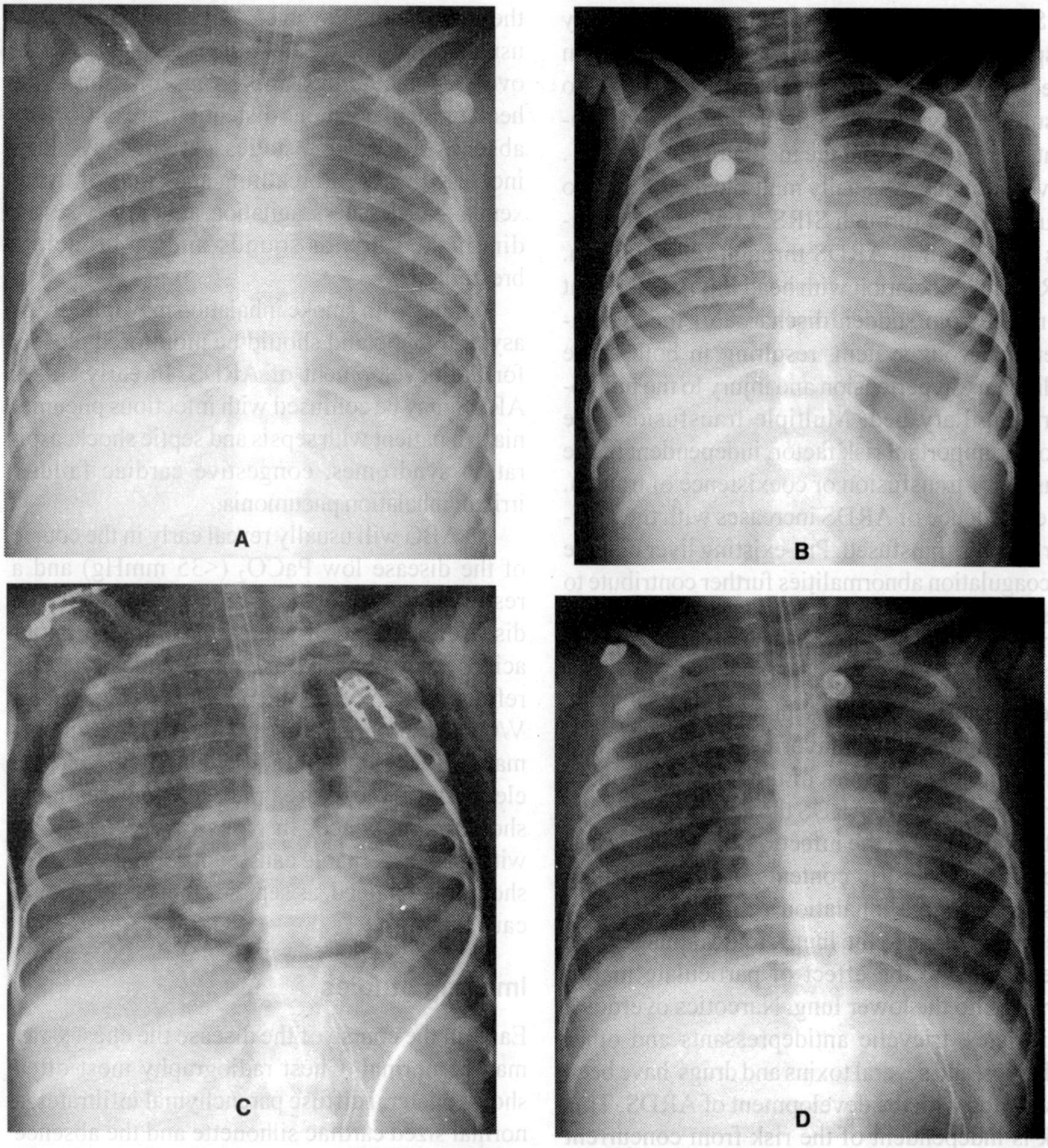

Fig. 24.2: X-ray showing (A) Pneumonia progressing to (B) white-out of both lungs consistent with ARDS (C) Airleaks with ARDS and (D) At recovery in same patient

some decrease in mortality over the past decade, the death rate remains about 25-40 percent.

All patients with significant risk factors for the development of ARDS, as listed above, should be admitted to the hospital, and those with dyspnea or tachypnea should be admitted to an intensive monitoring unit. A consultation with an Intensivist is mandatory for all such patients, particularly, those having high inspired oxygen requirement to ensure early identification of patients with

ARDS. ICU admission is mandatory for patients with respiratory alkalosis, hypoxia or findings on CXR.

Management of the patient is largely supportive. An IV line should be started and the patient should receive fluids if hypotensive. Intensive respiratory support and hemodynamic monitoring are essential. Patient should be attached to a cardiac monitor, pulse-oximeter and non-invasive BP cuff monitor. As volume overload in the presence of ARDS may significantly worsen pulmonary edema, volume status must be continually assessed and maintained at the lowest level that is consistent with adequate systemic perfusion.

Patients should be placed on sufficient supplemental O_2 to keep the oxygen saturation above 90%. If the oxygen saturation drops or the patient develops fatigue or hypercarbia, endotracheal intubation should be performed. Mechanical ventilation is needed invariably. The ventilator settings should aim to maintain oxygenation and ventilation, while minimizing the effects of barotrauma on the lung. If oxygen saturation cannot be kept above 90% after institution of mechanical ventilation, PEEP should be added in small increments (2 cm H_2O at a time). As higher airway pressures may decrease venous return and lead to hypotension, care should be taken to monitor and treat the patient's hemodynamic status.

Mechanical Ventilation

When considering approaches to mechanical ventilation in these patients it is useful to understand the underlying alterations in pulmonary mechanics that are characteristic of ARDS. The *Functional Residual Capacity (FRC) is reduced* and Closing Capacity is above FRC. This results in airway closure during normal tidal breathing leading to *alveolar collapse, V/Q mismatch*, and progressive hypoxemia. Resistance is normal or near normal as is anatomic dead space. The defect is usually one of oxygenation rather than ventilation. The *total compliance of the lung is reduced.* The involvement is non-homogeneous, patchy and transient, with wide variation in regional time constants and occurs primarily in dependent portions of the lung. As little as 25% of the lung may be participating in gas exchange. Those areas that remain are normally compliant and therefore are subject to overdistension when subjected to excessive inflating pressures.

Some basic assumptions must be accepted while setting up mechanical ventilation in ARDS. First, the high positive pressures causes pulmonary injury (barotrauma) and alveolar hyperinflation causes volutrauma. Peak alveolar pressures are probably most important in producing overdistension and injury. Second, very high oxygen concentrations are injurious to the lung. The higher the concentration the greater and more rapid the lung injury. Third, repeated closing and reopening (stretching) of collapsed alveoli may be injurious to the lung independent of overdistension or oxygen concentration ("shear" injury). And fourth, an increase in dead space to tidal volume ratio precludes the use of high rates to compensate for small tidal volumes.

In summary, lung damage may occur from regional over distention of lung units related to high ventilatory volumes and pressures and from cyclic closing and reopening of collapsed alveoli with resultant shear injury. Ventilation strategies should therefore be such that avoid regional overdistention and alveolar collapse with each assisted breath, and allow reopening of collapsed alveoli and keeping alveoli open (recruitment). This is done by avoiding high peak positive pressure or volume and through use of PEEP.

Traditionally ventilatory strategies were aimed at correction of hypoxia and avoidance of hypercarbia and respiratory acidosis. But lately, controlled hypoventilation with permissive hypercapnia ($paCO_2$>100 mmHg and pH >7.2) is being practiced to avoid need for high peak airway pressures and FiO_2 >0.6 as part of lung protective strategy (Also see Chapter 7).

Table 24.2: Possible adverse effects of permissive hypercapnia

Adverse Effect	*Mechanism*
Impaired oxygenation	-Decreased airway pressures -Effect on alveolar gas equation -Shift of O_2 dissociation curve
Haemodynamic (Increased HR, PVR, SVR)	-Catecholamine surge
Increased intracerebral pressure	-Direct vasodilation
Increased need for sedation/paralysis	-Increased ventilatory drive -Uncomfortable ventilatory modes
Delayed weaning	- Skeletal muscle weakness
Decreased oxygen delivery	- Myocardial depression
Renal failure	- Decreased renal blood flow
Less responsive to inotropic drugs, cardioversion and antibiotics	- Intracellular acidosis
Decreased seizure threshold	- Intracellular acidosis

Optimal Ventilatory Mode

The volume regulated pressure controlled ventilation is most appropriate way to maintain safe pressure and volume limits. Intermittent mandatory ventilation is preferred by some over and above the assist control mode because of the decreased risk of barotrauma. Ventilation strategies designed to limit airway pressures and tidal volumes (7-8 ml/kg) have been shown to decrease mortality when compared with a more conventional approach. These ventilation strategies are frequently associated with hypercapnia and may lead to as yet uncertain adverse effects (Table 24.2).

FiO_2

AV shunt is the major cause of hypoxemia in ARDS. Hence, increased FiO_2 does not markedly improve PaO_2. On the contrary, inspired O_2 more than 60% can convert areas of low ventilation - perfusion ratio (Va/Q) to areas of pure shunt and cause further lung injury. Therefore FiO2 must be kept below 0.6 as far as possible.

Ventilatory Settings

Tidal volume (VT) 10-12 ml/kg especially in patients with severe lung injury who have plateau pressure >40 cmH_2O; large VT (12-15 ml/kg) cause alveolar overdistension and injury whereas low VT (<6 ml/kg) increase the atelectatic segments due to alveolar collapse. *Low tidal volume (6 ml/kg) in conjunction with an inspiratory plateau pressures <30 cmH_2O is recommended.*

PEEP: PEEP is initially set at 5-6 Cm H_2O and then increased in steps of 2 cm H_2O at a time till SaO_2 >90% is achieved with an acceptable mean airway pressure and FiO_2< 0.6. On an average PEEP of 8-12 cmH_2O are needed, but PEEP as high as 15-20 cm H_2O, have been used. PEEP helps in recruitment of nonventilated lung units and maintenance of patency of recruited lung and achieve a QS/QP ratio <15%. Very high PEEP can be tolerated by children with ARDS without hemodynamic compromise.

PIP: Should be < 35 cm H_2O as far as possible because rising PIP is proportional to amount of surfactant depletion and barotrauma.

I:E ratio:1:2 or even 1:1 with inspiratory hold, if needed. In certain situations inverse ratio ventilation is preferred for optimal oxygenation as long as a minimum expiratory time of 0.5 seconds is maintained.

High-frequency Oscillatory Ventilation

High-frequency oscillatory ventilation benefited children with severe ARDS. High-frequency oscillatory ventilation patients had significantly better outcomes than conventional ventilation patients. In addition high-frequency oscillatory ventilation was found to achieve improved oxygenation without hemodynamic compromise.

Fluids and Diuretics

Fluid restriction has been found beneficial, improves lung compliance, gas exchange and length of time on ventilator. However, use of diuretics is risky; may compromise hemodynamic status, and systemic oxygen transport.

Surfactant Therapy

In ARDS there is an imbalance between the synthesis, release and consumption of surfactant as a result of damage to type II pneumocytes leading to serious surfactant deficiency. There is inactivation of the surfactant by plasma proteins that pass into the alveolus; inhibition or damage to the protein component or phospholipid component of the surfactant by mediators of inflammation, such as lipases, proteases, or oxidants; incorporation of the surfactant into hyaline membranes. The loss of surfactant is proportional to the phasic volume and pressure changes of the alveolus. Hence while ventilating such patients pressure fluctuations should be kept to a minimum.

Surfactant therapy moderately improves oxygenation in some children with severe acute respiratory distress syndrome secondary to pulmonary or systemic disease however, studies do not show whether surfactant changes the prognosis of children with ARDS.

Other therapies

Trials of NO, partial liquid ventilation and prone positioning have shown that these interventions can improve oxygenation but not survival. Prone position improves V/Q relationship by directing blood flow away from previously dependent atelectatic areas.

Routine or prophylactic use of antibiotics or corticosteroids have not proven beneficial, though some advocate use of pulse methylprednisolone to prevent progression to fibrotic phase. Use of methylpredmisone (2 - 3 mg/kg), 7 -14 days after onset of illness may offer survival benefit.

Neuromuscular blockers should be avoided if possible because of risk of 'critical care neuropathy/myopathy'. In severe cases these may be needed to decrease work of breathing, CO_2 production and PIP. If used, whether as continuous infusion, or boluses, depth of blockade should be monitored with 'train of four' monitoring.

Chapter twenty-five

Pneumonia in ICU Patients

Pneumonia in Critically ill patients receiving Intensive care is not uncommon. These children are at risk of various nosocomial pneumonias as well as aspiration. Salient features of both these are discussed here.

ASPIRATION PNEUMONIA

Etiology

Aspiration pneumonia is seen in patients who are unable to protect the airway. The common predisposing conditions are those associated with ***impaired consciousness level*** (head injury, coma, anesthesia, use of sedatives and neuromuscular blocking agents, seizures etc.), ***impaired gag/ cough reflexes*** (bulbar palsy ,Guillian-Barre, pharyngeal trauma, recent extubation) and large nasogastric tube feeds. Continuous microaspiration of infected gastric fluid past the cuff of an endotracheal tube in intubated patients probably accounts for many of the nosocomial pneumonias.

Pathophysiology

Aspiration of large volume of solid material may block a major bronchus and cause atelectasis. This will require bronchoscopic removal. Aspiration of gastric acid may result in a severe chemical pneumonitis, particularly if the pH of the gastric contents is <2.5. It carries a high mortality.

Gastric fluid is usually sterile because of low pH. Increases in pH resulting from antacid or H2 – antagonist therapy, which may lead to overgrowth of stomach contents with intestinal microorganisms, in patients who are hospitalized. Aspiration of such material, although not causing such severe pneumonitis, delivers a considerable inoculum of pathogens into the lungs, Patients present with pneumonia/respiratory failure. The changes may be diffuse.

Clinical Features

Clinical features of a large aspiration or highly acidic gastric contents include dyspnea, bronchospasm, pulmonary edema, hypoxia and shock. Patients who are on antacid or H2–antagonist therapy may not show features typical of pneumonitis (aspiration, pulmonary edema, shock). In these development of respiratory failure may be insidious.

Management

- Head down on the right side, and clearing of oropharynx.
- Respiratory failure should be dealt with appropriately. Supplemental oxygen should be given to keep normal SpO_2.
- Intubation and CPAP may be needed if the level of consciousness is impaired.
- Continuous monitoring cardio-respiratory function, including pulse oximetry, and ECG.
- Nasogastric tube placement to empty stomach.
- Treatment of bronchospasm with nebulized β2- agonists.
- A baseline chest X-ray shoud be obtained.
- Therapeutic bronchoscopy is indicated if there is any clinical or radiological evidence of lobar/ lung collapse. Therapeutic lavage is not useful.

- Prophylactic antibiotics should be avoided if there is no reason to believe that the stomach contents included pathogenic bacteria. If it is necessary to treat before bacteriological confirmation, a third generation cephalosporin (eg, cefotaxime) + cloxacillin + metronidazole or a carbipenem (eg, imipenem) is a suitable.
- Broad-spectrum antibiotic should be started to provide cover against anaerobes, *S. aureus* and Gram-negative species, including Pseudomonas in ICU patients who are on antacid or H2–antagonist therapy.

NOSOCOMIAL PNEUMONIA

Nosocomial pneumonia is defined as pneumonia diagnosed after at least 3 days of hospitalization. In contrast to other hospital patients, nosocomial pneumonia is the second most common nosocomial infection in the critically ill and has the highest morality among hospital-acquired infection. The risk factors include:

1. Intubation and ventilation
2. Impaired airway protection, due to CNS dysfunction, sedative drugs and nasogastric tube
3. Surgery factors, broad spectrum antibiotic therapy
4. Severe underlying disease
5. Immunosuppression
6. Malnutrition
7. Raised gastric pH because of antacids, H2 blockers etc. causing bacterial overgrowth of stomach.

Loss of normal host defenses, colonization of the oropharynx by Gram-negative bacilli and the presence of an endotracheal tube that provide ready passageway for organisms to enter the lower respiratory tract, all contribute to pathogenesis of nosocomial pneumonia. Endotracheal tube impairs mucociliary flow and allows pooling of subglottic secretions. Pooled secretions provide a culture medium that can be aspirated and lodged in the distal airways. Lastly, the inner lumen of the tube may become covered with a biofilm of organisms that may be either aspirated or mechanically displaced into the lower respiratory tract by suction catheter.

Diagnosis

Patients with Ventilator associated pneumonia (VAP) will have fever, leukocytosis, purulent tracheal secretions, and new or worsening pulmonary infiltrates, though these signs are very sensitive these are not highly sepcific.

Quantitative or semi-quantitative culture of tracheal aspirate may improve the overall accuracy of the diagnosis. Clinically significant pulmonary infections usually contain 10^5 or more organisms per mL.

Prevention

Proper infection control practices including hand washing, cleaning and disinfecting respiratory equipment, and clearing of pharyngeal secretions around endotracheal tube when the patient is extubated or the tube is repositioned. Additional measure that can decrease the incidence of nosocomial pneumonia include semirecumbent positioning, limiting reintubation, avoiding unnecessary antibiotics, and restricting acid-neutralizing stress ulcer prophylaxis to high-risk patients.

Therapeutic approaches have been used in an attempt to modify the development of VAP and prevent the development of antibiotic resistance. A rotation of empiric antibiotics from one class to another and continuous suctioning of subglottic secretions can lower bacterial colonization of the respiratory tract.

Antibiotic Therapy

Treatment must be started on the basis of the clinical circumstances, previous antibiotic therapy, urgent Gram stain of sputum, and the antibiotic policies of the unit and hospital. The organisms commonly involved in nosocomial pneumonia, along with their antibiotic sensitivities, are listed on Table 25.1. The suggested regimens must be adjusted according to the frequency and patterns of resistance of organisms isolated in the given hospitals.

In general, monotherapy with a third-generation cephalosporin is reasonable; an aminoglycoside may be added to the β-lactam. If Pseudomonas is likely, it is necessary to provide anti-pseudomonal antibiotic coverage. *P. aeruginosa* in the lung is best treated with combination therapy consisting of an aminoglycoside plus an anti-pseudomonal penicillin or a third or fourth-generation cephalosporin (ceftazidime or cefepime).

Table 25.1: Empirical antibiotic therapy for nosocomial pneumonia

Early	**Community organisms** Streptococcus pneumoniae, Staphylococcus aureus, Hemophilus spp.	Cefotaxime + gentamicin; add cloxacillin if *S. aureus* is suspected, add clindamycin if aspiration
Middle	**Intestinal flora, Gram-negative bacilli** including Klebsiella spp., Pseudomonas spp. MRSA	Third–generation cephalosporin (eg. Cefotaxime, ceftriaxone); ciprofloxacin or ceftazidime or piperacillin/tazobactam if pseudomonal coverage required; vancomycin for MRSA
Late	**Resistant/opportunistic organisms** Acinetobacter spp., Fungi	Microbiological advice Often colonization rather than true infection.

Chapter twenty-six

The Multiple Organ Dysfunction Syndrome

The Multiple Organ Dysfunction Syndrome (MODS), is now known to accompany a diverse group of disorders including severe sepsis, trauma, severe burns, and hemorrhagic pancreatitis. The clinical course of MODS follows a predictable pathway, irrespective of the inciting event. The first sign of organ dysfunction is usually cardiovascular (hemodynamic alterations) and pulmonary dysfunction with the appearance of acute lung injury (ALI) or acute respiratory distress syndrome (ARDS). Hypoxemia and the other pulmonary manifestations of ALI or ARDS are followed by hepatic dysfunction, disturbance of gastrointestinal function, renal failure, and "brain failure". Alterations in consciousness or mentation may occur early or late while bone marrow failure and myocardial dysfunction are usually late manifestations. Prognosis is most directly related to the number of ailed organs. Mortality in a patient with single-organ failure is 20% and as the number of additional organ system failures rise, mortality progressively increases.

The onset of organ dysfunction is also associated with a variety of metabolic and endocrine abnormalities. There are rapid increases in the plasma concentration of catecholamines, adrenocorticotrophic hormone (ACTH), growth hormone (GH), and corticosteroids including cortisol. One manifestation of these changes is hyperglycemia. Following the initial phase, catabolism exceeds a shift to fat as a primary energy source.

PATHOGENESIS

A number of factors play a role in the development of MODS. These include excessive systemic activation of macrophages, alterations in endothelial cell adhesion molecules, failure of the gut mucosal barrier, and microcirculatory ischemia and reperfusion injury. Cytokine-induced prothrombotic abnormalities in the microcirculation appear to play a major role in this process. Coagulation abnormalities in patients with severe sepsis are clearly related to the development of organ dysfunction and death. Laboratory changes support this direct relationship.

Endothelial Cell Activation and Injury

The endothelium of microvasculature serves as an interface between the systemic circulation and the tissues. It modulates microcirculatory blood flow and cell trafficking. Release of NO by endothelial cells dilates small blood vessels while endothelial adhesion molecules help to localize an inflammatory focus.

Sepsis is associated with endothelial activation. Progression of the process results in endothelial injury or apoptosis. Following stimulation by cytokines such as IL-1, TNF-α, and by components of complement, subsets of endothelial cells may respond by a shift to a prothrombotic phenotype, upregulation of adhesion molecules, release of vasoactive substances, and secretion of inflammatory mediator such as IL-6. The goal of these responses is to localise an infectious process. The activated endothelium is eventually damaged. Dysfunctional endothelial cells may produce a capillary leak syndrome and be unable to finely regulate the blood supply through the micro-circulation. Other factors that may contribute to endothelial cell dysfunction in patients with sepsis include toxic oxygen free radicals from reperfusion injury, superoxide and proteases from adherent neutrophil, and endothelial cell apoptosis.

Evidence of these changes includes increase in the circulating levels of adhesion molecules, soluble thrombomodulin (sTM), von Willebrand factor, IL-6, and activated coagulation factors. Manifestations of dysfunctional endothelium include coagulation activation, impaired fibrinolysis and disturbed microcirculatory blood flow.

Coagulation Activation

Hemostatic activation appears to be almost universal in patients with severe sepsis. Cytokines (TNF, IL-1, or IL-6, TF) activate coagulation. This is followed by an immediate decrease in the levels of Factor VII antigen and Factor VIIa with an increase in plasma levels of Factor I-II and thrombin-antithrombin (TAT) complexes. Extrinsic pathway of coagulation is activated with conversion of prothrombin (PT) to thrombin. Subsequently, thrombin amplifies the initial thrombotic response by activating the intrinsic system through the conversion of factor XI to XIa and VIII to VIIIa. Natural inhibitors of the hemostatic system that localize coagulation and maintain homeostasis include antithrombin (AT; antithrombin III), Tissue Factor Pathway Inhibitor (TFPI, and Protein C (PC). Antithrombin levels decline early in patients sepsis. During sepsis, TFPI levels remain stable or increase, presumably due to release from endothelial cells. Generation of APC occurs in rough proportion to thrombin formation. Levels of PC decline early in sepsis due to consumption and decreased production.

Fibrinolysis is an essential element in microcirculatory homeostasis. Tissue plasminogen activator (tPA) activates fibrinolysis by converting plasminogen to plasmin. Additional inhibition of fibrinolysis occurs from the actions of α_2-antiplasmin and thrombin-activatable-fibrinolysis inhibitor (TAFI).

Clinical and laboratory signs suggestive of organ dysfunction are shown in Table 26.1.

Most of the organ failure syndromes are discussed in separate chapters. Remaining ones are discussed below:

ORGAN DYSFUNCTION SCORES

Organ dysfunction is a marker of disease severity and significant contributor to overall mortality. Presence of increasing numbers of organ failures has a cumulative effect on mortality. The lungs and kidney are the most frequent organ dysfunctions. To describe disease severity, a number of organ dysfunction scores have been developed (See Appendix). Since the degree of organ dysfunction varies over time and will be assessed in multiple patients, it is important that these scores utilize objective simple and routinely analyzed parameters.

ACUTE ADRENOCORTICAL INSUFFICIENCY

Adrenocortical insufficiency is the lack of sufficient glucocorticoids (cortisol) or mineralocorticoids (aldosterone) to meet the demands of the cells. Adrenocortical insufficiency may be primary or secondary and if acute may precipitate adrenal crisis.

Primary adrenocortical insufficiency results from disease of the adrenal gland itself. In critically ill patients particularly in those with severe sepsis, septic shock, and meningococcemia it may occur because of destruction or hypofunction of the adrenal cortex leading to a decreased production of cortisol and aldosterone.

Table 26.1: Clinical and laboratory signs suggestive of organ dysfunction

Organ System	*Clinical Signs*	*Laboratory/Monitoring*
Respiratory	Tachypnea, laboured breathing Cyanosis Need for Mechanical ventilation	PaO_2 <70 mm Hg SaO_2 <90% PaO_2/FIO_2=300
Renal	Oliguria, Anuria Need for Renal replacement therapy	Elevated creatinine (>1.0 mg/dl)
Hepatic	Jaundice	Hyperbilirubinemia Increased AST, ALT, LDH Increased alkaline phosphatase Hypoalbuminemia Increased PT, INR
Cardiovascular	Tachycardia Hypotension Arrhythmias HR:MAP ratio Need for Hemodynamic support	Altered CVP, PAOP
Hematological	Bleeding Thrombotic episodes	Thrombocytopenia Abnormal WBC count Increase PT or aPTT Decreased Protien C Increased FDPs, Increased D-dimer
Gastrointestinal	GI bleeding or perforation lleus Intestinal ischemia or infarction Acalculous cholecystitis Acute pancreatitis Intolerance of enteral nutrition	Decreased pHi
Neurological	Altered consciousness Impaired mentation Confusion, Psychosis, Delirium GCS <15	
Endocrine	Weight loss	Hyperglycemia Decreased cortisol Hypertriglyceridemia Hypoalbuminemia
Immune	• Pyrexia • Nosocomial Infection	Leukocytosis Abnormalities of T cell subsets Impaired leukocyte function

Adapted from Balk RA, CCM, 2000; 16: 337-52.

In may occur. Secondary adrenocortical insufficiency results from a pathological condition outside the adrenal glands.

The primary function of cortisol is to raise the blood sugar and make glucose available for energy and an anti-inflammatory effect providing against potentially harmful toxins. The primary function of aldosterone is to maintain salt and water balance. Manifestations of acute adrenal insufficiency therefore, are hypoglycemia and, hyponatremia, hypovolemia, hypotension and hyperkalemia.

Diagnosis

In patients 'at risk', particularly those in fluid and catecholamine refractory shock, a high index of clinical suspicion is helpful. Presence of biochemical features—hypoglycemia, hyponatremia with hyperkalemia are highly suggestive. Low random cortisol and/or loss of cortisol response to ACTH (ACTH stimulation test) is diagnostic.

Management

1. Cardiovascular support: Correction of hypovolemia and extracellular fluid (ECF), deficit with 0.9% saline; large volumes may be required. It should be guided by measurement of CVP and hourly urine output.
   Vasopressors may be necessary in severe cases; high doses may be required.
2. Corticosteroid and mineralocorticoid replacement therapy: Hydrocortisone 50 mg IV every 6 hours and fludrocortisone 50-100 micro g orally or by nasogastric tube daily.
3. 50% dextrose as necessary to treat hypoglycemia.
4. Treatment of precipitating cause.

An Addisonian crisis will usually only develop when the stress response fails to develop in response to an appropriate stimulus.

BLEEDING AND COAGULOPATHY

Bleeding and coagulopathy are commonly seen in critically ill children, often as consequence of the primary illness or part of multiorgan dysfunction because of disruption of physiological process of hemostasis. Hemostasis is accomplished through the balancing of coagulation and anticoagulation sequences.

Normal Hemostasis

The first response to bleeding is vessel spasm at the site of injury, which is mediated through myogenic, neuorgenic, and humoral mechanisms. Then, platelets aggregate at the site adhering to each other and to blood cells and trapping plasma, loosely plugging the area. The process is aided by von Willebrand's factor, factor VIII, and by release of adenosine diphosphate, thrombin, thromboxane, and other substances from platelets. Formation of clot follows, in which a fibrin network, which traps red cells, platelets and plasma is formed. This is accomplished through sequential activation and inhibition of procoagulation factors. Both, the intrinsic and the extrinsic pathways (that respond to tissue damage) end in a common pathway that produces thrombin and fibrin to form an insoluble clot (Fig. 26.1). Following vessel-wall repair, plasma protein plasminogen (profibrinolysin) is converted to the proteolytic enzyme plasmin (fibrinolysin) by activators formed in vessel endothelium, liver and kidneys. Plasmin interrupts the clotting mechanism by digesting clotting factors (fibrinogen and factors V and VIII) and the fibrin clot. This prevents vessel occlusion.

Bleeding disorders may occur due to defective or diminished platelets (thrombocytopenia), deficiencies of clotting factors, their precursors or catalysts, or increased consumption of clotting factors. A coagulopathy is a disorder in which the primary cause of bleeding is a problem with the formation, stabilization, or lysis of the fibrin clot. Since all but three clotting factors (III, VIII, XIII) are synthesized in the liver and the clotting sequence requires both calcium and vitamin K coagulopathy may occur in liver disease, impaired synthesis or storage of vitamin K (destruction of intestinal flora with antibiotic therapy, impaired fat absorption), drug effects or side effects (anticoagulants, nonsteroidal anti-inflammatory drugs, chemotherapeutics), or calcium deficiency.

Hypercoagulation states may be due to increased platelet activity (trauma), slowed blood flow (immobility, shock), and increased clotting activity or decreased anticoagulant activity (drugs, malignancy, sepsis).

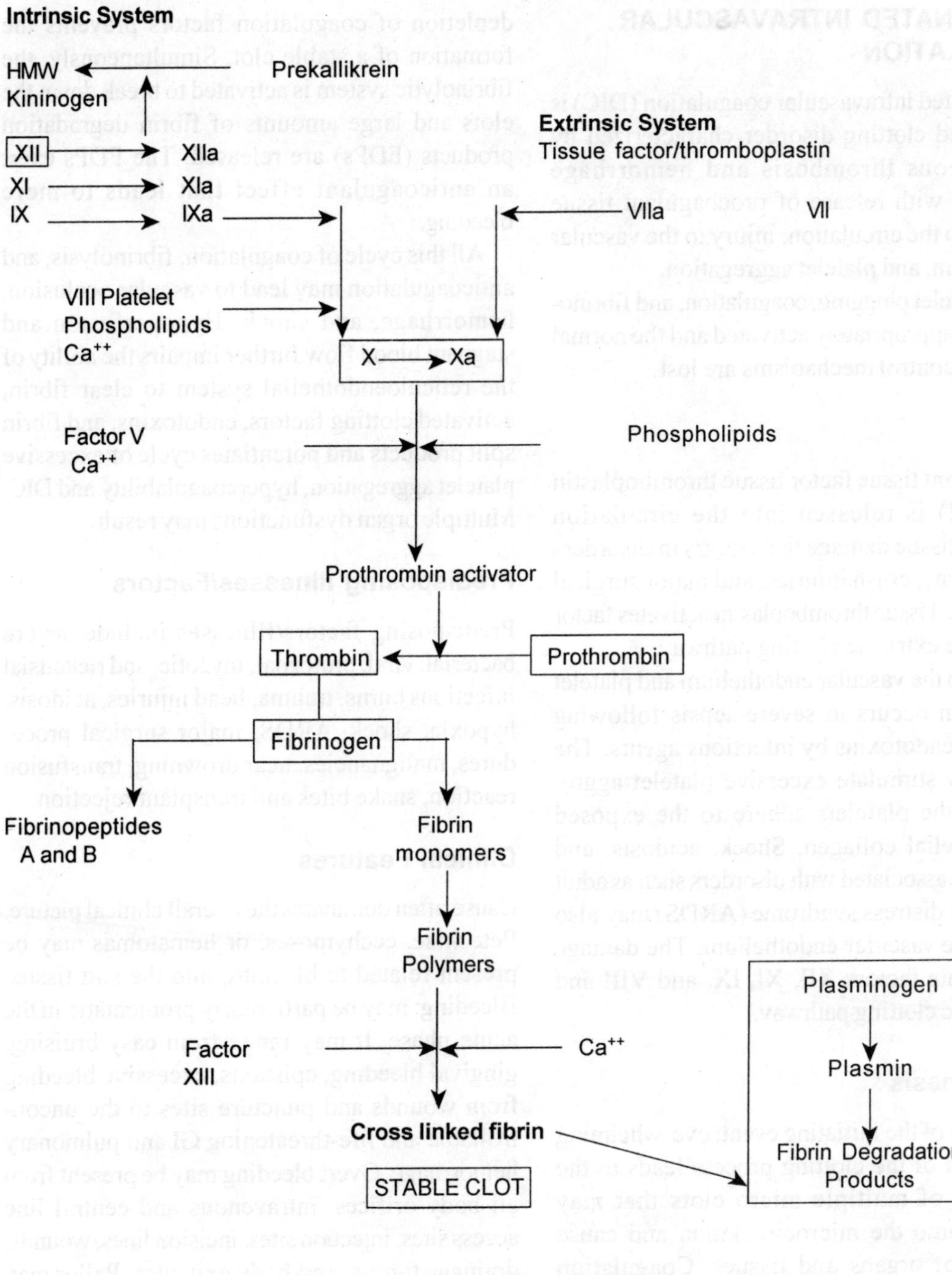

Fig. 26.1: Coagulation pathway

DISSEMINATED INTRAVASCULAR COAGULATION

Disseminated intravascular coagulation (DIC) is an acquired clotting disorder characterized by simultaneous thrombosis and hemorrhage associated with release of procoagulant tissue factors into the circulation, injury to the vascular endothelium, and platelet aggregation.

The platelet plugging, coagulation, and fibrinolysis are inappropriately activated and the normal inhibitory control mechanisms are lost.

Etiology

Procoagulant tissue factor tissue thromboplastin (factor III) is released into the circulation following tissue damage that occurs in disorders such as burns, crush injuries, and major surgical procedures. Tissue thromboplastin activates factor VII and the extrinsic clotting pathway.

Injury to the vascular endothelium and platelet aggregation occurs in severe sepsis following release of endotoxins by infectious agents. The injury may stimulate excessive platelet aggregation as the platelets adhere to the exposed subendothelial collagen. Shock, acidosis, and hypoxemia associated with disorders such as adult respiratory distress syndrome (ARDS) may also damage the vascular endothelium. The damage may activate factors XII, XI, IX, and VIII and the intrinsic clotting pathway.

Pathogenesis

Regardless of the initiating event, overwhelming stimulation of the clotting process leads to the formation of multiple micro clots that may embolize into the microcirculation and cause ischemia of organs and tissues. Coagulation factors such as prothrombin, platelets, factor V, and factor VIII are rapidly consumed. Clotting factors are consumed faster than they can be replaced by the liver and bone marrow. The depletion of coagulation factors prevents the formation of a stable clot. Simultaneously, the fibrinolytic system is activated to break down the clots and large amounts of fibrin degradation products (FDPs) are released. The FDPs exert an anticoagulant effect that leads to more bleeding.

All this cycle of coagulation, fibrinolysis, and anticoagulation may lead to vascular occlusion, hemorrhage, and shock. Hypoperfusion and stagnant blood flow further impairs the ability of the reticuloendothelial system to clear fibrin, activated clotting factors, endotoxins, and fibrin split products and potentiates cycle of excessive platelet aggregation, hypercoagulability and DIC. Multiple organ dysfunctions may result.

Predisposing Illnesses/Factors

Predisposing factors/Illnesses include severe bacterial, viral, protozoal, mycotic, and rickettsial infections burns, trauma, head injuries, acidosis, hypoxia, shock, ARDS, major surgical procedures, malignancies, near drowning, transfusion reaction, snake bites and transplant rejection.

Clinical Features

Cause often dominates the overall clinical picture. Petechiae, ecchymoses, or hematomas may be present related to bleeding into the soft tissue. Bleeding: may be particularly problematic in the acute phase. It may range from easy bruising, gingival bleeding, epistaxis, excessive bleeding from wounds and puncture sites to the uncontrollable and life-threatening GI and pulmonary hemorrhage. Overt bleeding may be present from all body orifices, intravenous and central line access sites, injection sites, incision lines, wounds, drainage tubing, and body exit sites. Pallor may be present, related to significant blood loss. Hypotension out of proportion to blood loss may be seen as result of myocardial depressant action of FDP's. Microvascular thrombosis may be seen in late stage; the levels of clotting factors and platelets may be normal at this stage representing a balance between increased production and consumption. Organ dysfunctions including renal failure, adrenal hemorrhage, cerebral hemorrhage, digital ischemia may occur secondary to primary cause, hypotension, microvascular thrombosis etc. Jaundice may be present because of microemboli in the hepatic circulation. DIC may need differentiation from coagulopathy associated with liver failure, and thrombotic thrombocytopenic purpura.

Laboratory Diagnosis

1. Thrombocytopenia (90% of patients will have a platelet count less than 150,000/mm^3)
2. Prolonged prothrombin and partial thromboplastin times (> 60-90 seconds)
3. Hypofibrinogenemia (< 75-100 mg/dL)
4. Evidence of fibrinolysis:
   a. FDPs
   b. Elevated D-dimers
   c. Shortened euglobin clot lysis time
5. Decreased factors V and VIII
6. Antithrombin II >60% normal activity
7. Red cell fragmentation on blood film due to microangiopathic hemolysis; this may be the only abnormality in chronic DIC states.

Management

The process may be prevented by early blood pressure and oxygen utilization goal-directed hemodynamic resuscitation in patients with severe sepsis, septic shock, trauma etc. Once ongoing coagulation has consumed clotting factors (including fibrinogen), anti-thrombotic factors (Antithrombin III and Protein C), and platelets the therapeutic strategies must restore a homeostatic milieu by removing or inhibiting Tissue Factor activity and replacing anti-coagulant factors, pro-coagulant factors and platelets. The steps in management include the following:

1. Transfusion of fresh blood may be needed in life threatening massive bleeds.
2. Treatment of the predisposing cause.
3. Restoration of clotting factors and fibrinogen (to about 100 mg/dL): FFP contains most of the pro-and anticoagulant factors in plasma, and is the standard first-line treatment for bleeding complications. Initial dose is12-15 ml/kg. Cryoprecipitate is more concentrated preparation and is rich in factor VII and fibrinogen. It is useful adjunct to FFP therapy to boost fibrinogen levels.
4. Platelet transfusion: This is not well established but some advocate maintaining platelet count higher than 50,000/ mm^3, or higher if patient is uremic.
5. Heparin is used to switch off the coagulation cascade. It is often used along with FFP use in acute hemorrhagic phase and is indicated in chronic DIC. It is started at a low dose, e.g., 5-10 IU/ kg per hour.
6. Antifibrinolytic Aprotinin, a serine protease inhibitor is well established in open-heart surgery to reduce fibrinolysis and blood loss. All antifibrinolytics increase risk of thrombosis. The loading dose is 2,000,000 units followed by 500,000 units/ hour.
7. Pentoxyfilline has been shown in a randomized controlled trial to improve survival in very low birth weight children with septic shock in part through prevention and reversal of DIC.

Debate continues on whether specific therapies (e.g. anti-thrombin III, protein C, heparin, activated protein C, TPA), non-specific therapies (FFP and platelet replacement, or plasma exchange) or a combination of both (plasma exchange + antithrombin III, or protein C, or activated protein C with TPA added for life or limb threatening thrombosis) is best.

Thrombocytopenia

Thrombocytopenia is defined as a platelet count 150,000/μL. Thrombocytopenia that is clinically significant corresponds to a platelet count < 100,000/μL. A structural lesion in the absence of platelet counts down to 5000/μL can be tolerated without evidence of bleeding.

Thrombocytopenia in the ICU

The causes of Thrombocytopenia most likely to be encountered in the ICU are systemic sepsis, Disseminated intravascular coagulation, Thrombotic thrombocytopenia, and some commonly used drugs (such as heparin, paracetamol, rifampicin, co-trimoxazole). An approach to diagnosis and management of thrombocytopenia is shown in Figure 26.2.

Heparin Induced Thrombocytopenia (HIT)

Heparin can combine a heparin-binding protein on platelets to form an antigenic complex that induce the formation of IgG antibodies. These antibodies then bind to platelets and form cross-bridges that result in platelet aggression. If

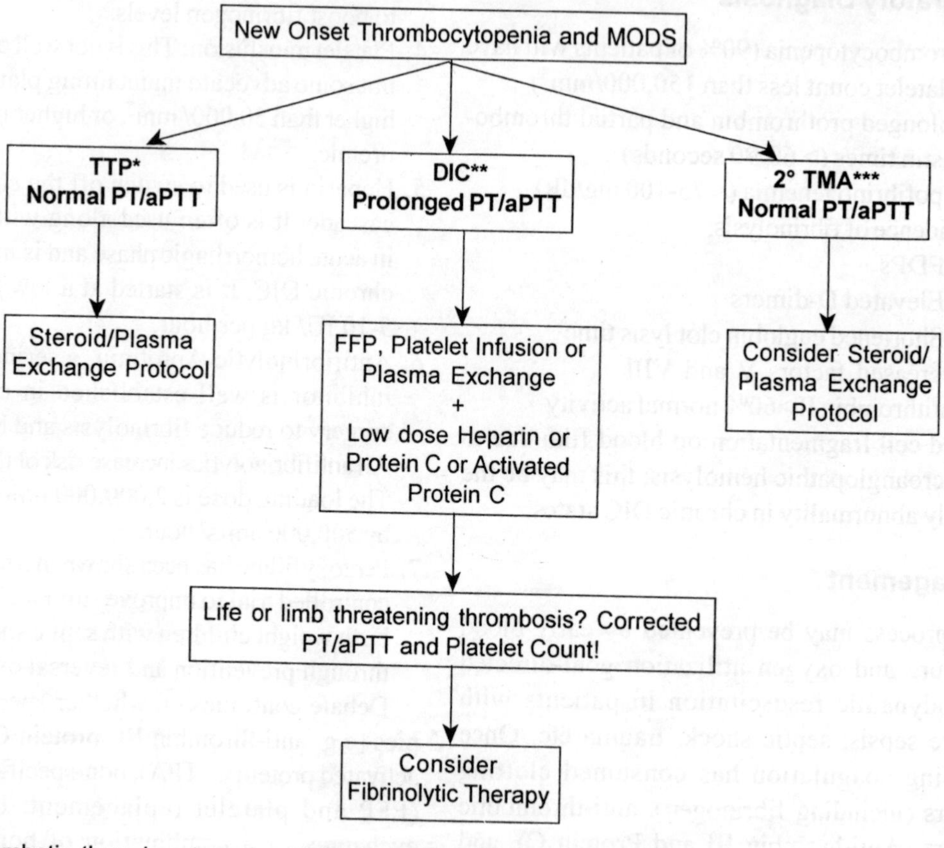

***TTP**-Thrombotic thrombocytopenia, ****DIC**-Disseminated Intravascular Coagulation, *****TMA**-Thrombotic micro-angiopathy

Fig. 26.2: Flow chart showing treatment options in a child with thrombocytopenia and multiorgan dysfunction syndrome

severe enough this process can result in a consumptive thrombocytopenia and clinically apparent thrombosis. The risk of HIT is greater with unfractionated heparin (UFH) than with low molecular weight heparin (LMWH). HIT can appear with very low doses of heparin. This includes heparin flushes and small amounts on heparin coated catheters.

The major complication of HIT is thrombosis including deep vein thrombosis of the lower extremities and upper extremities, acute pulmonary embolism, arterial thrombosis involving a limb and thrombotic stroke.

The diagnosis of HIT required a high-probability clinical scenario; suspect any thrombocytopenia that develops 5 to 10 days after starting heparin.

Thrombocytopenia Associated MOF

Thrombocytopenia associated MOF (platelet count < 100,000 or a 50% drop in platelet count from baseline) is often attributable to purpura fulminans and disseminated intravascular coagulation. But in one autopsy study only 20% of patients had DIC. Eighty per cent of these patients showed thrombotic thrombocytopenia (normal PT/PTT, normal Tissue Factor activity, elevated Plasminogen Activator Inhibitor Type I activity, normal or elevated fibrinogen, ultra large vWF multimers, and reduced vWF cleaving protease) or Thrombotic micro-angiopathy. They had had a hypercellular bone marrow with platelet and fibrin thrombi observed in the microvasculature.Following algorithm may be considered in the management of children with thrombocytopenia associated MODS.

Plasma exchange (centrifugation based- 11/2 volume exchange × 1 followed by daily 1 volume exchange × 2 weeks) reversed coagulation abnormalities in patients with thrombotic thrombocytopenic purpura in one study. Specific therapies for the treatment of thrombotic microangiopathy include heparin, antithrombin III, and protein C to inhibit thrombosis.

Thrombotic Thrombocytopenia pupura

Thrombotic thrombocytopenia purpura (TTP) is a rare but life threatening condition caused by immune-mediated platelet aggregation with widespread microvascular involvement. It is classified as one of the thrombotic microangiopathies.

Clinical features

The clinical presentation of TTP is characterized by five clinical features: fever, change in mental status, acute renal failure, and thrombocytopenia and microangiopathic hemolytic anemia. All 5 clinical features are required for the diagnosis. Patient usually experiences fever and depressed consciousness that can progress rapidly to coma to coma and generalized seizures thrombocytopenia the microangiopathic hemolytic anemia is detected by the presence in the blood smear.

Management

The treatment of choice for TTP is plasma exchange. Acute fulminant TTP is almost always fatal if untreated.

Chapter twenty-seven

Management of Death in ICU

During the course of ICU management many patients will be identified who are best treated by shifting goals from cure to comfort. This may be the emotionally most demanding and time consuming. This process can be broken into four parts. The first step is deciding whether the patient is dying. Determine on basis of co morbidities, number of organ systems in failure, level of response to therapy of the acute illness etc. Second step is addressing this realization with the family and communicating this to the patient and family. This will enable the physician to help with decisions to withhold or withdraw life support. Third is engaging in a compassionate process to address the concerns of family. The objective of patient care should be changed from cure to comfort. The change of goals should be undertaken with same zeal.

Comfort

In a dying child the management is directed to treat pain, relieve dyspnea, allay anxiety, minimize interventions, increase family access, and support grieving so as to ensure that when withdrawal occurs, the patient is comfortable. Remove as many technological connections as possible and increase human contact. In up to 90% of patients who die in ICUs following withdrawal of life sustaining measure, exemplary care helps to ease the transition.

BRAIN DEATH IN ICU

Brain death constitutes irreversible cessation of all brain function, and is considered, medically, and legally, to be the death of the individual. Criteria for the diagnosis of brain death have been established.

Condition 1: Cerebral Functions are Absent

The patient must be deeply comatose, with no spontaneous movement and no response to external stimuli such as noise, bright light, or pain. Spinal reflexes may be present, but decorticate or decerebrate posturing cannot. Rarely, brainstem lesions may leave the patient paralyzed but with intact cognition ('locked-in'), requiring additional studies such as electroencephalography to evaluate cerebral function.

Condition 2: Brain stem functions are absent. Brain stem reflexes are absent

Following reflexes are examined:

- **Respiratory drive** is examined by disconnecting the patient from the ventilator for long enough to ensure that the $PaCO_2$ is above the threshold for stimulation of the respiratory center (normally 60 mm Hg). (Figs 27.1 and 27.2). The patient must not be hypotensive during the test.
  1. Preoxygenate with 100% oxygen for 10 minutes.
  2. Disconnect the patient from the ventilator.
  3. Look for respiratory effort while repeating blood gas analysis to ensure that the $PaCO_2$ threshold has been passed. The $PaCO_2$ will increase at approximately 3 mmHg/min.
  4. Hypoxemia must be prevented during the test. If hypoxemia develops during the above

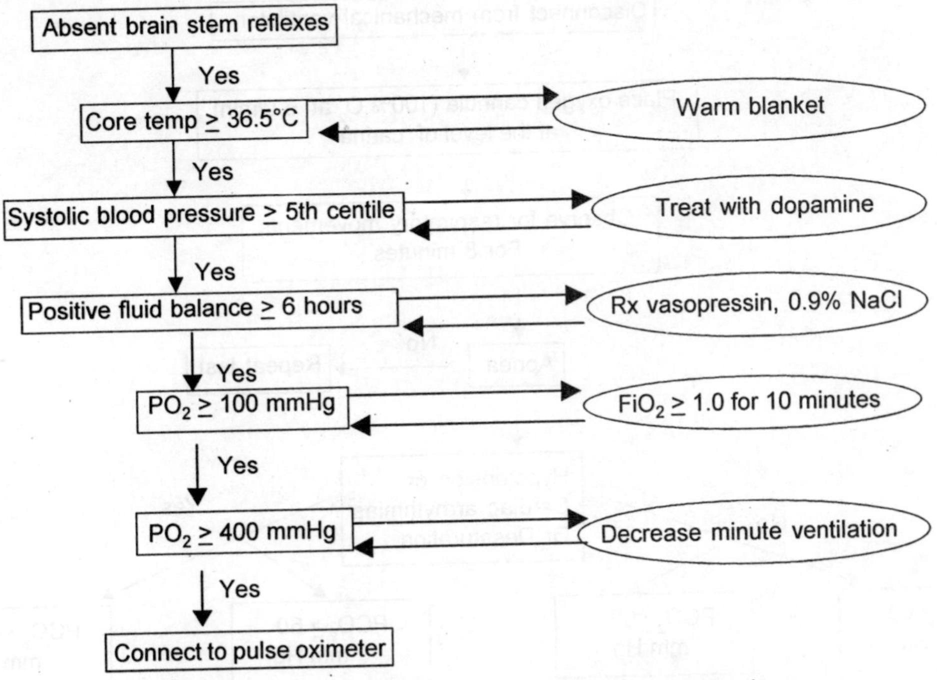

Fig. 27.1: Precautions for the apnea test in brain death

protocol, the two approaches may be used after first restoring oxygenation. One strategy is to hypoventilate the patient with 2-4 breaths per minute of 100% oxygen, allowing a more gradual rise in $PaCO_2$. Alternatively, hypoxemia may be prevented through the administration of O_2 6 L/min by passive flow into the trachea.

- **Pupillary reflex to light** (tests II and III cranial nerves)–The pupils are fixed in diameter and do not respond to light. Local trauma may prevent examination of pupillary reflexes.
- **Corneal reflex** (tests V and VII nerves)–Local trauma may prevent examination of corneal reflexes.
- **The cold caloric vastibulo-ocular reflex** (tests III, IV, VI, VIII nerves)–Clear access to the tympanic membranes must be established by direct inspection. The reflexes are considered to be absent when no eye movement occurs during or in the 30-sec period after the slow irrigation of the external auditory meatus with 20-ml. of ice-cold water. Local trauma may render this test impossible.

Condition 3: Cessation of brain function is irreversible

All three of the following must be present to establish this criterion (Fig. 27.3).

1. ***The cause of the coma is established***, and sufficient to explain the loss of brain function. Most causes of loss of brain function can be readily determined though a comprehensive history and physical examination, computed tomography of the brain, basic biochemical laboratories, and drug screening. However, some causes-for example, viral encephalitis or unusual drugs or toxins-may not be obvious, and may require additional testing.
2. ***There is no possibility of recovery of any brain function***. Important causes of reversible loss of brain function include hypothermia

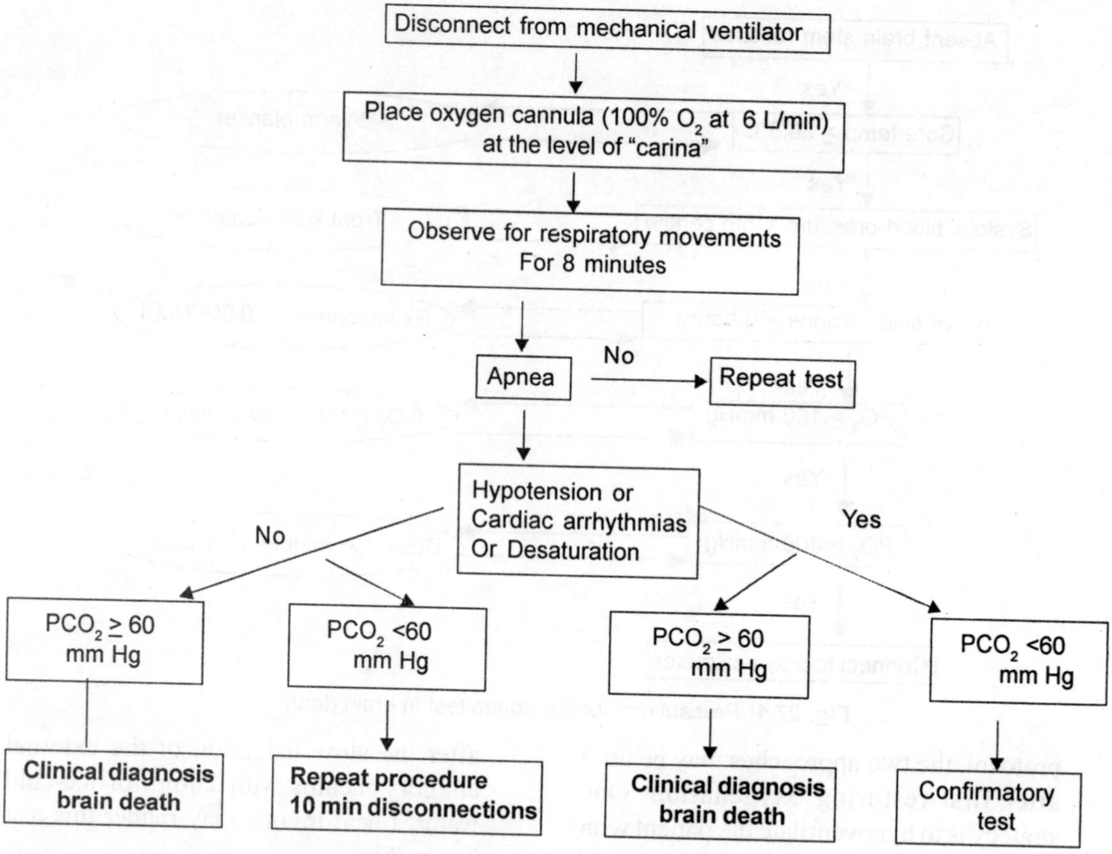

Fig. 27.2: Procedure for the apnea test in brain death

(<35°C), drug intoxication, therapeutic barbiturate administration, neuromuscular blockade, and severe hypotension. These must be ruled out.

3. ***Cessation of all brain function persists for an appropriate period of observation***, and despite (if possible) a trial of therapy. When the precise structural insult is known, 12 hours of observation is sufficient. Following a diffuse insult such as cerebral anoxia, 24 hours, observation is reasonable.

When the cause of the coma is not clear, or the neurological evaluation is necessarily incomplete (for example, severe facial trauma), additional testing may be helpful. Electroencephalography and cerebral blood flow studies (Transcranial Doppler sonography, cerebral angiography, etc.) may be helpful in selected patients.

It may be difficult to assess brain death in patients having trauma to eyes, ears or face, 'locked-in' syndrome, brainstem encephalitis and unrecognized drug ingestion.

Brain Death and The Patient's Family

Many patients with critical illness are not able to communicate or are comatose, and other rapidly progress to brain death. Intensivist should anticipate a very complex physician-family relationship in the first 24 hours. The main goals are (a) clarification and explanation of the acute neurologic disorder (b) discussion of the level of responsiveness of the patient (c) estimation of the expected

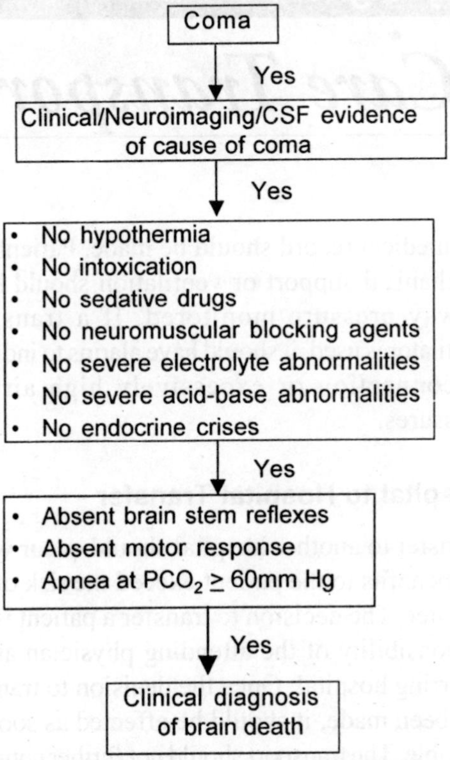

Fig. 27.3: Proposed guidelines for the clinical diagnosis of brain death

progression or improvement in the first 3 days (d) review of possible long-term outcome and expected level of functioning in dependence and independence. Coping of family members of patients with acute neurologic disorders varies from family to family and may vary within a particular family. Acute neurologic catastrophes may bring an acute stress reaction to some family members.

Very important patients and their families pose a particularly demanding problem. "VIP syndrome" loosely defined as unusual medical care and unconventional reactions by the attending physician.

One must realize that despite hard evidence to the contrary, the family's assessment of prognosis can be more optimistic than the physician's, initially. It is ill-advised to use platitudes or to express a sense of hope and optimism in the first 24 hours. The following day the significance of change (or no change) must be openly discussed.

When no improvement in the neurologic deficit is seen and the outlook for a meaningful recovery is remote, withdrawal of treatment and withdrawal of support must be discussed with the family. The decision of families to withdraw care is very difficult, and the responsibility enormous. Guilt plays an important role; nonetheless, reiteration of hopelessness, if applicable, may overcome this feeling. One should discourage the use of terms such as "miracles can happen" and be frank in prognostication. Opening of eyes, blinking, grimacing, grinding of teeth, and sleep-wake cycles are part of a developing vegetative state and must be explained as unpurposeful. When withdrawal is considered, a plan should be discussed with the family. There are several levels of withdrawal of support, from withdrawal of high technology ventilation support to withdrawal of medication antibiotics, vasopressors, insulin, antiarrhythmia agents and withdrawal of hydration and nutrition.

Discussion of a patient who fulfills the clinical criteria of brain death is very complex. Nonetheless, the intensivist should be crystal clear and not procrastinate. The family should be told in unequivocal terms that brain function has ceased and the patient is no longer alive, having passed away. Mechanical ventilation and pharmaceutical support are continued in the event the family agrees to donation of organs and tissue. Refusal of donation removes the rationale for further support. Infrequently, family members want continuation of mechanical ventilation and pharmacologic support because the concept of brain death is not understood. It is questionable whether family should be present during discontinuation of ventilation support. Some patients may have agonal breathing that suggests discomfort or have so-called Lazarus signs (reflex movements resulting in elevation of arms) during withdrawl of support. These decisions therefore, need to be individualized.

Chapter twenty-eight

Pediatric Critical Care Transport

Transport of a critically ill patient may be required within the hospital or to another health care facility because of need for additional care or investigations. The decision to transport, however, must be based on an assessment of potential benefits against the risk of transport. The need and role of optimum care of critically ill child during the transport is being more and more emphasized, as the period of transport is a period of potential instability. With all the personnel, gadgetry and equipment available in intensive care unit, patient and the attendants feel safe and comfortable to handle any situation. However, during transport one may have to face tremendous difficulties and multiple problems. Main emphasis of the pediatric transport system is to extend and deliver as far as possible the same advanced and skilled care during the process of transport as is available in intensive care units. Careful planning, use of qualified personnel and appropriate equipment can minimize the risk during the transport.

DECISION AND COMMUNICATION

Transport within the Hospital

Pre-transport Coordination and Communication

Pre-transport confirmation should be obtained from the area to which the patient is being transported (X-ray, operating theatre, nuclear medicine etc.) that it is ready to receive the patient and immediately begin the procedure or test for which the patient is being transported.

Documentation of the indications for transport and the patient's status during transport in the medical record should be made. Patients on mechanical support or ventilation should have airway pressure monitored. If a transport ventilator is used, it should have alarms to indicate disconnection or excessively high airway pressures.

Hospital to Hospital Transfer

Transfer to another hospital should occur when the benefits to the patient exceed the risk of the transfer. The decision to transfer a patient is the responsibility of the attending physician at the referring hospital. Once the decision to transfer has been made, it should be effected as soon as possible. The transport should not further compromise the patient's outcome. Resuscitation and stabilization should begin at the referring hospital.

It is always advantageous to communicate with the higher center in advance and provide brief summary of the illness, management and interventions done, vitals and state of condition at the time of transfer. The pediatrician at higher center should guide the referral physician regarding anticipated problems and necessary equipment and staff to handle the situation on the route. Any change in therapy however must be tailored to the facilities available at referring hospital. In most cases transported in our setup even the basic information is lacking and this delays the therapy at the higher center. Precious time is wasted in finding the details of illness and treatment from anxious and shocked parents.

Good medical practice requires that the patient or the legally authorized representative of an incompetent patient give an *informed consent prior to interhospital transport.* This must include a presentation of the risks *versus* benefits of transport with documentation in the medical record and a signed consent document.

Mode of Transport/Vehicle

In India as most of the places are well connected to each other with roads, this remains the most common means of patient transport. The vehicle used should be suitable to local terrain, safe, spacious, equipped with portable power supply and preferably air-conditioned.

The best handling and care of any critically ill child during transport requires proper organization. Emphasis should be on all the aspects viz. the team, the equipment, the mode of transport and the specific clinical situation. The child may be transported by:

i. *Local ambulance service with the specific instructions from the referring pediatrician:* Though financially advantageous the care during transport is far from being optimum.
ii. *Ambulance services with staff from referring hospital*: It may help the pediatrician to carry out the instructions reliably.
iii. *Specialized critical care transport:* Virtually a mobile ICU with well trained staff, portable equipment and necessary medications to handle any kind of emergency during the transport–this is usually the extension of the regional PICU center.

In India local ambulance services are the most common system of transport. The patient should be placed on a cushioned platform with head towards the front of the vehicle. The equipments must have proper fixed place and easily visible and handled. Regardless of its origin, the transport system should have proper communication, administration, trained team staff, reliable equipment, and safety program.

The Personnel

The composition of the transport team is important and may vary depending upon the clinical situation. At least 2 persons should accompany the patient. It should be determined by the pediatrician responsible for the transport and may include:

a. Physician
b. Nurse
c. Respiratory therapist
d. Emergency medical technician
e. Pediatric Intensivist.

Besides handling the individual field in appropriate and experienced manner each team member should be able to interact in a sensitive manner with parents and each other. The presence of physician is not a must in transport team. It may be possible to perceive the need and physician may accompany the team if patient has unstable cardio-respiratory or neurological status. Even though the skills may not be required enroute, judgment of the physician remains a unique contribution.

Capability and the performance of the team will be determined by the (a) level of training in critical care (b) knowledge of transport medicine and its physiological effects (c) managing the supplies and equipment and knowing its limitations (d) ability to withstand the stress and fatigue of transport (e) commitment to the care of the child. The level of knowledge, skills and responsibilities of individual team member are depicted in Table 28.1.

The Equipment

The team should carry equipment and drugs required for monitoring and stabilization of child en route. The equipment should be light weight, durable, portable, well secured and easily accessible even during the entry and exit of the vehicle.

Table 28.1: Pediatric critical care transport team: Guidelines for level of training, skills and responsibilities of individual team member

Team member	*Level of training*	*Skills*	*Desirable*	*Responsibilities*
Physician	Senior pediatric resident Pediatric intensive care fellow Pediatric intensivist	Airway Arterial line Venous access CVP/Cutdown	Constant exposure and 2 yrs experience in pediatric intensive care	Leads, coordinates team enroute, Stabilization; monitoring; management of child
Nurse	Pediatric training for (6 months) If team leader training for 1 yr (6 month as team member)	Of drug (sedative, pressors, anticonvulsant) Temp. control, Nursing	PICU training Airway management Assistance, knowledge of life saving procedures	Team leader, To coordinate activities, To follow norms and protocols
Respiratory therapist	Trained in pediatric critical care			Airway stabilization, Monitoring respiratory problems. Provide ventilation assistance.
Emergency technician	Training in cardiopulmonary resuscitation			Assists in cardiopulmonary resuscitation
Coordinator	Physician trained in pediatric critical care and transport medicine			Consulting peditrician for referring doctor Decides composition, mode, plan with team leader

Various life saving medicines and equipment should be arranged in different kits to give easy access.

The Respiratory Bag Should Contain

i. Ambu bag/silicon bag (200-250, and 450-500 ml).
ii. Oral airways (size 0-5), endotracheal tubes (2.5-8/0 mm ID).
iii. Nasal cannula, suction catheters, Ryle's tube.
iv. Laryngoscope with infant and children size blades and extra batteries.
v. Adhesive tape, manometer.
vi. Masks, tubes, assorted adaptors, Y connections, elbow.
vii. Oxygen tanks to lasts approx. 2 hrs at a rate of 6 L/min).
viii. Suction apparatus—foot operated suction machine may be used, catheter and sterile gloves.
ix. Pulse oximeter, portable nebulizer.

Desirable: Transport ventilator, end tidal CO_2 ($EtCO_2$) monitors.

The cardiovascular bag should have:

i. BP, heart rate, temperature monitor with digital display, BP cuffs of different sizes.
ii. IV cannula or catheters of different sizes (in sufficient number).

Butterfly needles	: 18 to 24 G
Over the needle catheter	: 18 to 24 G
Venous catheters	: 18 to 24 G (8 to 20 cm long)

iii. Venous cutdown set
iv. ECG monitor cum defibrillator

The Drugs

All the drugs should be packed in a different box and carry proper labels and strength of dilution. It is preferable to have charts indicating the dosage, route of administration and caution in the use of the drugs. It should include:

i. Adrenaline, Atropine, adenosine
ii. Fluids : sterile water for injection, 5%, 10%, 25% dextrose, Ringer lactate, N/2, N/5 saline, 5% to 20% albumin, dextran (if required, blood and plasma products)
iii. Soda bicarb solution, Potassium chloride, calcium gluconate, magnesium sulphate solution
iv. Diazepam, midazolam, phenytoin, phenobarbitone
v. Succinylcholine, pancuronium/ vecuronium
vi. Salbutamol (nebulization and IV use), dobutamine, aminophylline, dexamethasone
vii. Dopamine
viii. Mannitol, furosemide.

The team members should be well versed with the use of these drugs and should use these only under the guidance of physician.

Monitoring During Transport

The patient being transported should receive the same physiologic monitoring during transport as they are receiving in the ICU as far as possible. All critically ill patients being transported should have as a minimum level of monitoring, which should include following:

- Continuous monitoring with periodic documentation of electrocardiogram, pulse oximetry.
- Intermittent measurement and documentation of—air entry, colour, respiratory rate, chest expansion, pulse rate, blood pressure. In addition, selected patients based on clinical status, may benefit from monitoring capnography.
- Continuous measurement of blood pressure, intracranial pressure, intermittent measurement of central venous pressure may be needed in selected patients.

Stabilization

The key point for safe transport is optimal stabilization of the child prior to leaving the referring hospital. There is a tendency among some referring physicians to feel that the sooner a problem was of their territory, the better it was for all concerned. However, this has often resulted in hasty transfer of unstable patients who deteriorated enroute or were moribund on arrival. There is no place for hasty handover of an unstable patient in the back of an ambulance.

The stabilization process should include a thorough review of the history, clinical state of the patient and all laboratory data. Stabilization should concentrate on ensuring that the ABC's can be attended to reliably throughout transport identifying any potential cause of deterioration or system failure (see Chapter 3).

The most common cause of cardio-respiratory arrest in children is an unstable airway and respiratory system, irrespective of organ system primarily involved in the disease process. Quick assessment and stabilization of airway should be the first priority to prevent the further deterioration and improve chances of survival.

Great attention should be paid to stable airway, oxygen delivery, IV access, security of all tubes (endotracheal tube, nasogastric, chest catheters) and treatment to correct all abnormal physiological parameters. There should also be an assessment of treatment suggested by the transport coordinator which have been completed successfully and which is outstanding.

Stabilization of Respiratory System

The respiratory system must be evaluated objectively for any compromise. The child is usually unable to communicate the sensation of distress. Patient with respiratory compromise must be assessed for:

i. Undue anxiety
ii. Rate and pattern of breathing, apnea, gasps
iii. Color, cyanosis and saturation on pulse oximeter
iv. Grunting, stridor, accessory muscle use
v. Chest wall recessions and air entry.

Inspiratory stridor, suprasternal recessions and rates less than 50 per min usually indicate upper airway obstruction. Whereas predominantly lower airway involvement is manifested by rapid breathing, shallow efforts, crepts, rales and prolongation of expiration. Respiratory failure should be anticipated in certain pulmonary and non-pulmonary conditions (Table 28.2), if suspected (Table 28.3) and if present appropriate care during transport should be initiated (Table 28.4).

Table 28.2: Indications for respiratory system stabilization

1. PULMONARY
   - i. Upper airway obstructions: acute infections, foreign body, congenital anomalies, trauma.
   - ii. Lower respiratory tract disease
     - a. Small airways-asthma, bronchiolitis
     - b. Parenchymal-pneumonia
     - c. Respiratory muscle fatigue
2. NONPULMONARY
   - i. Neurological: abnormal breathing, head injury, status epilepticus, hypoxic insults, metabolic diseases, low Glasgow coma score
   - ii. Cardiovascular instability
   - iii. Severe sepsis/shock
   - iv. Inability to protect airway
   - v. Neuromuscular paralysis
   - vi. Poisoning

Table 28.3: Clinical features that should alert to possibility of respiratory failure during transport

a. Feeble cry, poor feeding and activity
b. Excessive drowsiness or agitation
c. Cyanosis or declining SpO_2
d. Severe bradycardia or hemodynamic compromise are present

Table 28.4: The major components of the respiratory care during transport

1. Provision and maintenance of a stable and patent airway
2. Respiratory support to maintain good oxygenation in a spontaneously breathing child oxygen, PAP and assisted ventilation if respiratory arrest
3. Associated hemodynamic or neurological care.

Provision and maintenance of airway: The child, if conscious should be with parents as far possible to allay the anxiety and fear of being driven away. Head and neck should be placed in position of maximum comfort and slight extension to maintain patency of airway. There should be proper support beneath and by the side of neck to cushion the jerks during the transport. Oropharynx should be cleaned beforehand and foot operated suction machine be used in the vehicle.

Oropharyngeal airway of proper size used in comatose child shall prevent the fall of tongue during jerks and keep airway patent. In semi-conscious children nasopharyngeal airway may be better tolerated but needs regular suctioning.

Endotracheal intubation may be required to maintain airway and assist ventilation if child has:

i. Apnea
ii. Upper airway obstruction
iii. Aspiration risk
iv. Raised ICP with low Glasgow coma scale < 8
v. $PaO_2 < 60$ mmHg with $FiO_2 > 60\%$, $PaCO_2 > 50$ mmHg
vi. Imminent cardiac failure
vii. Long duration of transport.

Though intubation should preferably be performed in the referring hospital the skill and necessities must be available in the vehicle to replace tube or intubate. It must be performed by an expert with the aid of sedation and muscle relaxants. Practice of rapid sequence intubation reduces the risk of acute complications such as laryngospasm, arrhythmias, bradycardia and raised intracranial pressure (ICP). Ketamine (1-2 mg/kg IV) may be used to induce brief anesthesia. Hypertension, raised ICP, head injury are the contraindications to its use. Thiopental (4-5 mg/kg IV) is the sedative of choice if there is no hypotension. It is contraindicated in status asthmaticus where ketamine is preferred. After preoxygenation with 100% oxygen and premedication with atropine (0.15 mg/kg), priming dose of muscle relaxant is given. Pancuronium/ vecuronium (1-2 mg/kg) 4 to 5 min after the initial priming dose (0.01 mg/kg) may be used. Alternatively succinylcholine (1 to 2 mg/kg) after the defasciculation dose of pancuronium may be administered. During awake intubation there is substantial risk of wide fluctuation of BP, heart rate, hemodynamic instability and increase in ICP. It should be tried only if the person is not familiar with the use of sedation and the protective reflexes of airway need to be preserved. After intubation it is mandatory to fix and secure the tube properly to prevent any life-threatening hazard on the way. Proper care to suction endotracheal tube must be taken.

Other procedures to establish the airways in the form of cricothyrotomy or tracheotomy are needed only under specific clinical situation viz. burns, trauma, and must be performed by a person with experience.

Oxygenation and respiratory support: Oxygenation of a spontaneously breathing child during transport can be achieved with the help of oxygen therapy. Various delivery systems, depending upon clinical condition and concentration of oxygen required may be used. Sufficient number of standard size cylinders with properly functioning regulators to last the journey should be carried. Usually cylinders with capacity of 1320 L are carried on ambulances. It can last for approximately 2 hours if supply is used at a rate of 6 L/ min.

If child is not breathing spontaneously, after intubation positive pressure ventilation should be started with proper size Ambu-bag. Use of reservoir will help in achieving the higher FiO_2. 'T' connection and manometer should be used to judge the pressure required. The monitoring during transport should include assessment of air entry, chest expansion, color and oxygen saturation by pulse oximetry. If available $EtCO_2$ monitor attached in the airway circuit may give valuable information about ventilation, tube displacement and block. A nasogastric tube must be put to avoid the risk of aspiration.

Transport ventilators may be used for patients not able to breathe or in respiratory failure. However, its use will require specialized and physician led teams.

Hemodynamic and Neurological Stabilization

Along with ventilation attention must be given to the hemodynamic state of the child to maintain adequate perfusion and oxygenation of vital organs particularly brain. Undue tachycardia, decreased urine output, cold extremities and hypotension indicate decreased cardiac output. Adequate replacement of volume and inotropic support must be instituted timely.

Neurological state of the child could be a reflection of cardiovascular compromise or hypoxia. However, vigorous measures should be taken in cases with raised intracranial pressure and seizures (Table 28.5). In such situations preparedness to handle any cardio-respiratory compromise is must beforehand, particularly while using anticonvulsants.

Table 28.5: Measures to stabilize raised intracranial pressure

1.	Position Head up 30°, with forward tilt
2.	Manual hyperventilation with bag
3.	Mannitol 0.25 – 0.5 g/kg stat IV

Sedation

Although to achieve calm and cooperative child is always the goal, it is usually not possible in critically ill child during transport. It may be very difficult infact to manage any anxious and restless child particularly during the associated stress of transport. The sedation of any child who is semi-conscious or awake will improve oxygenation, allay apprehension and facilitate procedures. Patient safety, side effects of drugs and interference with neurological assessment of the child are the limiting factors. Pharmacotherapy remains the mainstay, however in older children communication and comprehension of situation may be adjunctive. In case of infants and young children presence of parents makes them more comfortable and safe. Ideal sedative agent during transport should have following characteristics:

i. Rapid onset and predictable duration of action
ii. Multiple route of administration
iii. Wide therapeutic window and
iv. Minimum alteration of metabolism in various disease states.

The transport kit should have various sedative agents to be used as and when required. These should be preferably in ready to use from. There should be a display chart mentioning the strength, dilution, dose calculation, routes of administration and proper precaution during the use. The sedative agents, common in practice, and guidelines for their use are shown in Table 28.6. The use of any sedative in a sick child may result in serious and virtually life threatening complications particularly when the child is on a transport vehicle away from the intensive care setting.

The aim should never be to have a obtunded child; it should be to medically control the sensorium to a level of conscious sedation so that: (a) protective reflexes are well maintained (b) ability to maintain a patent airway is preserved (c) appropriate response to the verbal command of the physician is present. This level of sedation facilitates minor procedures and may increase oxygenation in the situations of respiratory distress.

Table 28.6: Chart depicting the common sedative agents dosage and precaution in use

Agent (Formulation)	*Route*	*Dose (mg/kg)*	*Duration (Effect)*	*Caution/comments*
Morphine 15 mg/ml	IV	0.1-0.3	1-3 h (sedation)	Respiratory depression leads to CO_2 retention
	IM	0.1-0.3	7 h (pain)	and raised ICP. Histamine release and bronchoconstriction
Diazepam 5 mg/ml	IV	0.1-0.3	6 h (sedation)	Cardiovascular and respiratory depression
	PO	0.1-0.3		
	R	0.2-0.3		Metabolism altered by hepatic disease
Midazolam (1 & 5 mg vial)	IV	0.05-0.15	1 h (sedation)	Dosage >0.25 mg/kg: anxiety and distress
	IM	0.05-0.15		Short acting: repeated administration
	PO	0.5-0.75		
	SL	0.2-0.5		
Trichloryl (500 mg/5 ml)	PO	50-75	1-2 h (sedation)	Reduces airway secretions. Rapid tolerance
Promethazine	PO	0.5-1	Variable	Receptor block: caution in hemodynamically unstable child, Dystonia, hallucinations, convulsions in large dose
Ketamine	IV	1-3	1-10 min	Excellent for short procedures. Reduces
	IM	2-10	(Dissociative	secretion, bronchodilator action
	PO	3-10	anesthesia)	Unusually causes laryngospasm, Bizarre
	R	5-10		memories
	SL	3-5		

Abbreviations: IV–intravenous, IM–intramuscular, PO–Oral, R–Rectal, SL–Sublingual

The deep sedation is needed for procedures like endotracheal intubation or cutdown and if anticipated these should be performed at the referral hospital itself. It should be practiced only rarely during the transport. Ketamine, opioids and benzodiazepines are the usual agents used. Deep sedation leaves a child non arousable and unable to maintain the airway patency because of loss of protective airway reflexes. Special attention, therefore, must be given to the vitals signs, airway patency and adequacy of ventilation before and during transport.

Before the use of any sedative one must check and record vitals signs, medical problems anticipated, relative risk and benefits of the sedation to the patient and aspirate the gastric contents. It is important to realize that aim of the sedation is to have a restful child and to minimize the discomfort of journey. One should choose a proper sedative agent considering particularly underlying disease process and possible complications. It can be administered by bolus injection or other suitable route. Care must be taken to repeat the dose once concentration reaches sub-therapeutic level to avoid child fighting with airway or oxygenation. Though infusion of opioids or benzodiazepines could be an alternative to repeated boluses, special precautions are needed to regulate the rate of drip. One must ensure that there is availability of positive pressure oxygen delivery system, airways and masks, foot operated suction, pulse oximeter and oxygen. A physician should preferably be a team member when sedation is used. If any antidote to the sedative agent used is available then it must be in the resuscitation kit.

To conclude, proper airway management is an essential part of pediatric transport. Once airway is secured, attention must be given to provide adequate ventilation and tissue oxygenation. The careful and judicious use of sedative agents will facilitate the achievement of these objectives during the transport.

Chapter twenty-nine

Organization and Setting up of a Pediatric Intensive Care Unit

Guidelines and standards for establishing PICU, and standards of care have been spelled out by specifically formed expert groups as well as individual experts. In the following discussion these recommendations have been incorporated from the stand point of needs in our country.

Do you need a PICU? The first consideration in establishing a new PICU is to document the need for such a unit. Otherwise it may be an unnecessary drain on the limited health service resources. Since PICU is an integral part of the health care services being offered in a particular set up, an assessment of its need should primarily be based on the existing patient load and type of illnesses cared for in that set up. Conditions that often require intensive care are shown in Table 29.1.

Availability of committed and appropriately trained staff, and adequate resources are other important considerations. An institution providing pediatric intensive care should be capable of providing 24 hours accessibility to a broad range of pediatric subspecialities as these are essential for optimal care.

PHYSICAL FACILITY

Size

There are no clear standards or methods to determine ideal size of a PICU. It is felt that a multi-speciality hospital requires about 5% of beds for critical care, out of which 1-2% should be in ICU. A unit smaller than 6 beds risk inefficiency and units larger than 16 beds may be difficult to manage.

Location

Location of PICU should be such that there is no thorough traffic passing through the area, and transport of patients to and from the unit for diagnostic and therapeutic procedures is minimised. Keeping this in mind a PICU should be located adjacent to or within direct access to pediatric emergency room, children wards, radiology department and operating and recovery rooms. It is also desirable for critical care units to be close to each other.

Space

Adequate provision of space is essential. The patient care area should have approximately 20 m^2 space available per patient with 3-3.5 meters separating each patient. There must be provision for enough floor space around the head end of the bed to assemble necessary personnel and equipment for resuscitation. In addition, space should be provided for nursing and clerical activity, equipment, store, doctors' duty rooms, nurses' locker room, conference room, toilets, offices of nursing superviser and consultant physician, laboratory, storage area for supplies, linen and patients belonging, and a clean and soiled work room. An intermediate care area to allow for continuing care of patients, and waiting room for families should also be provided immediately

Table 29.1 : Electrical, illumination, oxygen suction and physical environment requirement for a PICU

Electrical requirements

1. *Electric outlets*–16-18 per bed, for spot light, call bell alarms, monitoring equipments, vacuum, exhaust fan, air-conditioning, T.V.
2. *Special electric outlets*–Two, for ventilator and portable X-ray machines.
3. *Earthing*–All the outlets must be properly earthed, and have earthing circuit breakers to protect against electrocution.
4. *Voltage stabilization*–For all the outlets. Voltage fluctuations may damage sensitive monitoring equipment.

Illumination (Lighting)

1. *Background lighting*–low intensity lighting below the patient's bed level to keep a minimum illumination at all times.
2. *General and additional illumination*–during active patient care. For procedures needing extra brightness, additional lights are needed. Full size fluorescent tube lights- fixed in ceilings, 4 per patient, 2 for general and 2 for additional illumination is minimum requirement.
3. *One spotlight* to give high-level illumination for procedures, examination and treatment. This may be fixed in ceiling or may be a portable one.

Compressed air: One outlet per bed, provision of double filtered air at a line pressure of 50-55 psi.

Oxygen outlets: Two per bed, supplied from a central source, should have distinct colour for identification, alarm for low pressure, and shut-off valve between the main and the outlet to close the flow if needed.

Suction-vacuum: Two per bed minimum; a third outlet may be desirable. The pressure should be adjustable to varying needs such as nasogastric suction, thoracostomy tube drainage, endotracheal suction etc.

Physical environment

1. *Temperature:* adjustable between 22°–26° C.
2. *Relative air pressure* inside as compared to adjacent area.
3. *Air-exchanges*: at least 6 per hour; at least 2 of outdoor air. Recirculated air must pass through a two-bed filter.
4. *Air conditioning system* must allow for the above requirement for air exchange and filtration.

adjacent to the unit. The total area needed is about 3 times the size that is needed for beds alone. Floor plan of an optimum sized PICU is shown in Figure 29.1.

Design/Lay-out

Of central importance in the design of patient care area is a provision for adequacy of observation and easy access to the patient. A central station for observation, record keeping and charting, preparation of medications and other functions is therefore necessary. The patient care area may have an open ward design or multiple enclosed room design (each room serving l-2 patients). Both the designs have their advantages. However, in our setup with shortage of nurses, it is better to opt for an open ward design. For a 6-8 bed unit, a big room serving 4-6 patients, and two smaller rooms (25-30 m^2) serving l-2 patients are adequate. These rooms are required for isolation and dialysis. An area for intermediate care may be designed adjacent to PICU, to look after patients 3-4 who require intensive monitoring but are not on life supporting therapeutic intervention. Each room should have adequate shelf space (cabinet), and gowning and hand washing facility. Presence of glass covered windows is helpful in providing adequate light and for patients to maintain day-night orientation. Attractive colourful designs on walls and ceiling may be helpful.

Each bed side must be provided with appropriate electrical, illumination, suction, air and oxygen supply outlets (Table 29.1). Appropriate air conditioning, heating, ventilation, plumbing and fire safety features must be observed (Table 29.1).

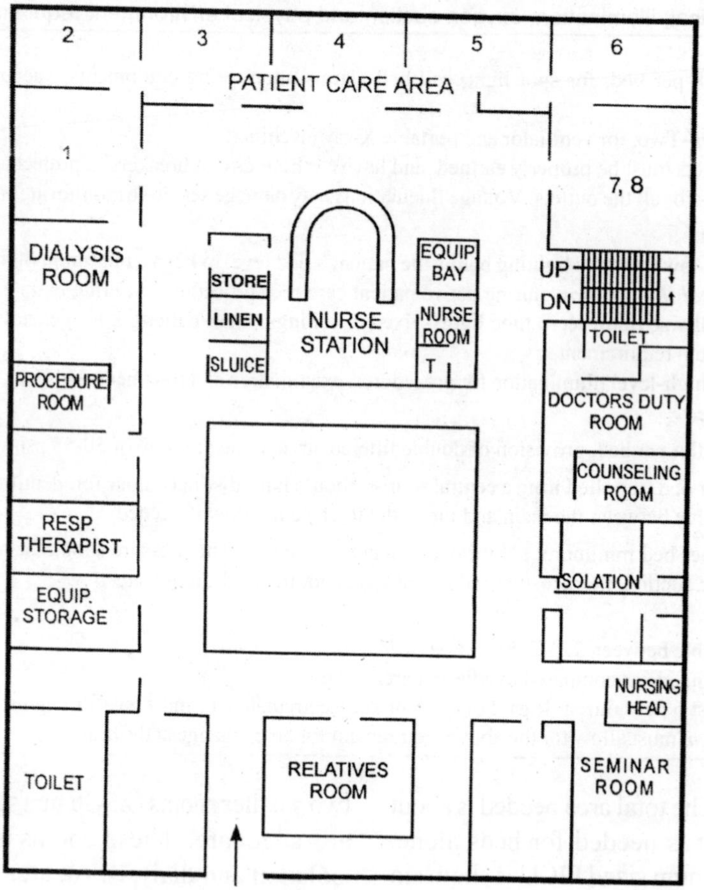

Fig. 29.1: Floor plan of Pediatric Intensive Care Unit at PGIMER

PERSONNEL

1. Physician Staff

i. ***Medical director/consultant incharge:*** The consultant incharge of the PICU should have special training and experience in the care of critically ill children including advanced skills in monitoring and life support techniques. He must be available full time for clinical, administrative and educational activities of the unit. These activities include supervision of regular care and resuscitation and life support measures to all patients, quality control and appropriateness of the care, coordination of multiple subspeciality services, maintenance, calibration and replacement of equipment, organisation of educational and research activities, staff development and improvement in standards of care, collection of statistical data necessary for evaluation of the unit's effectiveness, and implementation of policies and procedures.

It is desirable that the PICU consultant maintains regular participation in continuing education programme in the field, and scholarly activity.

ii. ***House-staff (resident)*** for 24 hrs in house coverage by a pediatric resident is a must. This person should be exclusively designated for PICU and should not be covering other areas such as the emergency department or other wards simultaneously. He/she must be trained in cardio-pulmonary resuscitation and intubation.
Formal recommendation for residency training programme in Pediatric Intensive Care are now available, and should be used as a guideline.
iii. On call coverage by subspeciality pediatrician, pediatric surgeons and anesthestist.

2. Nurses

Nurses are the most important staff in any PICU for actual delivery of critical care. It is essential to have high quality, specially trained nurses to provide 24 hours coverage. However, at present such specialized training is not available in India. A continuing education programme for nurses therefore must be developed within the unit. A common problem in our hospitals is frequent change of nursing staff and transfers. The incharge of PICU therefore must take up the issue with the concerned administrative authorities to ensure undisturbed availability of trained and experienced nurses. The ideal nurse patient ratio is l:l ; the minimum is one nurse per three patients in the unit all the time.

The nurses should have basic understanding of commonly encountered clinical conditions and should be trained in resuscitation techniques, respiratory care, electronic monitoring, PICU equipment and usage. They should be able to recognise and interpret changes in patient monitoring data, and results of common laboratory tests, perform venepuncture to obtain blood sample and establish IV line, and administer drugs and parenteral fluids and electrolytes. It is helpful to have written protocols for nursing care.

3. Respiratory Therapist

Respiratory therapist is a person trained in respiratory care. He has a knowledge of ventilation equipment and basic life support. Respiratory therapists have become an important part of ICU team in the developed countries. At least one respiratory therapist should be available round the clock.

4. Other Members

A biomedical and a laboratory technician, a unit clerk to handle patient and administrative paper work, and a physiotherapist, should be assigned specifically for PICU. Adequate coverage by a nutritionist, and a social worker should be available. A social worker is valuable in socio-psychological evaluation and family support.

SERVICES THAT SHOULD BE AVAILABLE

Monitoring

An essential part of successful intensive care is the anticipation and treatment of critical problems. A PICU must therefore, have capability to monitor on continuous basis the following:

1. *Cardiac and Hemodynamic indices:*
   i. Heart rate and rhythm
   ii. ECG
   iii. Blood pressure (non-invasive and invasive)
   iv. CVP and pulmonary artery pressure
   v. Cardiac output
2. *Respiratory functions:*
   i. Respiratory rate
   ii. Oxygen saturation of hemoglobin (SpO_2)
   iii. Blood gases
   iv. Inspired oxygen and end-tidal CO_2 monitoring for ventilated children.
3. *Temperature:* including core temperature.
4. *Cerebral functions:* Following monitoring should be available as and when needed.

i. Intracranial pressure
ii. EEG
iii. Evoked potential
iv. Cerebral blood flow.

Therapeutic or Diagnostic Modalities

Besides the usual facilities available in pediatric wards following specific services should be available:

1. Emergency resuscitation
2. Respiratory support
   i. Tracheostomy
   ii. Mechanical ventilation
   iii. Tube-thoracotomy, thoracocentesis
   iv. Bronchoscopy
3. Cardiac support
   i. Defibrillation
   ii. Temporary cardiac pacing
4. Infusion pumps and pressure infusion devices
5. Dialysis-Peritoneal/Hemodialysis, CVVH
6. Desirable
   i. Left heart support
   ii. Intra-aortic ballon assist
   iii. Extracorporeal membrane oxygenation
   iv. Hyperbaric oxygen.

Support Services Necessary for PICU

1. **Radio-diagnosis and imaging facility**
   - 24 hours coverage for portable X-rays of chest, abdomen
   - Ultrasound
   - CT-Scan
   - Echo cardiography
   - Angiography, lung scan.
2. **Laboratory service**
   It is necessary to have 24 hours a day availability of following services:
   - Hematocrit, Hb, blood counts
   - Blood glucose, urea and electrolytes
   - Prothrombin time, PTT and platelets counts
   - Body fluid analysis (CSF, urinanalysis)
   - Arterial blood gases (result within 1/2 hour)

   Other facilities that should be available are:
   - Microbiology
   - Blood biochemistry (Ca, PO_4, Mg, liver functions)
   - Toxicology and drug level measurements (digoxin, theophylline, aminoglycoides, phenobarbitone etc.).
3. Centralized O_2, compressed air, and suction facility.
4. Blood bank and pharmacy.
5. Physiotherapy and occupational therapy.
6. **Transport system:** An ambulance team with a nurse, and a resident trained in evaluation and stabilisation of critically ill patient and resuscitation equipment, drugs and basic monitoring equipment.
7. **Equipment maintenance and care:** Services of a biomedical engineer/technician should be available for regular and frequent servicing of equipment to keep it in good working order. For costly equipment regular maintenance contract should be made with the manufacturing firm if possible.

Ancillary Services

i. Housekeeping: related to cleaning, water, electrical, air-conditioning, linen-cleaning, central sterlization services.
ii. Communication: within ICU and outside through telephone, paging and intercom system. A direct outside telephone line should be available in PICU.
iii. Computerised record keeping is desirable.
iv. Social service.

EQUIPMENT

Equipment required for Intensive care is costly and needs reliable maintenance. While acquiring equipment especially the imported ones, it must be ensured that there is an Indian agency which is capable of providing high-level back-up and maintenance service. These days there are several Indian agencies offering highly sophisticated and expensive instruments, but their maintenance services are very unreliable. It may be kept in mind that high technology can not replace human skills and usually increase the work load. A list of various equipments required for monitoring and therapeutic or diagnostic purposes is given in Table 29.2.

Most of the intensive care monitors available in India offer continuous monitoring of heart rate, ECG, respiratory rate, BP, and two pressure lines (for CVP, direct arterial blood pressures, or end pulmonary artery pressure). Some also have option for cardiac output determination. All monitoring equipment should have high and low visible and audible alarms for heart and respiratory rates and all the pressures. It should also be reliable and electrically isolated from the patient.

Table 29.2 : List of equipment required for a PICU

General
Adjustable beds, cribs, incubators; emergency resuscitation trolley, laryngoscope and Ambu bag and mask for each bed, endotracheal tubes and tracheostomy tubes, spot light, suction machine, electronic thermometers with low reading facility, stethoscope for each bed, ophthalmoscope, weighing scale, oxygen cylinders, and flow meters, humidifiers, equipment for venous and arterial access, BP instruments.
Monitoring equipment
Monitors for ECG and heart rate, oscillometric blood pressure (noninvasive), central venous pressure, direct arterial blood pressure, Pulmonary artery pressure.
Respiratory rate and depth with continuous wave form.
Oxygen saturation monitor (pulse oximeter)
Oxygen-analyzers
Temperature (skin and core temp)
Intracranial pressure monitoring
EEG and cerebral function monitors
Transcutaneous pO_2
End-tidal pCO_2 measurement
Simultaneous monitoring of 3 or more pressures
Cardiac output
Equipment for therapeutic and diagnostic purposes
Ventilators with specific capabilities
Defibrillators
Infusion pumps and pressure infusers
Dialysis equipment
Temporary pace-makers
Bronchoscope–fiberoptic and regular
Optional
Pulmonary function measuring device
Intraortic balloon pump
ECHMO

There are a number of ventilators available in Indian market. While choosing one, physical size and developmental characteristics of infants and children must be kept in mind. Some of the ventilators may be suitable for adults but not for very young infants and children. Small infants need a time cycled, pressure control ventilator. Volume control ventilators for a PICU should be capable of delivering small volumes (range 15-2000 ml). Pediatric ventilators should have the following capabilities:

i. Should be able to deliver mechanical breaths via a variety of modalities: assist control, synchronous intermittent mandatory ventilation (SIMV), pressure support ventilation and controlled mechanical ventilation (CMV)
ii. PEEP
iii. Humidification and warming of gases
iv. Oxygen pressure, volume and apnea alarm
v. Adjustable flow rate and inspiratory/expiratory ratio
vi. Control of inspired O_2 concentration.

MANAGEMENT

Administration

A permanent committee consisting of PICU consultant, nursing sister/nursing supervisor, administrator, pediatrician, pediatric surgeon, and pediatric superspeciality representative should be formed for PICU administration. This committee should act as an advisory body for major equipment purchase, structural and design changes, formulation of patient care policies and procedures, and training and education programme.

There must be well defined mechanism for identification of ongoing needs and problems, as well as for providing remedial measures and improving the care.

The consultant incharge (medical director) of the unit should have the ultimate authority over admission, discharge and transfer of patients in the PICU.

Financial Management

Ideally there should be integration of finance and function with management. Financial requirement can be assigned under three heads: physical facility, equipment and personnel. Recurring expenditure should include service contract for equipment and anticipated repairs and spare parts.

Budgetary needs must be estimated per bed, from collected statistics, under recurring and non recurring expenditure, and subheadings of drugs, consumables, replacements. The overall financial management should be under the advise and supervision of a PICU committee, but PICU Incharge must have a say in deciding the priorities.

Chapter thirty

Critical Illness Neuromuscular Weakness

Critical illness neuromuscular weakness is the term given to those NMDs that are acquired *de novo* during the treatment of critical illnesses. This condition was first reported in adults with sepsis and multiorgan failure and was called critical illness polyneuropathy (CIP). Intensive care acquired NMDs are infrequent in children.

The term critical illness neuromuscular weakness includes critical illness neuropathy and myopathy (CIP &CIM). Each of these categories may occur in pure form or in combination. The spectrum of illness varies from isolated nerve entrapment, which presents with focal pain or weakness, to severe myopathy or neuropathy with associated severe and prolonged weakness.

Incidence and Prevalence

The prevalence of critical illness neuromuscular weakness is likely to be higher than generally recognized. Prospective studies have found that CIP or CIM was present in more than halt of adult patients remaining in the ICU for >7 days and in about two-third patients with sepsis or systemic inflammatory response syndrome In children, the incidence of critical care illness-associated muscle weakness appears to be lower.

Risk Factors

A number of risk factors have been identified. These include severe sepsis, systemic inflammatory response, multiorgan failure, mechanical ventilation use of corticosteroids, neuromuscular-blocking drugs (NMBAs), and amino-glycosides hyperosmolality, parenteral nutrition and hyperglycemia.

Pathogenesis

The pathogenesis is not fully understood. CIP is likely to be another end-organ manifestation of multiple-organ dysfunction. Various cytokines and inflammatory mediators may have a role in pathogenesis by damaging myelin, oligodendrocytes, and even axons in septic shock. Paralysis of arteriolar vasoreactivity lack autoregulation and impaired microcirculation in blood vessels supplying peripheral nerves may cause nerve energy failure. Both hypoxia and ischemia impair axonal transport of proteins. An alternative mechanism involves hyperglycemia and hyperosmolality, both of which increase endovascular resistance. Microvascular permeability may aggravate endoneural edema.

The mechanism that underlies CIM is not clear. *Acute necrotizing myopathy* occurs in sepsis and multiorgan dysfunction. It is fulminant and is associated with increased serum creatine kinase, myoglobulinuria, and myopathic changes on electromyography. *Thick-filament myopathy* is associated with the use of corticosteroids, and concurrent neuromuscular blocking agents (NMBAs) augment damage. In some patients, thick-filament loss and myonecrosis both may be present, which suggests a spectrum of muscle injury between the two types.

Clinical Features

Prolonged neuromuscular transmission blockade has been described in those who receive muscle relaxants for several days or weeks. These patients become ventilator dependent and have persistent paralysis and areflexia long after the drug is discontinued. Renal failure, hypermagnesemia and metabolic acidosis are important risk factors in prolonging neuromuscular blockade.

CRITICAL ILLNESS POLYNEUROPATHY (CIP)

CIP is characterized by acute, generalized neuropathy occuring after overwhelming sepsis and multiorgan dysfunction. Clinical signs usually develop 2–3 weeks after the onset of sepsis. Rapid development of flaccid, quadriparesis or paraparesis with hyporeflexia/areflexia occurs. The symptoms of polyneuropathy are not identified early because these patients are usually sedated to facilitate mechanical ventilation. The problem is recognized when an obvious difficulty is encountered in weaning from mechanical ventilation. During recovery, some patients may complaint of painful paresthesia and some may develop weakness after discharge. Loss of sensation in glove-and-stocking distribution is seen. These patients fail to grimace or move their limbs in response a painful stimulus. Clinically, the cranial nerves appear to be spared, but they may show abnormal electrophysiology. Bladder and bowel function is usually preserved. Limb edema, a common occurrence in critically ill patients, may obscure distal atrophy.

Critical Illness Myopathy (CIM)

CIM is a more common cause of critical illness neuromuscular weakness than CIP. Exposure to corticosteroids or NMBAs appears to be the major risk factor; other risk factors include sepsis and multiorgan failure. Patients have flaccid tetraparesis or tetraplegia. Deep-tendon reflexes are either normal or diminished but usually are not completely lost. The cranial nerves are intact on examination, although facial weakness may be mild. Sensation is preserved. Painful stimulation elicits facial grimacing without limb withdrawal, unlike the finding in CIP. Weaning from mechanical ventilation is difficult.

Diagnosis

The diagnosis of *critical illness neuromuscular weakness* is not easy, mainly because of limitations imposed by concurrent therapy and because the patient is usually deeply sedated and immobile. The laboratory findings are unhelpful, as these may merely reflect critical illness. Elevated creatine phosphokinase may suggest a possible toxic or inflammatory cause of myopathy. GBS can be confused with CIP/CIM. However, it can be distinguished from these by careful observation of the clinical presentation, cranial nerve involvement, and any evidence of demyelination on nerve conduction studies.

ELECTROPHYSIOLOGIC STUDIES

Nerve conduction studies and electromyography can be performed at the bedside. CNS and non-neurologic causes can be excluded, and the cause of weakness can be localized to either muscle or nerve in most cases. In a cooperative patient, CIP can be distinguished from CIM with these procedures.

The salient features on electrophysiologic studies are as follows:

CIP—The features of CIP include decreased amplitude of CMAP in response to motor nerve stimulation, with preserved motor conduction velocity and some loss or absence of sensory nerve action potential on sensory nerve stimulation, along with preserved sensory nerve conduction velocity. Phrenic nerve stimulation also yields reduced amplitude of diaphragm. Electromyography findings may show fibrillation potentials or normal or large polyphasic motor unit potentials with a reduced recruitment pattern. Findings are suggestive of axonal loss only, most severe distally, without any features of demyelination (e.g., conduction blockade or temporal dispersion nerve slowing).

CIM—Nerve conduction is usually normal. However, CMAP may be reduced with preserved sensory nerve action potential. The electromyography yields either no or a less-intense spontaneous fibrillation, but small motor unit potentials with an early recruitment pattern is seen.

Neuromuscular transmission defect—Pseudomyopathic findings with a decrement in response to repeated stimulation is seen.

TISSUE BIOPSY

Nerve biopsy in patients with CIP show acute axonal degeneration that involves both sensory and motor nerve fibers and is more pronounced in distal rather than proximal segments. No features of inflammation are seen. In the chronic stage, the nerve shows severely reduced numbers of myelinated large-diameter fibers indicative of thin myelin in almost all fibers, and cluster formation of myelinated small-diameter fibers, which indicates primary axonal degeneration with regeneration. Muscle biopsy from patients with CIP shows chronic denervation and myopathic changes.

In CIM, atrophy of type II fibers is seen with occasional atrophy of type I fibers. Muscle fiber necrosis is also seen. Electron microscopy and immunohistochemical studies demonstrate the loss of thick myosin filaments.

Treatment and Prevention

No specific treatments have been recommended. Early physiotherapy and good nutrition should help recovery. Studies have shown that glutamine, glutathione supplementation, and branched-chain amino acid supplementation is associated with improved survival and shorter ICU stay. Avoidance of prolonged immobilization and oversedation, glycemic control, and minimization of dosages and duration of corticosteroids and NMBAs can prevent, to some extent, development of this devastating complication of critical illness that requires prolonged ICU stay.

Outcome

The development of CIP/CIM affects both the short-term and long-term outcomes. It increases duration of mechanical ventilation, prolongs ICU stay and hospitalization, and increased healthcare cost. Much of the data on outcome in *critical illness neuromuscular weakness* is related to patients with CIP. Mortality is high in adults and much less in children. Chronic disability is a common. Some may be left with tetraplegia or paraplegia. Milder disabilities have been reported in patients with full functional recovery and include hyporeflexia or areflexia, sensory abnormalities, muscle atrophy, and footdrop. The time course of recovery varies greatly. Neuromuscular abnormalities may continue for 5 years after illness. Weakness and/or neuropsychologic changes may also persist for 5 years. Some patients may never become fully functional, affecting their quality of life. It is generally thought that patients with CIM recover faster and have better prognosis than those patients with CIP.

Appendices: Procedures

Appendix-1

Universal Precautions and HIV Exposure in PICU

In 1985, The Center for Disease Control introduced a strategy for blood and body fluid precautions known as universal precautions. The following recommendations apply to ICU procedures:

1. Use protective double gloves for all vascular cannulations.
2. Use sterile gloves for all cannulations except those involving the introduction of a short catheter into a peripheral vein.
3. Caps, gowns, masks and protective eyewear if splashes of blood/body secretions are anticipated (e.g., in a trauma victim). [These measures do not reduce the incidence of catheter-related sepsis].
4. Avoid needle stick injuries
   - i. Do not recap needles or manually remove needles from syringes.
   - ii. Place all sharp instruments in puncture–resistant containers immediately after use.
   - iii. If a needle stick injury is sustained during the procedure, follow the recommendations.

Accidental HIV Exposure

Risk and management

Risk of HIV transmission in the ICU is very low. Percutaneous Exposures to a single needle-stick injury with blood from an HIV-infected patient carries an average 0.3% risk of HIV seroconversion. The likelihood is higher from a deep skin puncture, visible blood on the needle, and injury from a needle that was placed in an artery or vein of the source patient. A single exposure of broken skin or mucous membranes of blood from an HIV-infected patient carries an average 0.09% (0.9 per 1000) risk of HIV seroconversion.

Postexposure Prophylaxis and Management (CDC recommendations)

After possible exposure to HIV from a needlestick injury or blood splash to the face the major decision is whether or not to begin prophylactic therapy with antiretroviral agents. If HIV infection is proven or suspected in the source patient treatment is recommended. If the HIV antibody status of the source patient is unknown perform a rapid HIV-antibody test on a blood sample from the source patient. A positive result must be confirmed by another test such as Western blot. When the source is HIV negative or HIV is unlikely in source patient no drug is needed. Two drugs regimen is given if the source patient is HIV positive but asymptomatic or HIV status is not known but it is likely in source patient. Three-drug regimen is used if the source is HIV positive and symptomatic or exposure from a asymptomatic HIV patient is severe.

The recommended two-drug regimen is zidovudine (200 mg TID) plus lamivudine (150 mg BID) for 4 weeks. A third antiretroviral agent is added if there is evidence for symptomatic or advance HIV infection in the source patient, or if the HIV exposure is severe.

Postexposure Surveillance: Antibody responses to acute or primary HIV infection can take 4 to 6 weeks to become evident. Therefore anyone with documented exposure to HIV infection should have serial tests for HIV antibodies at 6 weeks, 3 months, and 6 months after the exposure.

Appendix-2

Protocol of Hand Hygiene

HANDWASHING

Handwashing with soap and water is recommended when hands are visibly dirty or contaminated with or are visibly soiled with blood or other body fluids. An antiseptic solution rather than plan soap and water is recommended for most instances of handwashing. Among antiseptic agent Idophors (Betadine) have broad spectrum of activity, slow onset of action, and must be left in contact for few minutes to be effective; it can irritate the skin. Chlorhexidine has good residual activity and relatively narrow spectrum of activity

A waterless alcohol gel (such as Sterillium) is recommended if the hands are not visibly *soiled. Alcohols Rubs have rapid onset of action, broad spectrum of activity but little residual activity.*

Indication for Handwashing with an antiseptic preparation

1. Before and after direct contact with patients
2. After contact with body fluids, secretions, excretion, mucous membranes, wound dressing, and contaminated items.
3. Before donning sterile gloves to insert central intravascular catheters, before inserting urinary catheters, venous catheters, or other invasive devices.
4. When moving from a contaminated body site to a clean body site during a patient's examination.

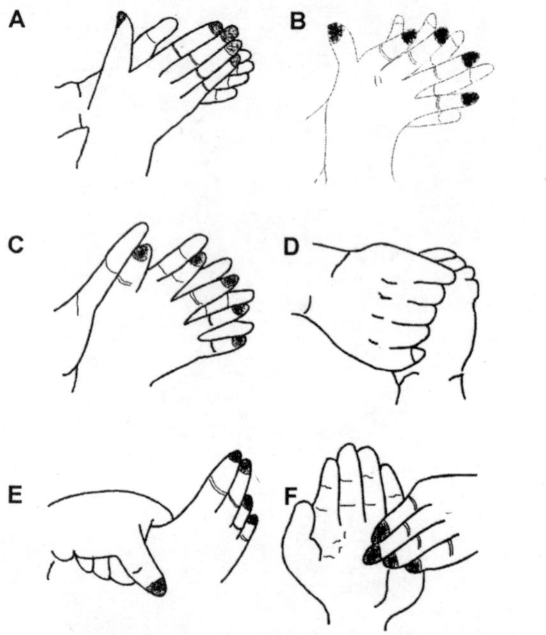

Fig. A2.1: Procedure for Effective Hand Hygiene (A) Palm to palm (B) Right palm over left dorsum and left palm over right dorsum (C) Palm to palm fingers interlinked (D) Backs of fingers to opposing palms and fingers interlocked (E) Rotational rubbing of right thumb clasped in left palm and vice-versa (F) Rotational rubbing backwards and forwards with clasped fingers of a right hand in left palm

ROUTINE HAND HYGIENE

1. This process is mandatory for all medical, nursing and paramedical personnel who come in contact with the patient.
2. All such individuals should wash their hands and distal forearm with water and 2% chlorhexidine surgical scrub solution at the

beginning of their duty hours and after every break away from the unit.

3. No watches or jewellary must be worn during this wash. This wash must last for a minimum of two minutes.
4. The hands must be dried with a sterile, dry towel or with disposable paper tissue.
5. The process must be repeated after any accidental unprotected contact with the body fluids of a patient.
6. A hand rub (with alcohol or chlorhexidine in alcohol) should subsequently be used:
   - Before and after every contact with the patient.
   - While moving from one bed to another.
   - While moving to common areas (refrigerator /store/telephone).
7. The hand rub is also required before gloving and after degloving for any non-procedural contact that involves handling of IV lines fluids, blood draws or contact with body fluids or wounds.
8. The use of gloves does not preclude the need for the hand hygiene techniques described above.

PROCEDURAL HAND HYGIENE

1. This process is indicated before every procedure including, but not limited to, central venous access, PA catheter and arterial line placement.
2. The process is a full surgical scrub using running water and 4% chlorhexidine scrub solution from the fingertips to the elbow.
3. Care must be taken to ensure drainage of water away from the fingers and hands, towards the elbows.
4. No watches, rings or jewellary must be worn during the scrub.
5. There is no advantage to the use of sterile disposable brushes or sponges in the process.
6. The scrub should be performed for a minimum of two to three minutes.
7. Hand drying should be only with the use of sterile (autoclaved) towels.
8. This scrub always precedes gowning and gloving for the procedure.

Table A2.1 : Recommendations for Glove Use in the ICU

I. Sterile gloves

1. Recommended for the following procedures

A. Central venous catheterization
B. Peripherally inserted central catheters (PICC)
C. Arterial catheterization
D. Placement of drainage catherters in a closed space (pleural, pericardial, or peritoneal cavities)
E. Insertion of epidural catheters (for analgesia), intraventricular catheters, ICP transducers for intracranial pressure montioring

II. Nonsterile gloves

1. Should be used for contact with any moist body substance - blood, body fluids, secretion, excretions, nonintact skin, and mucous membranes. Clean (unsoiled) gloves should be used for contact with nonintact skin and mucous membranes
2. Can be used for insertion of peripheral venous catheters as long as the gloved hands do not touch the catheter.

III. General recommendations

1. Gloves should be changed between tasks and procedures on the same patient if there has been contact with material that may be infectious.
2. Gloves should be removed immediately after use, before contact with noncontaminated objects in the environment, and before going to another patient.

Appendix-3

Organization of CPR

CPR is simple when one or two rescuers are providing basic support. However, effective advanced CPR requires maticulous organisation. The following responsibilities must be assigned clearly and rehearsed on regular basis.

1. Team leader: The physian most experienced in CPR should assume this role. He should have overall command and coordinate the efforts.
2. Nurse: Should support physician's effort by obtaining drugs and other material.
3. Airway manager: Should be the person most skilled in airway management. He provide 100% O_2 by positive pressure ventilation via a bag and mask or an endotracheal tube.
4. A fourth person should administer chest compression

Finally a record keeper should document all events, drugs and vital signs during CPR.

Appendix-4

Sequence of Actions for Foreign Body Airway Obstruction

In a witnessed or seriously suspected foreign body aspiration, if the child is breathing spontaneously, he should be encouraged to persist with spontaneous coughing and breathing efforts as long as the cough is forceful. Intervention is necessary only if the cough becomes ineffective, if breathing is inadequate or if the child loses consciousness.

A. For an Infant

1. *Perform upto five back blows:* by holding the infant in the prone position straddling on one's forearm, with the head being held firmly by holding the jaw in a position lower than the trunk (Fig. A4.1). Back blows are given using the heel of the hand to the middle of the back between shoulder blades. If this fails to dislodge the foreign body, one should proceed to perform the chest thrusts.
2. *Perform up to five chest thrusts:* at the same location as for chest compression after turning the infant as a unit into supine position. The technique for chest thrusts should be sharper and more vigorous than compressions and carried out more slowly (5 thrusts in 15 seconds).
3. *Remove the foreign body from the mouth* if it is seen.
4. *Open airway*: by head tilt-chin lift maneuver and reassess breathing.
5. *Provide upto 2 rescue breaths* if child is not breathing.
6. *Repeat five back blows and five chest thrusts* and rescue breathing cycles until the airway is cleared and rescue breathing a successful.

B. For a Child

Abdominal thrusts (Heimlich maneuver) are used to generate an artificial cough to clear the airway in the following sequence :

a. *When the child is conscious:* With the child standing or sitting, one stands behind him and the arms are wrapped around the child just below the lower margin of the rib cage . Clasping the hands tightly together, a series of up to five quick upwards thrust are given over the victims abdomen in the midline slightly above the navel and well below the tip of the xiphoid process (Fig. A4.2). The series of five thrusts should be continued until the foreign body is expelled or the patient loses consciousness. If the child loses consciousness, the airway is opened and rescue breathing attempted, as described for infants and Heimlich maneuver is repeated as described below.

b. *When the child is unconscious:* With the child lying down, the rescuer kneels beside the victim's hips. Both hands are placed on top of

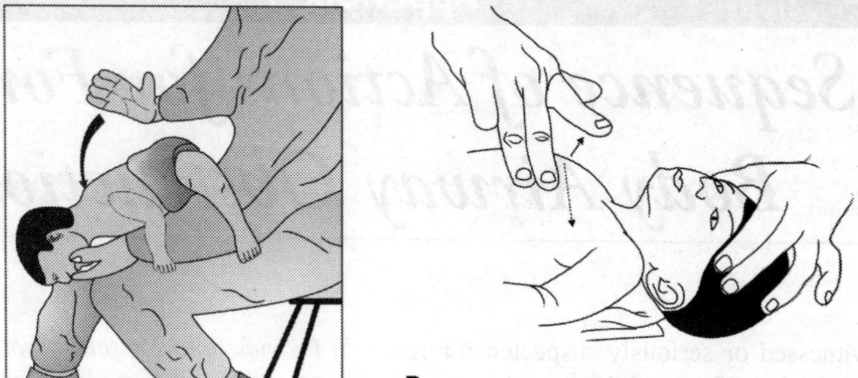

Fig. A4.1: Position for relieving foreign body obstruction in infant (A) By back blows (B) By chest thrust

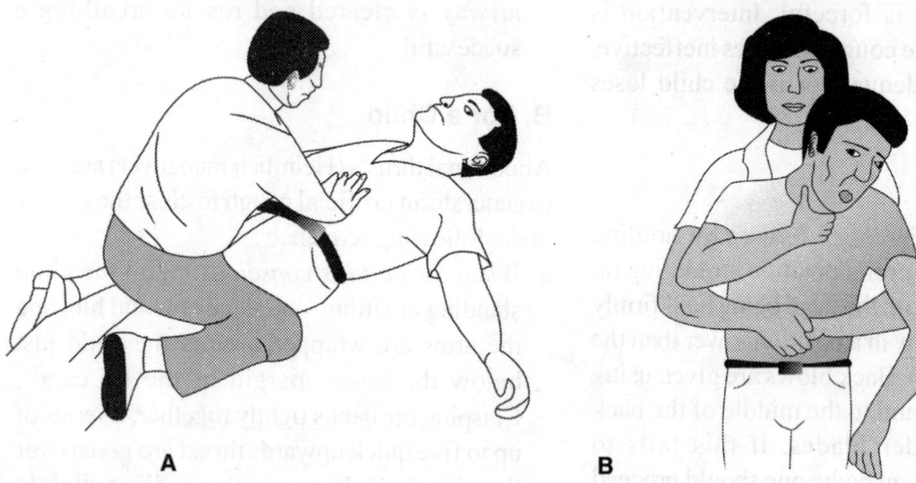

Fig. A4.2: Position for relieving foreign body obstruction in older children (A) Abdominal thrust in unconscious patient lying flat (B) Abdominal thrust (Heimlich Maneuver) in conscious patient sitting or standing

each other with the heel of one hand at the same site as described for conscious child.

Rest of the sequence is same as for conscious child.

Appendix-5

Chest Compression

Chest Compression in the Infant

The area of compression is the lower half of the sternum. The technique of compression is as follows:

1. Maintain the infant's head position using one hand unless it is under the child's back.
2. Compress the chest using other hand. Place the index finger of that hand on the sternum just below the level of infant's nipples. Place the middle fingers on the sternum adjacent to the index fingers. Perform sternal compression approximately one finger-width below the level of the nipples. Avoid compression of the xiphoid process because it may injure the liver, stomach or spleen.
3. "Push hard" Compress the sternum upto a depth of 1/2 to 1 inch which corresponds to approximately one third to one half the anteroposterior width of the chest.
4. At the end of each compression, release pressure to allow the sternum to return briefly to its normal position. Compression should be rhythmic with equal time for compression and relaxation.
5. "Push fast" Perform about 100 compressions per minute and co-ordinate compressions with ventilations in a 15:2 ratio.
6. Administer drugs after approximately 1 minute of CPR (20 cycles).
7. Continue chest compression if heart rate is less than 60/min and peripheral pesrfusion is poor.

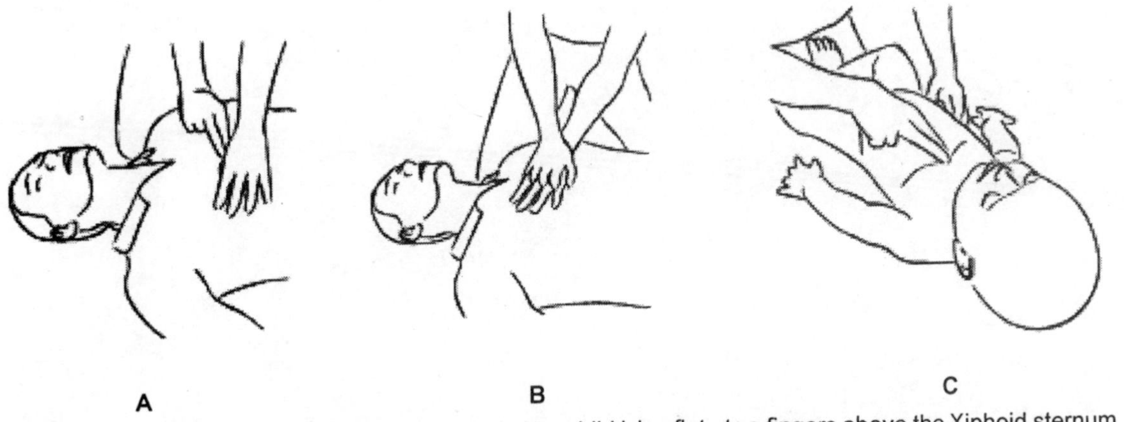

Fig. A5.1: Landmarks for Chest Compression (A) In a child lying flat - two fingers above the Xiphoid sternum, place heel of the hand. (B)In a child lying flat–as in 'A' bring other hand interlock the fingers and apply downward compression 2.5 to 3.5 cms. with heel of both the hands (C) In an infant lying flat–compression with two fingers at the lower of half of sternum.

Chest Compression in the Child

1. Maintain the head position using one hand.
2. Place the heel of the hand over lower half of the sternum (below the nipple line), avoiding the xiphoid process. The long axis of the heel is over the long axis of the sternum.
3. Compress the chest to about 1-1.5 inch in children.
4. Allow the chest to return to its resting position after each compression. Compression and relaxation should be of equal duration.
5. Administer medications after one minute of CPR.
6. Continue chest compression if heart rate is less than 60/min and peripheral perfusion is poor.

Frequently reassess the breathing, pulse and circulation to determine response to basic life support.

Appendix-6

Intubation and Extubation

INDICATIONS

Please refer to chapter 5.

EQUIPMENTS

1. Suction machine/central suction source
2. Suction catheter
3. Bag valve mask device
4. Oxygen source
5. Endotracheal tubes of assorted size
6. Laryngoscopes, straight blade and curved blade
7. Tape
8. Medicine and supplies
9. Pulse Oximeter and ECG Monitor.

RAPID SEQUENCE INTUBATION: STEPS

1. Preoxygenate with 100% oxygen, connect with a saturation monitor and vital sign monitor for BP.
2. Atropine 0.02 mg/kg (max. 1 mg, minimum 0.1 mg) IV.
3. Optional priming/defasciculation dose (avoid in hyperkalemia, raised ICP)
   Priming–vecuronium 0.01 mg/kg IV.
   Defasciculation–Pancuronium 0.01 mg/kg IV.
4. Keep self-inflating bag and mask for ventilation ready.
5. Apply cricoid pressure to occlude oesophageal lumen (separate person).
6. Muscle relaxant
   - Vecuronium 0.1 mg/kg IV (4 min after priming dose)
   - Succinylcholine 0.1 mg/kg (infants) IV, 1.5 mg/kg IV (children) 1-3 minutes after defasciculating dose (Avoid in hyperkalemia, raised ICP).
7. Sedation agent–Problem specific
   - **No hypotension/hypovolemia:** Thiopental 4-5 mg/kg IV or diazepam 0.2 mg/kg IV + Morphine 0.1 mg/kg IV.
   - **Mild hypotension/hypovolemia** with suspected head injury or raised ICP: thiopental 2-4 mg/kg IV slowly.
   - **Mild hypotension / hypovolemia** without raised ICP or head injury: no sedative or ketamine 1–2 mg/kg + diazepam 0.2 mg/kg IV.
   - **Status asthmaticus:** Ketamine 1-2 mg/kg. plus Midazolam 0.2 mg/kg.
8. Monitor BP and oxygen saturation.
9. Intubate when full relaxation is achieved.
10. Release cricoid pressure.
11. Assess the position of tube: ensure it is in trachea, not in right bronchus.
12. Fix the tube/Get check X-ray.
13. Reversal of vecuronium if desired – Atropine 0.02 mg/kg, and Edrophonium 0.5 mg-1.0 mg/kg IV.

TECHNIQUE OF EXTUBATION

- Withhold feeds for at least 4 hours and empty stomach
- Thorough physiotherapy, postural drainage and endotracheal suctioning
- Withdraw tube during positive pressure inflation of 'Ambu' bag

- Place child with head elevated and oxygen as required.

POST EXTUBATION COMPLICATIONS

- *Stridor:* usually self limiting, rarely will require steroids, nebulized adrenaline for extended period.
- *Upper lobe atelectasis:* treat with physiotherapy, humidified O_2
- *Reintubation:* rare.

Trouble shooting problems with intubation

Problem	*Suggested approach for solution*
1. Copious secretion prevents visualization	Suction prior to attempt Place suction catheter in oropharynx through left side of mouth and have assistant apply suction.
2. Tube seems too big to fit through vocal cords	Verify correct size for ideal patient weight Decrease angle of neck extension. Apply traction rather than leverage to blade. Select next smaller size tube
3. Vocal cords are closed	Await spontaneous breath. Apply gentle pressure over suprasternal area. Give Succinylcholine (2 mg/kg); ventilate.
4. Unsure of appropriate depth for insertion	Insert tube only just past vocal cords. Determine length of ET tube at lip. Obtain radiograph with head in neutral position and document position relative to carina and thoracic inlet.
5. Hard to ventilate through tube after insertion	Verify that tube is intratracheal. Verify that tube is not in bronchus. Consider airway obstruction.
6. Return of blood via ET tube in absence of lung disease.	Remove tube and evaluate for perforation or trauma.
7. Tube slips into right bronchus	Avoid neck extension. Keep tape secure. Maintain appropriate lip-to-tip distance.
8. Unplanned extubation	Regularly verify correct lip-to-tip distance Keep tape secure and replace as often as necessary. Support neck whenever moving infant. Avoid neck flexion or traction on tube. Secure hands of infant.

(Adapted from Ramesh S. Indian J Practical Pediatrics 1999; 11: 35-40).

Appendix-7

Central Venous Catheter Insertion

INDICATIONS

1. Inadequate peripheral venous access- Inability to cannulate peripheral veins.
2. Administration of incompatible mediations through a multilumen catheter.
3. Administration of irritating , caustic, or hypertonic solutions.
4. Hemodynamic monitoring.
5. Infusion of resuscitation fluids and vasoactive drugs.
6. Access to central circulation (endocardial pacing, hemodialysis, pulmonary artery catheterization).

Sites for Insertion of Central Venous Catheters

Subclavian vein	Popular choice with the inexperienced High rate of pneumothorax (up to 20%) Bleeding from punctured subclavian artery difficult to control. Generally comfortable for patients (although awkward for treatment of shoulder contractures in neurological/ neurosurgical patients) Probably lowest infection rate Suitable for tunneling.
Internal jugular vein	Reliable access to superior vena cava (SVC) and right atrium. Risk of damage to neck structures (hematoma from punctured carotid artery can cause life-threatening airway obstruction), lower risk of pneumothorax than subclavian vein, less comfortable for patient.
Basilic vein (ante-cubital fossa)	Avoids damage to structures of thoracic inlet, neck. Maneuvering past clavi-pectoral fascia may be difficult, but correct placement in up to 90% of patients in experienced hands. Risk of damage to brachial artery and median nerve. Thrombophlebitis is common, Traditionally performed using single-lumen 'long lines'.
Femoral vein	Long-lines required to allow CVP measurement. Useful when clotting is deranged or when patient will not tolerate head-down position. Convenient site for large-bore devices (eg, dialysis catheters). Higher risk for infection.
External jugular vein	May be difficult to find. Potentially less damaging to neck structures and lung. May be awkward to pass guide wire into SVC because of tortuous route Useful for temporary emergency access.

Table A7.1 : Catheter Size Chart

French size	Gauge	Inner Diameter	Outer Diameter
1	27	0.0007 in or 0.1 mm	0.016 in or 0.4 mm
2	23	0.012 in or 0.3 mm	0.025 in or 0.6 mm
3	20	0.020 in or 0.5 mm	0.037 in or 0.9 mm
4	18	0.025 in or 0.6 mm	0.047 in or 1.2 mm
5	16	0.035 in or 0.7 mm	0.065 in or 1.7 mm

Equipment

Single-lumen or multilumen central venous catheter or insertion kit

General supplies

1. Sterile central venous catheter, guidewire, 20-21 gauge thin-walled central venous needle.
2. Syringe, scalpel, dilators, suture, syringes and infiltrating needles.

3. Tape.
4. Sterile 2 × 2 and 4 × 4 gauge sponges.
5. Medication for local anesthesia and sedation
6. Sterile gloves, gown, mask, cap and drapes for universal precautions.
7. Povidone iodine.
8. Supplemental oxygen (cannula, mask, other as appropriate).
9. Pulse oximeter.
10. ECG monitor.
11. Intravenous tubing and fluid.
12. Resuscitation chart available.

Technique

General—Modified Seldinger technique

- Inform patient if conscious
- Assure peripheral intravenous access if possible and if not previously done
- Apply oxygen monitor pulse oximeter and ECG and monitor
- Position patient (see specific site below)
- Don mask and cap
- Wash hands
- Don sterile gown and gloves
- Create sterile field
- Identify anatomical landmarks
- Establish the needle entry site and the angle/ depth of insertion
- Assemble equipment
- For internal jugular and subclavian vein cannulations, estimate the length of central venous catheter needed by comparing to the patient's anatomy by laying the catheter over cava and right atrium (approximately at the second intercostals space)
- Infiltrate local anesthetic
- Advance 20-21-gauge needle at specific angle and direotion to predetermined depth while applying suction to the syringe
- Entry into the vein will be signaled by rapid flush of venous blood into the barrel of the syringe
- If a rapid flush of blood does not occur as the needle is advanced to the predetermined depth, continue to apply suction to the syringe and withdraw the needle slowly along the same pathway. Often, a flush of venous blood will occur during withdrawal, indicating that the needle collapsed the vein and perforated both anterior and posterior walls during advancement
- If the vein is not encountered, do not change needle direction midcourse; rather, retract the needle tip to a subcutaneous position and redirect the tip
- Once in the central vein, immobilize the needle with free hand
- Remove the syringe from the needle and cover hub of needle with thumb of the hand holding the needle
- Some needle/ syringes units are made to insert the guidewire directly through the syringe (see package insert of specific equipment in use)
- Advance guidewire through needle ; minimal to no resistance should be met
- Many guidewires are long enough to reach the heart and cause ectopy ; monitor the ECG carefully during passage of the guidewire
- When guidewire is in place, withdraw needle from the insertion site over the wire, leaving guidewire in place
- Use scalpel and dilator to open skin and dilate subcutaneous tissue
- Using a rotating motion, advance catheter over the guidewire into the vein to predetermined depth
- Remove guidewire, aspirate free flow of venous blood through the catheter to confirm catheter tip is within vessel lumen, then connect IV tubing and fluid
- If the catheter is correctly positioned, blood should be easily aspirated from all ports of a multilumen catheter
- Secure the catheter with suture and apply sterile dressing

- Obtain a chest radiograph to confirm position for internal jugular and subclavian vein catheters.

Note: During subclavian and internal jugular line placement, aspiration of air into the venous circulation is possible while syringes, tubing and guidewires are exchanged and connected. This is a particular risk in patients who are breathing spontaneously and are not on positive-pressure ventilation. Care should be taken to occlude intravascular catheters any time syringes and line are being connected so as to minimize the risk of air entrainment and embolization.

Internal Jugular Vein (Central Approach)

- Position patient in a 15° head – down (Trendelenburg) position to ensure filling of the internal jugular vein.
- Stand at the head of the bed.
- Turn patient's head away from the side to be cannulated.
- Both right and left internal jugular veins can be cannulated; however, the right side has several advantages over the left:
  - More direct route to the superior vena cava
  - The apex of the left lung is higher than the right, making the possibility of pneumothorax greater on the left
  - The thoracic duct is on the left, making the possibility of thoracic duct injury greater on the left
  - The medial (sternal) and lateral (clavicular) bellies of the sternocleidomastoid muscle from a triangle with the clavicle at the base
  - The internal jugular vein lies within the carotid sheath just beneath the apex of the triangle formed by the bellies of the sternocleidomastoid
  - The carotid artery also lies within the carotid sheath just medial and deep to the internal jugular vein.
- The skin is punctured at the apex of the triangle; the needle tip is directed caudally at a 45° to 60° angle to the frontal plane and laterally toward the ipsilateral nipple (Fig. A 7.2).
- The needle is advanced to a depth of 3 to 4 cm, depending on patient size.
- If the vein is not entered, redirect the needle tip slightly more medially and repeat; do not direct the needle tip across the midline as the carotid artery may be punctured.
- When the vein is entered, proceed as above for passage of the guidewire and catheter.

Subclavian Vein (Infraclavicular Approach)

- Position patient in a 15° head-down (Trendelenburg) position to ensure filling of the subclavian vein
- Stand at the side of the bed
- Turn patient's head away from the side to be

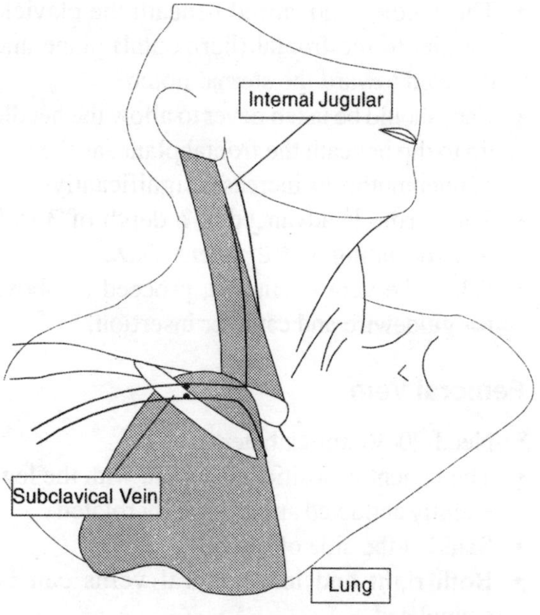

Fig. A7.1: Site for subclavian approach, its relationship with lung

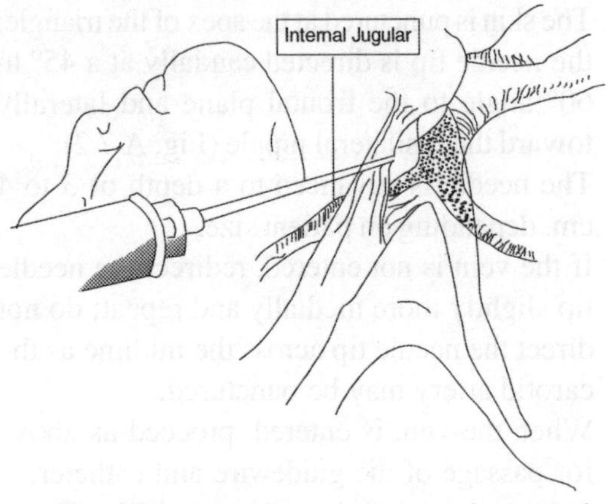

Fig. A7.2: Internal jugular—central approach

cannulated. Place a rolled towel vertically between the scapulas

- Both right and left subclavian veins can be cannulated
- The skin is punctured at the junction of the medial and middle thirds of the clavicle (Fig. A7.1)
- The needle is advanced beneath the clavicle parallel to the frontal (horizontal) plane and directed toward the sternal notch
- Care should be taken never to allow the needle tip to dip beneath the frontal plane, as the risk of pneumothorax increases significantly
- The needle is advanced to a depth of 3 to 5 cm, depending on the patient's size
- When the vein is entered, proceed as above for guidewire and catheter insertion.

Femoral Vein

- Need 20-30 cm catheter
- The patient is positioned supine with the legs slightly abducted and externally rotated
- Stand at the side of the bed
- Both right and left femoral veins can be cannulated
- Palpate the anterior superior iliac spine and the pubic tubercle. These bony landmarks delineate the course of the inguinal ligament. The abdominal compartment lies cephalad to the inguinal ligament, the leg caudal. Do not attempt venous access cephalad to the inguinal ligament
- The femoral artery runs directly beneath the inguinal ligament. It should be identified by palpation of its pulse and its course determined
- The femoral vein lies medial and parallel to the femoral artery
- The skin is punctured 1 to 2 cm below the inguinal ligament
- The needle is advanced at an approx. 20-45° angle and directed cephalad
- The needle is advanced until venous blood is freely aspirated
- When the vein is entered, proceed as above for guidewire and catheter placement.

V. Precautions/Complications

Central Venous Pressure: sources of variability

CVP can be misleading as measures of ventricular preload. Body position at the time of CVP measurement may be a source of variability. Central venous pressures should not be recorded when patients are placed in lateral positions. The zero reference point for venous pressures in the thorax is a point on the external thorax where the fourth intercostal space intersects the mid-axillary line. This point corresponds to the position of the right and left atrium when the patient is in the supine position.

Changes in thoracic pressure may also affect CVP. The physiologically important vascular pressure is the transmural pressure i.e., the difference between the intravascular and extravascular pressures. The intravascular pressure is an accurate reflection of the transmural pressure only when the extra-vascular pressure is zero. When vascular pressures are recorded in the thorax, changes in thoracic pressure can be transmitted across the wall of blood vessels, resulting in a discrepancy between intravascular and transmural pressures. Therefore intravascular pressures should be measured at the end of expiration, when they are equivalent to the transmural pressure. However, if the patient is on PEEP, intravascular pressures measured at the end of expiration will exceed the transmural pressure. Therefore, *when external PEEP is applied, intravascular pressures should be measured at end-expiration when the patient is briefly disconnected from the ventilator.* In the presence of intrinsic PEEP, accurate recording of intravascular pressures can be difficult.

Complications of venous puncture

- Pneumothorax, hemothorax, chylothorax (subclavian and internal jugular approaches)
- Ectopic placement and delivery of fluid (e.g. into pleural cavity)
- Arterial puncture.

  Note: If a large catheter is inadvertently placed in an artery, it should be left as is and expert consultation obtained
- Local subcutaneous tissue, nerve, artery, and vein damage. Damage to larynx, thyroid, thoracic duct, esophagus, endotracheal tube, brachial plexus, recurrent laryngeal nerve
- Thrombosis and thrombophlebitis
- Infection-Catheter-related sepsis
- Erosion through SVC/Right atrium
- Catheter, guidewire embolism
- Cardiac arrhythmias
- Hemorrhage
- Air embolism.

Appendix-8

Technique for Radial Artery Puncture

- Explain the process to patient/parents
- Perform modified *Allen's Test* (see below)
- Clean the site with spirit
- Local anesthesia is optional
- Use 21 gauze needle with syringe
- Flush syringe and needle with heparin
- Palpate artery with one hand and enter skin at 45 degree angle (Figs A8.A and B)
- Obtain 2-3 ml of blood preferably without aspiration
- Withdraw syringe and needle and give firm pressure at site of puncture
- To maintain anaerobic conditions eliminate air bubbles and seal syringe with a cap
- Perform the analysis as soon as possible or place sample immediately in ice sluch if delay is likely.

The Allen Test

The Allen test evaluates the capacity of the ulnar artery to supply blood to the digits when the radial artery is occluded.

1. Occlude the radial and ulnar arteries with the thumb and index finger.

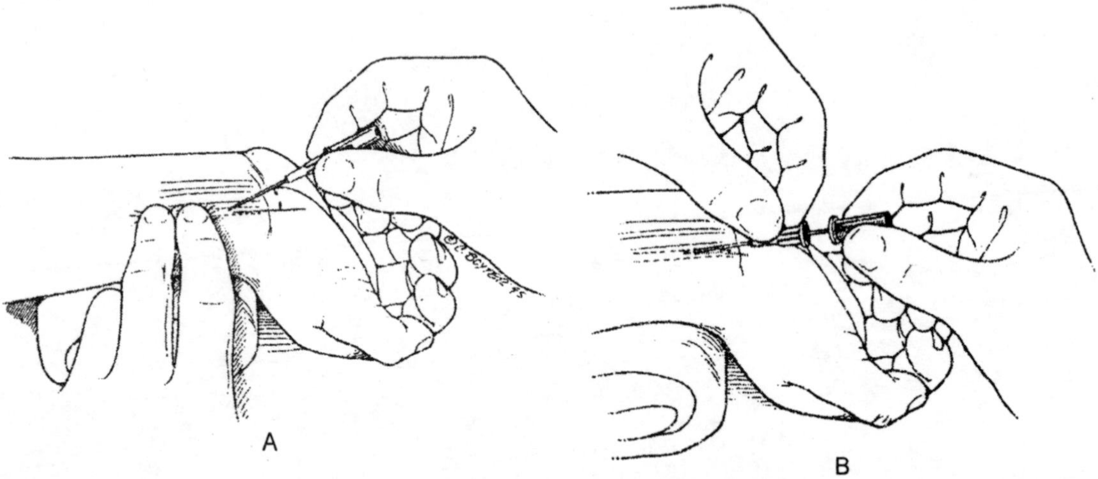

Figs A8.A and B: (A) After extending and immobilizing the wrist, the radial artery is localized by palpation. The needle is inserted at a 20° to 45° angle. (B) After the artery is entered, advance the catheter over the needle and withdraw the needle

2. Raise the patients wrist above the head and to make a fist repeatedly until the fingers turn white.
3. Release the ulnar artery and record the time required for return of the normal color to the fingers.

A normal response time is 7 seconds or less, and a delay of 14 seconds or greater is evidence of insufficient flow in the ulnar artery.

A positive Allen test is generally a contraindication to radial artery cannulation. This test is not possible in infants as patient's cooperation is needed to perform the test.

Appendix-9

Arterial Catheter Insertion

I. Indications

A. Continuous assessment of systolic, diastolic, and mean blood pressures

B. Frequent arterial blood gas measurements.

II. Equipment

A. Radial artery cannulation

1. 20-22 gauge catheters over the needle
2. 20-24 gauge radial artery catheterization kit with guidewire (preferred).

B. Femoral artery cannulation

1. 20 gauge catheter over the needle
2. 20 gauge, 6 inch femoral artery catherization kit with guidewire (preferred).

C. General

1. Arterial catheter or kit (above)
2. Tape
3. Sterile 2 × 2 and 4 × 4 gauge sponges
4. Medication for local anesthesia
5. Medication for sedation, if necessary
6. Sterile gloves, gown, mask, cap, drapes, eye protection for universal precautions
7. Povidone iodine
8. Pressure transducer, tubing, pressure monitor.

III. Technique

Radial Artery

- Complete aseptic technique
- Inform patient
- Assure intravenous access
- Position patient as shown in Figure A9.1
- Don mask, cap and eye protection
- Wash hands and don sterile gloves
- Create sterile field
- Identify anatomic landmarks
- Assemble equipment
- Palpate radial artery at head of the radius
- Infiltrate anesthetic
- Insert needle over radial artery ~ 1 cm distal to radial head (Fig.A9.1A)
- Advance needle at ~ 20° to 45° angle
- Entry into artery will be signaled by appearance of pulsating arterial blood
- Once in artery, immobilize needle with free hand
- Catheter over the needle – advance the catheter with a rotating motion to hub and remove needle
- Modified Seldinger technique (Fig. A9.1B)
- Advance the guidewire
- Pass arterial catheter over the guidewire
- Remove needle and guidewire
- Connect tubing to pressure transducer
- Secure the catheter to the skin with suture and apply sterile dressing.

Femoral Artery Cannulation

- Complete aseptic technique
- Inform patient
- Assure intravenous access
- Position patient
- Don mask, cap and eye protection

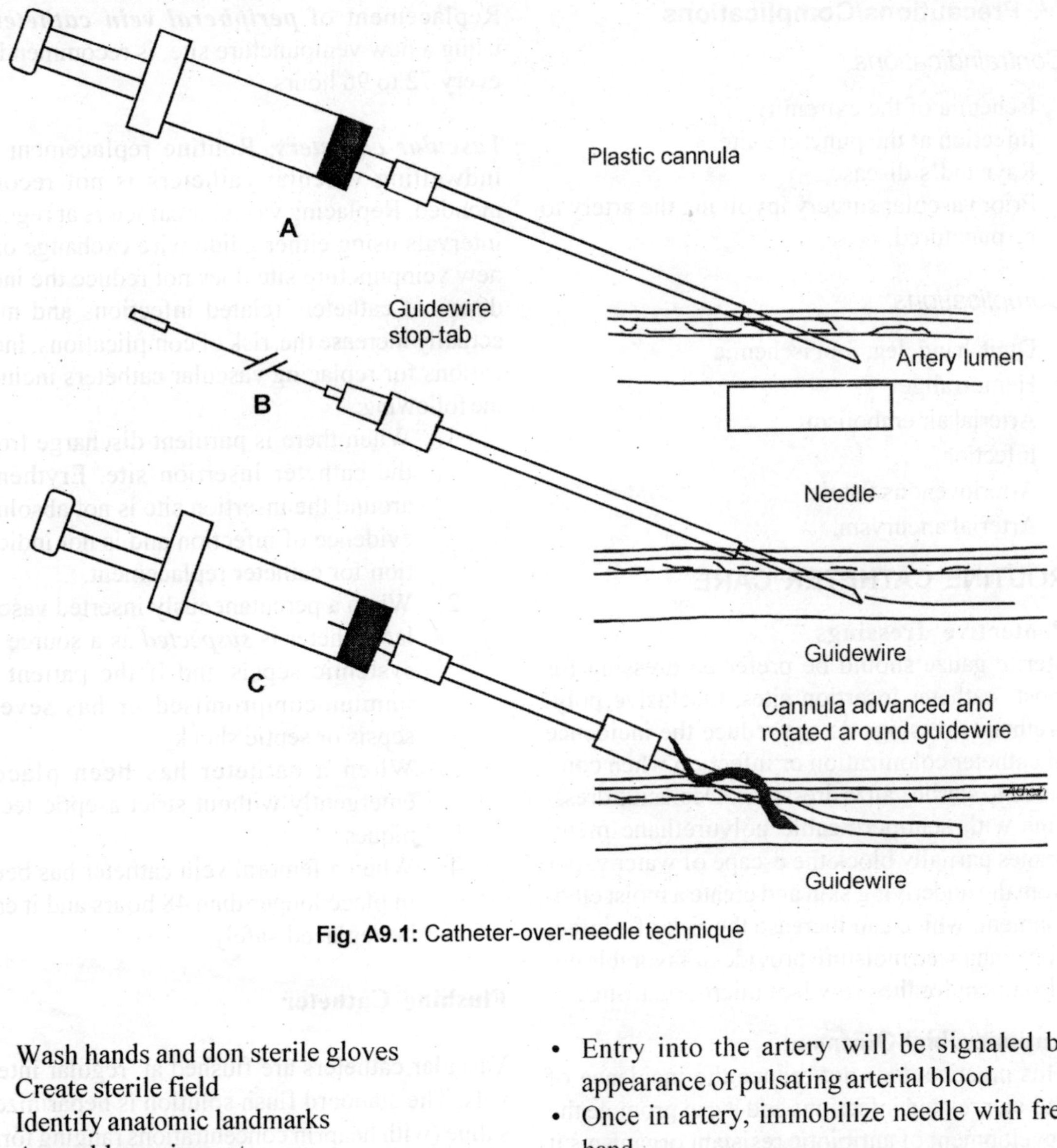

Fig. A9.1: Catheter-over-needle technique

- Wash hands and don sterile gloves
- Create sterile field
- Identify anatomic landmarks
- Assemble equipment
- Palpate femoral artery below the inguinal ligament
- Infiltrate anesthetic agent
- Enter skin over femoral artery ~ 1 to 2 cm below the inguinal ligament
- Advance needle at approximately a 45° angle
- Entry into the artery will be signaled by appearance of pulsating arterial blood
- Once in artery, immobilize needle with free hand
- Advance guidewire through needle
- Remove needle, leaving guidewire in place
- Pass arterial catheter over the guidewire
- Remove guidewire
- Connect tubing to pressure transducer
- Secure the catheter with suture and apply sterile dressing.

IV. Precautions/Complications

Contraindications

- Ischemia of the extremity
- Infection at the puncture site
- Raynaud's disease
- Prior vascular surgery involving the artery to be punctured.

Complications

- Digit, hand, leg, foot ischemia
- Hemorrahge
- Arterial air embolism
- Infection
- Arteriovenous fistula
- Arterial aneurysm.

ROUTINE CATHETER CARE

Protective dressings

Sterile gauze should be preferred dressing for most catheter insertion sites. Occlusive polyurethane dressings do not reduce the incidence of catheter colonization or infection when compared to sterile gauze dressings. Occlusive dressings with semipermeable polyurethane membranes partially block the escape of water vapor from the underlying skin and create a moist environment, which can increase the risk of infection; enhanced moisture provides a favorable environment for the growth of microorganisms.

Antimicrobial Ointment

This practice does not reduce the incidence of catheter related infections and it can promote the development of antibiotic resistant organisms it is wise to avoid the use of topical antimicrobial ointments on catheter insertion sites

Replacing Catheters

Peripheral inserted central catheter (PICCs) can be left in place for 30 days or longer without an increased risk of catheter – related septicemia when compared with central venous catheters.

Replacement of ***peripheral vein catheters***, using a new venipuncture site, is recommended every 72 to 96 hours

Vascular catheters: Routine replacement of indwelling vascular catheters is not recommended. Replacing vascular catheters at regular intervals using either guide wire exchange or a new veinpuncture site does not reduce the incidence of catheter related infections and may actually increase the risk of complications. Indications for replacing vascular catheters include the following:

1. When there is purulent discharge from the catheter insertion site. Erythema around the insertion site is not absolute evidence of infection and is not indication for catheter replacement.
2. When a percutaneously inserted vascular catheter is *suspected* as a source of systemic sepsis and if the patient is immunocompromised or has severe sepsis or septic shock
3. When a catheter has been placed emergently without strict aseptic techniques.
4. When a femoral vein catheter has been in place longer than 48 hours and it can be replaced safely.

Flushing Catheter

Vascular catheters are flushed at regular intervals. The standard flush solution is heparinized saline (with heaprin concentrations ranging form 10 to 1,000 units/mL)

Arterial catheters are flushed continuously at a rate of 3 mL/hour using a pressurized bag to drive the flush solution through the catheter. 1.4% sodium citrate is a suitable alternative to heparinized saline for flushing arterial catheters. Saline alone is as effective as heparinized saline for flushing venous catheters.

Appendix-10

Prevention of Infections Associated with the Use of Vascular Catheters in an Indian ICU

(Summary of Recommendations made by the Indian Society of Critical Care, 2004)

SHORT PERIPHERAL INTRAVENOUS CATHETERS

Catheter Material

1. Use either non-PVC (polyvinyl chloride) plastic catheters or steel needles (e.g. scalp vein sets) to minimize the incidence of phlebitis. However, there is an increased potential for extravasation with steel needles (A).

Hand Hygiene

2. During catheter insertion, hand disinfection using an antiseptic rub is preferred to routine wash with unmedicated soap (A).
3. The use of clean gloves after hand hygiene is recommended (A).

Skin preparation

4. Prepare clean skin with 70% alcohol solution (A).
5. Use of acetone or ether is not recommended (A).
6. Once prepared, the site of insertion should not be palpated (A).

Dressings; types and frequency of change

7. Use either sterile gauze or sterile transparent dressing at the catheter site (A).
8. No recommendation can be made on the practice of direct application of adhesive plaster to secure catheters (Unresolved).
9. Keep dressings on for the duration of the catheter, unless it is soiled, loosened or moist (A).

Monitoring and Surveillance of site

10. Daily palpation over the intact dressing for signs of phlebitis is essential (A).
11. Routine removal of gauze dressings is not recommended for surveillance of the site (A).
12. The dressing should be removed if palpation through the gauze is not possible, or if tenderness warmth or swelling is noted during surveillance. Direct inspection of the site is essential in these situations.

Duration and Catheter replacement

13. Do not routinely replace catheters before 96 hours, unless there are signs of phlebitis, infection or malfunction (A).
14. In the absence of phlebitis, infection or malfunction, IVs may be left for longer periods with close surveillance of the site (B).
15. In children, IVs may be left in place as long as clinically necessary, unless there are signs of phlebitis, infection or malfunction (A).

Replacement of administration sets

16. Do not routinely replace administration sets before 96 hours (B).
17. Administration sets used to infuse lipid based parenteral solutions and blood products should not be left in place for longer than 24 hours (A).
18. No recommendation can be made from existing data on the practice of reusing administration sets in a given patient for discontinuous infusions (Unresolved). However, the consensus group discourages this practice (C).

Value of in-line filters

19. There is no value of in-line filters for the prevention of catheter infection (A).

Stopcocks and side ports

20. Catheters with injection side ports can be safely used with standard hygienic precautions (A).
21. Cap all stopcocks which are not being used (A).
22. Clean injection ports with 70% alcohol before access (A).

Cut-down

23. Do not routinely use cut downs for peripheral venous access (A).
24. In an emergent situation when no alternative route of venous access is possible, a cut-down approach to peripheral venous access may be attempted. Such a catheter should be removed within 24 hours (A).

Anticoagulant flush

25. In catheters at low risk for local complications, heparin is not recommended over normal saline flushes for the maintenance of patency or the reduction of phlebitis (B).

CENTRAL VENOUS CATHETER

Site preference

1. In adults, subclavian vein cannulation is preferred to the jugular or femoral sites to reduce risk of infection (A).
2. Any site (including the femoral vein) is acceptable in children as the infection risks are not significantly different (B).
3. In the selection of a site, weigh the non-infectious risks (haemorrhage, pneumothorax) against the benefits of reducing CRBSI (A).

Catheter material and type

4. Use Polyurethane or Teflon catheters rather than catheter made of polyvinyl chloride/polyethelene to reduce risk of infection (B).
5. The decision to use multi-lumen catheters and the number of lumens used should be influenced by the clinical needs of the patient, rather than by the marginally increased risk of infection associated with use of multi-lumen catheters (B).

Antibiotic coated catheters

6. Antibiotic coated catheters may be used for short term CVCs likely to remain in place for more than five days (A).
7. They may be considered in patients with high risk of infection (neutropenia, burns) (C).
8. The use of antibiotic coated catheters should not be a substitute for strict adherence to catheter insertion and maintenance protocols (A).

Hand hygiene

9. Hand hygiene procedures must be strictly followed (even when gloves are worn) before and after injection, blood sampling dressing or any contact with the CVC or insertion site. (A)
10. For the insertion of CVCs, full scrub (up to the elbows) with an antiseptic solution is recommended (A).

Aseptic technique

11. Use maximal sterile barrier precautions for the insertion of a central venous catheter (A). These include the use of cap, mask, sterile gloves, full-sleeved sterile gown, and large sterile drapes.

12. Pulmonary artery catheters should have a sterile protection sleeve (A).

Skin preparation

13. Aqueous or alcoholic chlorhexidine (0.5-2%) is preferred to povidone-iodine for cleaning the skin prior to CVC insertion (A).
14. If chlorhexidine solutions are not available, 10% povidone iodine is an acceptable alternative (B).
15. 5% povidone-iodine solution is not recommended for site preparation (B).
16. The antiseptic solution must be allowed to dry on the skin before insertion of the CVC. Povidine-iodine must remain on the insertion site for at least 2 minutes, if not dry before insertion (A).
17. Do not apply organic solvents (e.g. ether) to the skin before insertion of the catheter or during dressing changes (A).

Dressings; types; frequency of change

18. Use either sterile gauze or sterile, transparent, semipermeable dressing to cover the catheter site (A).
19. Do not replace dressings daily. However, any dressing that is moist, loosened, or soiled should be replaced (A).
20. A gauze dressing must be replaced every 2 days, whereas transparent dressings must be changed every 7 days (A).
21. When there is excessive perspiration over the catheter insertion site, or if the site is bleeding or oozing, a gauze dressing is preferred over a transparent dressing (C).
22. Do not use topical antibiotic ointments or creams at the insertion site (A).
23. No recommendations are made regarding use of povidone iodine ointment at the insertion site (Unresolved issue) except for haemodialysis catheters (A).

Monitoring and Surveillance of site

24. When gauze dressings are changed every 2 days, the site must be inspected for purulence and erythema and palpated for tenderness and induration (A).
25. In patients with transparent dressings, daily surveillance of the site should be performed without the removal of the dressing (A).

Systemic antibiotics

26. Administration of local or systemic antibiotics to prevent catheter colonization or BSI is not recommended, either prior to catheter insertion or during catheter maintenance (A).

Anticoagulant flush/lock

27. Heparin flushes and locks used to prevent catheter thrombosis are not recommended for the prevention of infection (A).

Catheter replacement

28. Routine (timed) replacement of CVCs is not recommended as a method of infection-control (A).
29. Do not routinely replace catheters in patients with fever explained by another focus of infection or non-infectious cause (B).
30. When a CVC has been placed with less than maximal sterile precaution (e.g. in an emergency) it should be replaced as soon as possible, and in any case, no later than 48 hours after insertion (C).
31. Replace any short-term CVC if purulence is observed at the insertion site (A).
32. Replace all CVCs if the patient is hemodynamically unstable and CRBSI is suspected (B).
33. Remove catheters as soon as they are not needed (A).

Over-the-guide wire exchanges

34. Routine replacement of CVCs over a guide wire is not recommended as an infection-control measure (A).
35. A CVC may be changed over a guide wire to replace a malfunctioning catheter or to convert an existing catheter (e.g. CVC to pulmonary artery catheter or vice versa) if there is no evidence of infection at the catheter site (B).

36. Maximal sterile barrier precautions must be used during an over-the-guide wire catheter exchange. After removal of the old catheter, a new set of sterile gloves must be used before handling the replacement catheter (B).
37. If CABSI is suspected or documented, guide wire-assisted exchange should not be undertaken (A). The old catheter must be removed and a new catheter inserted at a fresh site (A).

ARTERIAL LINES

Site preference

1. The preferred sites for insertion of arterial lines in adults are radial, dorsalis pedis and femoral (B). Axillary artery lines carry a high risk of infection.
2. The posterior tibial artery is an additional site in children.

Hand hygiene

3. All arterial line insertions using the Seldinger technique and all femoral arterial catheterizations should be performed using maximal sterile barrier precautions (masks, cap, sterile full-sleeved gowns, sterile gloves, and large sterile drapes) (A).
4. Placement of radial and dorsalis pedis arterial lines without a guide wire can be performed after hand hygiene using an antimicrobial soap/scrub and wearing of sterile gloves (B).

Skin preparation

Dressings; types; frequency of change

Monitoring and Surveillance of Site

Duration and Catheter replacement

5. Arterial catheter can safely be left in situ for 96 hours (A). Catheter may be left in place longer if clinically required with ongoing surveillance of the site (B).

Selection and replacement of pressure monitoring systems

6. Use disposable rather than reusable transducer monitoring systems whenever possible (A).
7. Replace the entire disposable transducer system at 96 hour interval (A).
8. Replace re-usable transducer system every 48 hour (B).

Care of pressure monitoring systems

9. Maintain patency using a closed continuous flush system rather than an open system to reduce risk of infection (A).
10. Keep all components of the pressure monitoring system sterile (A).
11. Minimize the number of manipulations and entries into the pressure monitoring system (B).
12. Do not administer dextrose containing solutions through the pressure monitoring circuits (A).
13. Sterilize reusable transducers according to manufacture's instruction if the use of disposable transducer is not feasible (A).

Appendix-11

Decontamination of the Alimentary Tract

Oral decontamination

The oral cavity in hospitalized patients is often colonized with pathogenic organisms. Colonization of the oral mucosa with aerobic gram-negative bacilli can be viewed as prelude to pneumonia as gram-negative aerobic organisms are the most common isolates in nosocomial pneumonia The change in microflora is directly correlated to the severity of illness.An average of 1 billion (10^9) microorganisms are present in each milliter of saliva so aspiration of even one microliter (10^{-3}) of saliva runs a risk of nosocomial pneumonia. This is the basis for a decontamination regimen that uses nonabsorbabale antibiotics applied locally in the mouth.

One regimen that has proven successful in ICU patients is use of a paste containing 2% genatamicin 2% colistin, and 2% vancomycin every 6 hours.This regimen will eradicate most aerobic bacteria and candida species from the mouth in about one week. Decontamination reduced the incidence of pneumonia and the mortality in adult patients. Centers for diseases Control (CDC) includes a recommendation for oral decontamination in their guidelines on preventing pneumonia in health-care settings. It can benefit patients with ventilator dependent for longer than one week, severely impaired lung function, increased risk of pulmonary aspiration and recurrent pneumonia in the ICU.

Selective Digestive Decontamination

Conditions in the ICU that might Benefit from decontamination of the Alimentary Tract include after liver transplantation, severe burn injuries, recurrent septicemia of unknown origin, neutropenia in the ICU that lasts 1 week and postgastrectomy patients with a prolonged ICU stay. The regimen that has been used is as follows:

Oral cavity: Paste containing 2% polymyxin 2% tobramycin 2% amphotericin applied to the inside of the mouth 6 hourly.

GI tract: A 10 ml solution containing 100 mg polymycin E, 80 mg tobramycin, and 500 mg ampoterican is given via a nasogastric tube every 6 hours and Intravenous cefuroxime, 1.5 g every 8 hours for the first four days of therapy. This regimens will eradicate most gram-negative aerobic bacteria and yeasts after one week..

Method to Administer Adenosine

Indication

Unstable narrow-complex tachycardia (supraventricular tachycardia) when vascular access has already been established.

Because adenosine has a very short half-life, it must be administered as rapidly as possible and followed immediately with a rapid saline fresh.

Procedures

1. Draw up the adenosine dose *(0.1mg/kg)* into a 1-ml syringe (or 3-mL if the dose is greater than 3 mg).
2. Draw up 2 to 3 mL of normal saline flush.
3. Locate the injection port nearest to the hub of the catheter (closest to the patient central venous access if a choice is available).
4. Place the needles of the adenosine syringe and the flush syringe into the injection port simultaneously.
5. Clamp the IV line just above the injection port so that the medication "will go directly in to the patient and not back up into the IV tubing.
6. Push the adenosine as rapidly as possible.
7. With the finger of one hand still maintaining pressure on the adenosine syringe, push the normal saline flush as rapidly as possible with the other hand.
8. When possible, maintain a record of conversion (attempted conversions) on a monitor strip recording paper.
9. If conversion is unsuccessful, double the dose of adenosine (0.2 mg/kg) and repeat steps 2 through 8.

Appendix-13

Defibrillation and Synchronized Cardioversion

Defibrillation is the untimed (asynchronous) depolarization of a critical mass of myocardial cells that allows a spontaneous organized beat to be initiated. The same principle is used in cardioverting the tachyarrhythmias, but the depolarization used then is timed (synchronous) so as to avoid the vulnerable period of the cardiac cycle.

Paddle size: The ideal paddle size of the pediatric patient is not currently known. The largest electrode size that allows good chest contact over its entire area and good separation between the two electrodes is preferred. Among currently available electrode paddles, the 4.5 cm diameter paddle is adequate for infants; the 8.0 and 13cm, for older children.

Since the skin acts as a resistor between the electrode paddles and the heart, a low-impedance interface medium (i.e., ECG electrode gel or cream) is recommended. Sonographic gels are unacceptable since they are poor electrical conductors; saline soaked pads are also best avoided since their conductivity is variable and they have a tendency to drip, thus potentially producing a short circuit. Alcohol pads are a fire hazard and can predispose to chest burns.

Electrode position: Effective defibrillation depends on an adequate current traversing the heart. The electrode paddles must be placed so that the heart is situated between them. An anterior-posterior arrangement, with one electrode on the anterior chest over the heart and the other on the back, is theoretically superior but impractical during resuscitation. The standard placement is one paddle on the upper right chest below the clavicle and the other on the left of the left nipple in the anterior axillary line. A mirror image is used in the case of dextrocardia.

***Energy dose*:** The optimal energy dose for the defibrillation of infants and children has not been conclusively established. The controversy over a relation between patient weight and optimal energy dose is recognized. Nevertheless, the available data in the pediatric age group suggest that a dose of 2 J/Kg be used initially. If defibrillation is not successful, the dose should be doubled and repeated twice, if necessary. If VF continues, attention should be turned to adequacy of ventilation, oxygenation, and correction of acidosis before another attempts made. An increase in energy is not required when the rhythm converts and then degenerates back into VF. Lidocaine is used in such instances to raise the fibrillation threshold.

***Defibrillator testing*:** There may be a significant variation between the stored and delivered energy, especially at the very low settings required for infants. All defibrillators should be checked periodically for safety, and the accuracy of the delivered energy dose should be checked against a 50-ohm resistance. It is important that defibrillators used for infants and children be checked at very low energy doses and that any variations be prominently displayed on the machine.

Defibrillation Sequence

If VF is seen on the monitoring system:

1. Continue CPR with as little interruption as possible.
2. Apply conductive medium to appropriately sized paddles.
3. Turn on defibrillator power and be sure that it is not in the synchronous mode.
4. Select the energy dose and charge the capacitor.
5. Stop chest compressions, place paddles in proper position on the chest.
6. Recheck rhythm on monitor.
7. Clear area to make sure that no personal are in contact with the patient of the bed: "I am clear, you are clear, everyone clear equipment clear."
8. Apply firm pressure to the paddles while depressing both discharge buttons simultaneously.
9. Reassess ECG and pulse:
   a. If VF persists, repeat counter shock using twice the energy
   b. If an organized rhythm has been established, check pulse and continue CPR as required
   c. If VF recurs, immediately repeat counter shock using the same pulse.

Synchronized Cardioversion Sequence

The procedures is the same as the outlined for defibrillation except as follows:

1. If the paddles are not of the monitoring type, the ECG must be connected to the defibrillator.
2. The synchronizer circuit must be activated (a light blinks and a marker is seen on the monitor with each QRS). On some older models, the QRS must be upright for proper activation.
3. The discharge buttons must be pressed and held until the countershock is delivered.

Appendix-14

Pericardiocentesis

Indication

A. Hemodynamically significant cardiac tamponade.

Equipment

A. Electrocardiogram machine, if available.
B. Sterile pericardiocentesis needle, guidewire, catheter, or 18 gauge spinal needle.
C. Sterile alligator clip.
D. Sterile syringes and infiltrating needles.
E. Table.
F Sterile 4 × 4 gauge sponges.
G. Medication for local anaesthesia and sedation.
H. Sterile gloves, gown, mask, cap, drapes.
I. Plovidone iodine.
J. Supplemental oxygen (cannula, mask, other as appropriate).
K. Pulse oximeter.
L. ECG monitor.
M. Intravenous catheter, tubing, and fluid.
N. Resuscitation cart.

Technique

- Prepare patient, sedate if necessary.
- Obtain intravenous access if not done previously.
- Apply oxygen, monitor pulse oximeter and ECG.
- Position patient
  - May be accomplished in supine position.
  - If time and circumstances allow, a semi-upright position enhances pericardial fluid pooling anteriorly.
- Don mask and cap.
- Wash hands.
- Don gown and gloves.
- Create sterile field.
- Subxiphoid approach (Fig. A14.1).
- Infiltrate local anaesthetic.
- Introduce needle tip left median between xiphoid and left costal margin (Fig. A14.1).
- Advance cardiac needle at 30° to 45° angle to the skin towards the left shoulder or left third intercostal space at midclavicular line while continuous suction is applied to the syringe (Fig. A14.2).
- Monitor ECG; ST or PR segment elevation or other "current of injury" suggests epicardial contact (if this occur, withdraw the needle several millimeters).

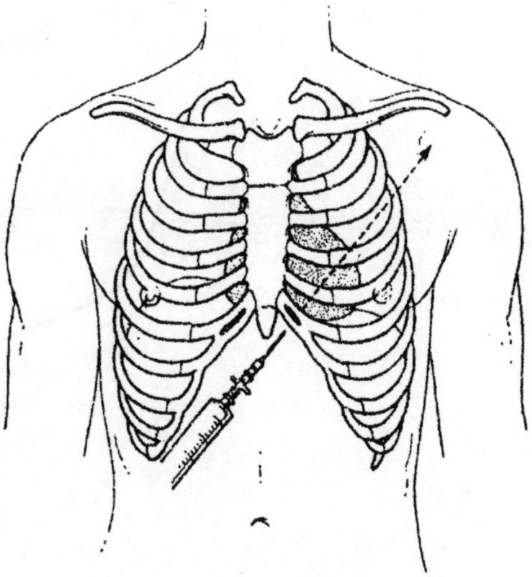

Fig. A14.1

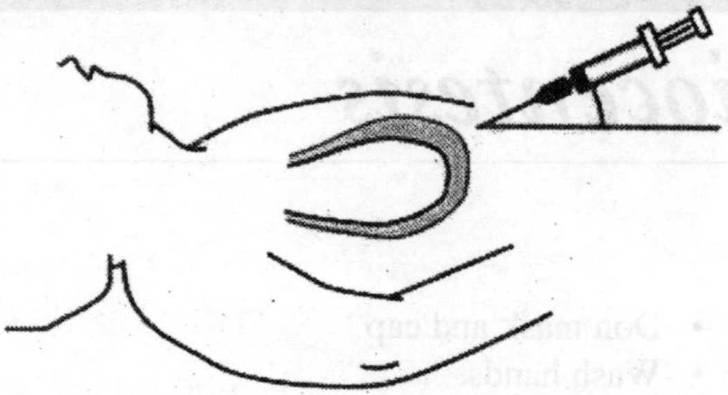

Fig. A14.2: Needle pericardiocentesis

- Withdrawal of as little as 50 mL of pericardial fluid is often all that is necessary to relieve cardiac tamponade (Fig. A14.3).
- Save fluid for analysis.
- Place guidewire through pericardiocentesis needle into pericardial space and remove needle. Reassess position of needle if resistance encountered when passing wire.
- Place pericardial catheter over guidewire into pericardial space.
- Remove guidewire.
- Attach drainage system and secure pericardial catheter with suture fixation.

Precautions/Complications

A. Pneumothorax, hemothorax.
B. Myocardial puncture and tamponade.
C. Cardiac arrhythmias.
D. Coronary or internal mammary artery laceration.
E. Liver laceration.
F. Infection.

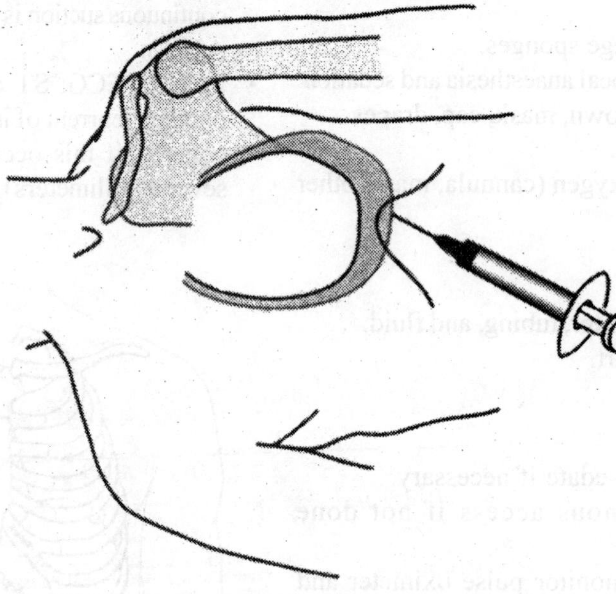

Fig. A14.3

Appendix-15

Temporary Transcutaneous Cardiac Pacing

Indications

Hemodynamically significant bradycardia unresponsive to pharmacologic management.

Conduction delay [second-degree (Mobitz II), or third-degree atrioventricular block] usually in the setting of myocardial infarction.

Equipment

- Cardiac packing electrode pads
- Pulse generator
- Connecting leads
- Medication for sedation, if necessary
- Supplemental oxygen (cannula, mask, other as necessary)
- Pulse oximeter
- ECG monitor
- Intravenous catheter, tubing, fluids
- Resuscitation cart.

Technique

- Recognize cardiac rhythm, determine severity
- Prepare patient
- Obtain intravenous access if not done previously
- Apply oxygen, monitor pulse oximeter and ECG
- Attempt pharmacologic management including atropine and/or dopamine where appropriate
- Assemble equipment
- Apply electrode pads in an anterior-posterior orientation
  - Anterior electrode cathode { - } to left of sternum as close as possible to maximal cardiac impulse.
  - Posterior electrode anode { + } directly behind anterior electrode to left of thoracic spine.
- Connect leads to pulse generator
- Set rate 60-100 beats/min
- Adjust pulse generator output upward until mechanical ventricular capture occurs (usually 20-200 joules)
- Assess efficacy of mechanical capture – obtain blood pressure or palpate pulse
- Arrange for temporary or permanent transvenous pacemaker as necessary.

Bradycardia with Hypoxemia

- Bradycardia in children is most often secondary to hypoxemia
- Pacing for bradycardia rhythms secondary to hypoxemic insult may be considered after airway management, oxygenation, ventilation, chest compressions, epinephrine bolus and infusion and possibly bicarbonate infusion have been accomplished

- The effectiveness of cardiac pacing in this setting is unproven
- Even if electrical capture of the heart is accomplished, contractility and myocardial blood flow may not improve without mechanical capture.

Precautions/Complications

- Inability to capture (~ 20% of patients), usually related to any delay in attempting to pace
- Painful skeletal muscle contraction
- Should be considered a temporizing measure only prior to transvenous pacing.

Appendix-16

Steps in Initiation of Ventilation

Mechanical ventilation demands unique skills and knowledge. It is associated with significant disruption of normal cardiopulmonary function and is not without risk. The process of initiating ventilation can be divided into four steps:

- Patient preparation
- Ventilator preparation
- Selection of ventilator parameters
- Setting up alarms.

Patient Preparation

1. Gain control of airway and ventilation
   a. The patient is intubated—secure it well to prevent unplanned extubation.
   b. Synchronize manual ventilation with the patient's respiratory efforts and gradually take over his ventilation.
2. Achieve cardiovascular stability:
   - Optimize preload: leg elevation, fluids, maintain a slow respiratory rate
   - Increase cardiac contractility: Use inotropes if required
   - Control of arrhythmias, if any
   - Correction of electrolyte abnormalities if any
   - Control of hypertension if any.
3. Establish monitoring:
   - Pulse oximetry
   - ECG
   - BP—Invasive/non-invasive
   - Respiratory wave form
   - End tidal CO_2 monitor.
4. Laboratory data: Obtain
   - Baseline arterial blood gases
   - Hemogram
   - Serum electrolytes
   - Blood sugar
   - Renal parameters.
5. Adequate sedation:
   - Needed to allay anxiety and reduce ventilatory drive
   - A combination of narcotics and sedatives (benzodiazepine) is recommended
   - A muscle relaxant may be indicated in the early phase.

Preparation of the Ventilator

- Check electrical and gas connections, should be functional. Air and O_2 should be flowing
- Ventilator must be clean and patient's tubing sterilized
- Check inspired and expired gas tubing for leaks and disconnection
- Check functioning of accessories such as the compressor, blender and humidifier
- Fill the humidifier till the marked level with distilled water
- Connect tubings and establish connections and working using ventilator lung
- Set ventilation parameters: Mode, cycling (Volume preset/pressure limited). Respiratory rate, FiO_2, tidal volume, pressure limit, inspiratory expiratory time, PEEP.

Alarm Settings

FiO_2: set it 5-10% above and below the set FiO_2, e.g. set FiO_2 - 0.5, alarm limits - Low = 0.4, High = 0.6.

In volume preset-expired minute ventilation: The expired minute ventilation is monitored rather than the inspired minute ventilation to detect any leaks in the circuit. Alarm limits are set at 10-20% above and below the expired minute ventilation.

Low-pressure alarm set at 5-15 cm of water.

Peak pressure alarm set at 30-45 cm of water (5 cm above desired peak pressure).

Initiating Ventilation

Once the patient is ready and the ventilator is set and tested, connect the patient to the ventilator and for the next 15-20 min. closely observe the patient. Chest wall movement should be adequate (but no excessive).

- Check that there is visible chest expansion with each inspiration
- Confirm the air entry and that it is bilaterally equal
- The ventilator and the patient should be in synchrony. If there is dyssynchrony, commonly referred to as "fighting the ventilator", it could either be due to equipment malfunction or patient factors such as intolerance of the ventilator mode, endotracheal tube displacement, pain, hypoxemia, hypercarbia, endotracheal secretions
- Maintain hemodynamic stability
- Confirm that the oxygen saturation and the end-tidal CO_2 are within acceptable limits
- After 30 min do an arterial blood gas
- Aim for a $PaCO_2$ between 35-45 mmHg by increasing the tidal volume in increments of 2 ml/kg. If the peak airway pressure is high, increase the ventilation by increasing the respiratory rate. If the $PaCO_2$ is <35 mm of Hg reduce the respiratory rate first. Reduce the tidal volume only if the peak airway pressures are high
- Aim for a SpO_2 >92%, PaO_2 >70 mmHg. If the PaO_2 is <70 mmHg. First, increase the FiO_2 to 0.6. If this is not enough, add a PEEP in increments of 2 cm of water. If after the above measures the PaO_2 is still less evaluate the patient's condition and accordingly decide which of the two evils is more acceptable viz. O_2 toxicity or pulmonary barotrauma. Don't become too obsessed with matching the ventilator settings to blood gas results
- If the PaO_2 is >70 mm of Hg, reduce the FiO_2 upto 0.4 and if it still remains >70 mm of Hg. it is good for the patient
- The patient will require catheterization and the temperature needs to be monitored
- Do a chest X-ray to check the position of the endotracheal tube and the lung fields
- During ventilatory support, whenever there are problems like patient instability or mechanical problems the patient must be disconnected from the ventilator and manually ventilated.

Appendix-17

A Protocol for Positive End Expiratory Pressure (PEEP) Management

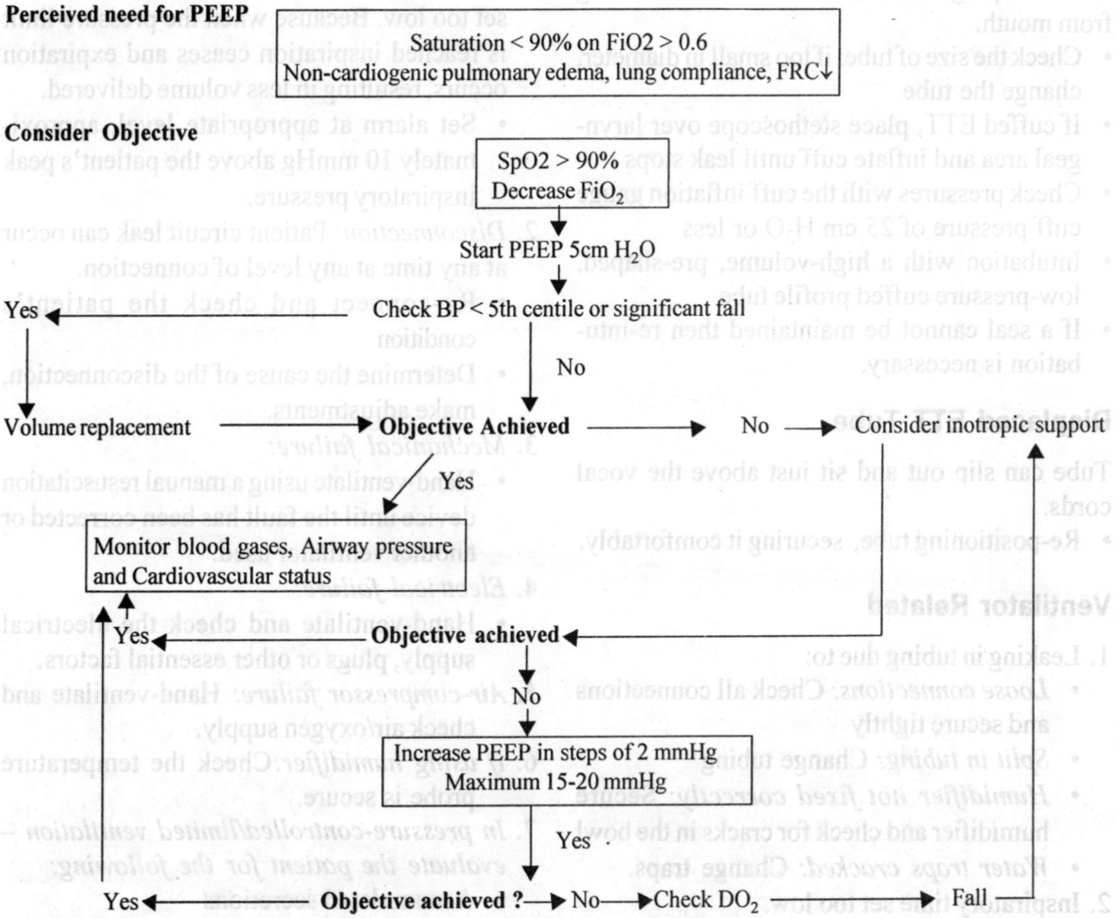

Appendix-18

Trouble Shooting on Ventilators

PROBLEM I–LOW TIDAL VOLUME / LOW MINUTE VOLUME

Patient Related: Peritubal/ Endotracheal Tube (ETT) Cuff Leak

Evaluate the cause of the leak. Air can be felt or heard escaping from the mouth or seen as frothing from mouth.

- Check the size of tube: if too small in diameter, change the tube
- If cuffed ETT, place stethoscope over laryngeal area and inflate cuff until leak stops
- Check pressures with the cuff inflation gauge cuff pressure of 25 cm H_2O or less
- Intubation with a high-volume, pre-shaped, low-pressure cuffed profile tube
- If a seal cannot be maintained then re-intubation is necessary.

Displaced ETT Tube

Tube can slip out and sit just above the vocal cords.

- Re-positioning tube, securing it comfortably.

Ventilator Related

1. Leaking in tubing due to:
   - *Loose connections:* Check all connections and secure tightly
   - *Split in tubing:* Change tubing
   - *Humidifier not fixed correctly:* Secure humidifier and check for cracks in the bowl
   - *Water traps cracked:* Change traps.
2. Inspiratory time set too low.

PROBLEM II–PATIENT NOT RECEIVING "TIDAL/MINUTE VOLUME"

1. *High airway pressure alarm setting too low:* Beware of potential volume loss resulting from the high airway pressure alarm that has been set too low. Because when the pressure limit is reached inspiration ceases and expiration occurs, resulting in less volume delivered.
   - Set alarm at appropriate level, approximately 10 mmHg above the patient's peak inspiratory pressure.
2. *Disconnection:* Patient circuit leak can occur at any time at any level of connection.
   - Re-connect and check the patient's condition
   - Determine the cause of the disconnection, make adjustments.
3. *Mechanical failure:*
   - Hand-ventilate using a manual resuscitation device until the fault has been corrected or another ventilator used.
4. *Electrical failure:*
   - Hand-ventilate and check the electrical supply, plugs or other essential factors.
5. *Air-compressor failure:* Hand-ventilate and check air/oxygen supply.
6. *If using humidifier:*Check the temperature probe is secure.
7. *In pressure-controlled/limited ventilation – evaluate the patient for the following:*
   - Accumulated secretions

- Bronchospasm
- Pneumothorax
- Decrease in lung compliance–because of evolving pulmonary edema, pneumonia.

PROBLEM III–LOW AIRWAY PRESSURE

1. *'Low exp. Minute volume alarm*/Correct tidal volume not delivered.
   An air leak may have occurred in the circuit or at patients level- check the tidal volume and minute volume, both of which will be low. Find the leak and adjust accordingly.
2. *Insufficient gas supply:*
   Changes may have been made in the ventilator settings. If changes have been made check the arterial blood gases to assess ventilatory status. If the patient is adequately ventilated then re-adjust the alarm limits.
3. *Disconnection:*
   - Re-connect and monitor.
4. *Improvement in patient's condition:*
   Not all changes in the ventilator observations indicate problems. It can be indication of improvement if patients oxygenation and CO_2 are maintained within acceptable range.
   - Improvement in airway resistance/bronchospasm
   - Improved lung compliance
   - General improvement in lung condition.

PROBLEM IV–HIGH AIRWAY PRESSURES

1. *Ventilator related:*
   A high pressure limit is intended to serve a dual purpose, it provides an indicator of elevated peak inspiratory pressure, as well venting off excessive volume and pressure to protect the airways from overdistension and barotraumas.
2. *The ventilator tubing is kinked/trapped:*
   Frequently with the amount of equipment around the bed, the tubing can be caught or kinked. Look for it, correct it or change the patient to a different ventilator.
3. *Secretions obstructing ETT:*
   This is *the most common cause*, secretions accumulate because of inability to cough, poor humidification and during resolution of pneumonia
   a. Apply suction and re-position both the patient and tube
   b. Apply suction, then listen for breath sounds to assess the need for further suction
   c. If secretions are thick then instill a few ml of normal saline to help loosen and remove the secretions
   d. Regular turning, physiotherapy and nebulizer will prevent the build-up of secretions.
4. *Coughing or gagging:*
   Secretions, movement of ETT, anxiety, turning or disturbing the patient in any manner may cause irritation of the trachea which results in coughing or gagging episodes.
5. *Bronchospasm:*
   Check the breath sounds, wheezes will be audible. If nebulizers are prescribed then administer these and seek help.
6. The patient develops a *pneumothorax:*
   Breath sounds will be unequal in the right and left lungs. Unequal chest movements occur. The patient's vital signs will deteriorate.
7. *Decrease in lung compliance:*
   It could be due to accumulation of secretions, evolving pneumonia, or pulmonary edema.
   Decrease in compliance will reduce the amount of volume delivered to the lungs. Hand-ventilate until assistance arrives. Get an X-ray and decide.

Appendix-19

Ventilator Evaluation

There are a number of ventilators available in Indian market. While choosing one, physical size and developmental characteristics of infants and children must be kept in mind. Some of the ventilators may be suitable for adults but not for very young infants and children.

All modern ventilators are time-cycled. In addition, these offer a pressure controlled mode and/or volume controlled mode. The modern "Microprocessor-controlled" ventilators are capable of providing various modalities of mechanical and spontaneous PPV-CMV, SIMV, PSV etc. and have flexibility to deliver tidal volumes needed to ventilate adult and pediatric patients.

Pressure and flow transducers are employed to monitor airway pressures (e.g., peak inflation pressure, gas flow rate, expiratory flow rate, Vt and minute volume). Calculated from these data are lung-thorax compliance, airway resistance and respiratory work. It is therefore possible to have 'Real-time monitoring' of a variety of ventilatory parameters, including ability to calculate and monitor: lung-thorax compliance, airway resistance, minute exhaled ventilation, mean airway pressure, respiratory work.

Computer controlled displays indicate all current ventilatory parameters, alarms and limits. Audible and/or visual alarms are used to indicate such things as sudden changes in the FiO_2, apnea, loss of CPAP, leak in the ventilator breathing circuit, and a peak inflation pressure limit.

Prior to purchasing and using a mechanical ventilator and evaluation checklist for documenting a ventilator's capabilities is advocated. It should address specific questions to ensure it suitability for infants and children:

1. Does the ventilator have options of CMV, IMV/ SIMV, PSV modes.
2. Does the ventilator possess adjustable peak pressure, PEEP, flow rate, inspiratory time or I:E ratio and volume capabilities, and other characteristics such as control of inspired oxygen concentration.
3. Is the ventilator too simple or too sophisticated for the needs? Does it work in tropical climate (20°-40°C temperature).
4. Does the ventilator have a comprehensive audible and visible alarm package: for oxygen, pressure, volume, apnoea package?
5. Are the monitoring capabilities enough and data displayed on pressures, tidal volume, oxygenation-concentration? Can compliance, airway resistance and respiratory work be monitored?
6. Is the ventilator too difficult to operate?
7. Can the ventilator be upgraded easily as improvements/innovations occur, or will the ventilator become obsolete in a short period of time?

9. What is the cost of the ventilator?

In general, it is more convenient to utilize pressure preset ventilators with variable flow rates (time cycled pressure limited) in infants under 1 year and volume ventilator in older children. Many modern ventilators provide both the options. However, if these options are not available any available ventilator may be used effectively if it is capable of delivering volumes adjustable in a range of 15-2000 ml.

10. While acquiring equipment must be ensured that the equipment has a battery backup for one hour.
11. An Indian agency which is capable of providing high level back-up and maintenance service. These days there are several Indian agencies offering highly sophisticated and expensive instruments, but their maintenance services are very unreliable. It may be preferable to have a service contract for 2-5 years after the warranty period.

Appendix-20

Peritoneal Dialysis for Acute Renal Failure

INDICATION

A. Clinical

1. Anuria for > 48 hours.
2. Severe central nervous system symptoms.
3. Fluid overload/refractory to medical management causing uncontrolled hypertension, congestive cardiac failure or pulmonary edema.

B. Biochemical

1. Severe azotemia (urea > 300 mg/dl, Serum creatinine >3mg/dl) or rapidly rising urea or creatinine.
2. Uncontrolled hyperkalemia (failure to keep potassium below 6.5 mEq/L using treatment for hyperkalemia).
3. Uncontrollable metabolic acidosis.

(The decision to dialyse should not be made on the basis of one isolated laboratory value—each case should be individualized).

TECHNIQUE

Details of technique for peritoneal catheter insertion are available in standard textbook on Pediatric procedures. The catheter should always be inserted with the help of nephrologist. The following steps are important:

1. Ensure a patent intravenous catheter for fluid infusion.
2. Vital signs of the patient should be stable and the patient should not be hypotensive.
3. Sedate the patient (phenergan 0.25 mg/kg IM, Diazepam IV).
4. Empty the bladder of any urine via catheterisation and prepare the abdomen.
5. The peritoneal fluid should be warmed to the body temperature.
6. Inject the warmed fluid (to which heparin 1000 units/L be added into peritoneal cavity through a 14 G needle while monitoring the patient's pulse, respiratory rate and blood pressure. The initial infusion is usually around 20 ml/kg.
7. Remove the needle and introduce peritoneal catheter after making a small nick. Rest the perforated end of the catheter in right iliac fossa, and ensure free outflow of dialysis fluid through the catheter.
8. Start with initial infusion volume of 15-30 ml/kg and increase as tolerated up to 50-70 ml/kg; usual amount of fluid exchange is 40-50 ml/kg).
9. Heparin (1000 units/L) may be added to the first 2 dialysate runs and discontinued if returns are clear.
10. Add no potassium to the dialysis fluid until serum K is less than 5 mEq-L. In patients with hyperkalemia, add no potassium to the initial 3-5 exchanges. Subsequently, add

2.5-3.5 mEq/L of potassium to the dialysis fluid.

11. Use 4.25% glucose solutions, when hypervolemia is the critical problem.
12. Run the dialysis fluid as fast as is tolerated and leave it in the peritoneal cavity for 30-45 minutes.
13. One cycle/hour is the standard practice—if you run the dialysate too rapidly hypernatremia and hyperosmolarity may develop.
14. Drain the dialysis fluid into the draining bottle (usual time 15-20 min).
15. Remove the dialysis catheter at the end of the dialysis (usually 20 exchanges). Reintroduce if peritoneal dialysis is required a second time.
16. Give maintenance intravenous fluid when peritoneal dialysis is going on.

MONITORING

A. Clinical

1. Continuous: Pulse rate, Temperature, Respiratory rate, Blood pressure
   Look for signs of dehydration.
2. Urine output (Strict monitoring) record.
3. Dialysis fluid 'IN' and 'OUT' volume record.

B. Biochemical

1. Serum sodium, potassium, blood urea, serum creatinine at the end of 3rd, 10th and 20th cycles.
2. ABG at the end of 3rd , 10th and 20th cycles.
3. Blood glucose—4 hourly dextrostix, more frequently if abnormal.

C. Infection Surveillance

1. Cell count, Gram staining and culture of the drained dialysis fluid after every 6 cycles.
2. Send the peritoneal dialysis fluid (from the bag), drained dialysis fluid after the last cycle and the catheter tip for fungal smear and culture.
3. Blood culture at the end of the dialysis.

ANTICIPATE PROBLEMS

A. Problems Suggested by Abnormal Fluid Colours

Pink	Minor bleeding
Bloody red	Bleeding into peritoneum from any site
Bilious/brown	Bowel perforation
Milky	Chylous ascitis

B. Problems Suggested by Abnormal Fluid Delivery Patterns

Fluid delivery patterns	Suggest
No inflow	• kinked catheter • fibrin-filled catheter • clotted catheter
Slow inflow	• Kinked catheter • All apertures not within the peritoneum • Partially clotted catheter • Fibrin-filled catheter
Slow outflow	• Kinked catheter • Fibrin-filled catheter • Clotted catheter • Omental tap

What to do?

Aseptically irrigate and aspirate the catheter to remove fibrin or blood clots. If this is insufficient, withdraw the catheter to see if the drainage improves. If still no improvement, replace the catheter.

Appendix-21

Scoring Systems: How to Use These

1. PRISM SCORE: PEDIATRIC RISK OF MORTALITY SCORE *(by Pollack MM et al. Crit Care Med 1989)*

PRISM is calculated from data collected during the admission day–within first 24 hours after physical admission to the intensive care unit. Worst of the readings is used. Readmissions are treated separately.

Data Needed

Collect the following 26 data points for 18 variables:

1. ICU outcome.
2. Age at admission (months).
3. Operative status (post operative = 1, non-operative =0).
4. Highest and lowest systolic blood pressure (mmHg).
5. Highest diastolic blood pressure (mmHg).
6. Highest and lowest heart rate (bpm).
7. Highest respiratory rate (breaths/min).
8. The occurrence of apnoea.
9. PaO_2/FiO_2 ratio (PaO_2 in mmHg and FiO_2 as a decimal. Do not record in patients with intracardiac shunts or chronic respiratory insufficiency).
10. $PaCO_2$ or capillary PCO_2 (mmHg).
11. Glasgow Coma Score (only record if there is known or suspected CNS dysfunction. Do not record during iatrogenic sedation, paralysis, anaesthesia, etc.).
12. Pupillary reactions (normal, unequal or dilated, or fixed and dilated).
13. Prothrombin time (PT) or partial thromboplastin time (PTT) and the associated control.
14. Highest total bilirubin (do not record for neonates).
15. Highest and lowest serum potassium (mEqL).
16. Highest and lowest serum Calcium (mgdL).
17. Highest and lowest plasma glucose (mgdL).
18. Highest and lowest serum bicarbonate (use measured values).

The PRISM score is obtained by adding the scores assigned to variables 4 to 18 in Table A20.1.

Calculation

The mortality risk (r) is given by

r= 0.27 (PRISM score) – 0.005 (age in months) – 0.433 (operative status) – 4.782.

The probability of death (which should be quoted in preference to the PRISM score or the mortality risk) is then given by

$POD = e^r, (1 + e^r)$

2. PEDIATRIC INDEX OF MORTALITY (PIM)

PIM is calculated from the data collected at or within one hour after first face-to-face contact between the patient and the ICU doctor from the unit being audited. The first value is used. The first contact may be in the PICU, emergency department, another ward in the same hospital or in a different hospital during a retrieval. Data on all children (less than 16 years old) admitted

Table A21.1: Score for PRISM variables

	Infants	Children	Score
Systolic BP	130 – 160	150 – 200	2
	55 – 65	65 – 75	
	> 160	> 200	6
	40 – 54	50 – 64	
	< 40	< 50	7
Diastolic BP		All ages	
		> 110	6
Heart rate	Infants	Children	
	> 160	> 150	4
	< 90	< 80	
Respiratory rate	Infants	Children	
	61 90	51 – 70	1
	> 90	> 70	5
	Apnoea	Apnoea	
PaO_2/FiO_2		All ages	
	200-300		2
	< 200		3
$PaCO_2$		All ages	
	51-65		1
	> 65		5
Glasgow coma score		All ages	
	< 8		6
Pupillary reactions		All ages	
	Unequal or dilated		4
	Fixed and dilated		10
PT/PTT		All ages	
	> 1.5 × control		2
Total bilirubin (mg/dL)			
	> 1 month		
	> 3.5		6
Potassium (mEq/L)		All ages	
	3.0-3.5		1
	6.5-7.5		1
	< 3.0		5
	> 7.5		5
Calcium (mg/dl)		All ages	
	7.0-8.0		2
	12.0-15.0		2
	< 7; > 15.0		6
Glucose (mg/dl)		All ages	
	40-60		4
	250-400		4
	< 40		8
	> 400		8
Bicarbonate		All ages	
	< 16		3
	> 32		

or retrieved to PICU is included. Readmissions are treated as separate patients.

Data Needed

If information is missing record zero; for systolic blood pressure it should be recorded as 120.

1. Bolded *admission to ICU after elective surgery or elective admission* to ICU for a procedure such as insertion of a central line or monitoring or review of home ventilation, no= 0, yes= 1.
2. Is there one of the recognised *underlying premorbid conditions* as shown in Table A21.2 (record the number in square brackets).
3. *Response of the pupils to bright light* Both > 3 mm and both fixed= 1. Other =0. unknown = 0.
   The pupil reactions are used as index of brain function; do not record an abnormal finding if this is probably caused by drugs, toxins or a local injury to the eye.
4. *Base excess* (mmol/L) in arterial blood (unknown= 0).
5. PaO_2 (mmHg) (unknown =0).
6. FiO_2 at time of PaO_2 (unknown =0).
7. *Systolic blood pressure* (mmHg) (unknown =120).
8. *Mechanical ventilation* at any time during the first hour (no = 0, yes = 1).
9. *Outcome of ICU admission* (discharged alive from ICU=0, died in ICU = 1).

Table A21.2: Premorbid conditions

0 None
1. Cardiac arrest out of hospital
2. Severe combined immune deficiency
3. Malignancy after completion of first induction
4. Spontaneous cerebral hemorrhage from aneurysm of AVM
5. Cardiomyopathy or myocarditis
6. Hypoplastic left heart syndrome < 1 month and requiring Norwood procedure
7. HIV infection
8. IQ probably < 35 (i.e. worse than Downs)
9. Neurodegenerative disorder (progressive ongoing loss of milestones)

Calculation

First work out PIM logit using coefficients given in Table A21.3.

Probability of Death = e PIM logit (1 + e PIM logit).

Table A21.3: Logistic regression coefficients to calculate probability of death

Elective admission Yes/no	-1.552
Specified diagnosis Yes/no	1.826
Pupils fixed to light Yes/no	2.357
Absolute 'base excess' mmol/L	0.071
100 × FiO_2/ PaO_2 (mmHg)	0.415
Absolute (SBP- 120) mmHg	0.021
Mechanical Ventilation Yes/no	1.342
Constant	- 4.873

3. PRISM III: PEDIATRIC RISK OF MORTALITY III *(by Pollack MM, Crit Care Med, 1996, Vol. 24, No.5)*

Data Collection

For each variable in the dataset, record the highest and lowest values in the first 12 and 24 hours after physical admission to the ICU. Readmissions are treated as separate patients. Do not record data for patients

- Routinely cared for in other hospital locations
- Staying in the PICU for less than 2 hours
- Admitted while receiving continuous CPR, and who do not achieve stable vital signs for < 2 hours.

Deaths of PICU patients occurring in the operating theatre are only included if the operation occurred during the PICU stay and was a therapy for the illness requiring PICU care.

Terminally ill patients transferred from the PICU for comfort care are included as PICU patients for 24 hours after PICU discharges or, if receiving technologic support, until 24 hours after the technologic support is discontinued.

PRISM III weight variables differently for four categories for age defined as follows:

- Neonate (0 < 1 months)
- Infant (≥ 1 month-12 months)
- Child (≥ 12 months-44 months)
- Adolescent (> 144 months).

Dataset

1. Systolic blood pressure (mmHg).
2. Temperature (oral, rectal, blood or axilla).
3. Mental status: *normal/stupor or coma.* Do not assess within 2 hours of sedation paralysis or anesthesia. If there is constant paralysis and/or sedation, use the time period without sedation, paralysis or anesthesia closest to the PICU admission for scoring. *Stupor or coma is defined as GCS < 8* or stupor/coma using other mental status scales.
4. Heart rate (bpm) (Do not assess during crying or iatrogenic agitation).
5. Pupillary reflexes: one fixed and one reactive or both fixed. Non-reactive pupils must be > 3 mm. Do not assess after iatrogenic pupillary dilatation.
6. Acidosis: total CO_2 or pH (pH may be measured from arterial, capillary or venous sites). If total CO_2 is not measured routinely then use calculated bicarbonate values.
7. PCO_2 (mmHg) 1 kPa = 7.5 mmHg (may be measured from arterial, capillary or venous sites).
8. PaO_2 (mmHg) 1 kPa = 7.5 mmHg (use arterial measurements only).
9. Glucose (serum or whole blood). Whole blood glucose measurements should be increased by 10%.
10. Potassium (serum or whole blood). Whole blood potassium measurements should be increased by 0.4 mEq/L.
11. Serum creatinine.
12. Blood urea nitrogen.
13. While blood cell count.
14. Platelet count.

Table A21.4: Score for PRISM III variables

A. Cardiovascular / Neurologic vital signs			
Systolic blood pressure MmHg			
Neonate	Score = 3	Score = 7	
Infant	40-55	< 40	
Child	45-65	< 45	
Adolescent	55-75	< 55	
Else score = 0	65-85	< 65	
Temperature			
All ages	Score = 3		
Else score = 0	< 33^{0}C (91.4^{0}F) or > 40^{0}C (104.^{0}F)		
Mental Status			
All ages	Score = 5		
Else score = 0	Stupor/coma (GCS < 8)		
Heart rate (bpm)			
Neonate	Score = 3	Score = 4	
Infant	215-225	> 225	
Child	215-225	> 225	
Adolescent	185-205	> 205	
Else score = 0	145-155	> 155	
Pupillary reflexes			
All ages	Score = 7	Score = 11	
Else score = 0	One fixed + one reactive	Both fixed	
B. Acid based blood gases			
pH or total CO_2-mmol/L	Score = 2	Score = 6	Score = 3
All ages	pH 7.0-7.28 or pH 7.48-7.55	pH < 7.0 or	pH > 7.55
Else score = 0	or total CO_2	total CO_2	
$PaCO_2$ (mmHg)			
All ages	Score = 1	Score = 3	
Else score = 0	50.0-75.0	> 75.0	
PaO_2 (mmHg)			
All ages	Score = 3	Score =6	
Else score = 0	42.0-49.9	<42.0	
C. Chemistry Tests			
Glucose (see dataset)			
All ages	Score = 2		
Else score = 0	> 200 mg/dl (11.0 mmolL)		
Potassium (see dataset)			
All ages	Score = 3		
Else score = 0	> 6.9 mmolL or mEq/L		

Contd.

Contd.

Creatinine			
Neonate	Score = 2		
Infant	> 0.85 mg/dL or > 75 μmol/L		
Child	> 0.90 mg/dL or > 80 μmol/L		
Adolescent	> 0.90 mg/dL or > 80 μmol/L		
Else score = 0	> 1.30 mg/dL or > 115 molL		
Blood Urea Nitrogen			
Neonate	Score = 3		
All other ages	> 11.9 mg/dL or 4.3 mmo/L		
Else score = 0	> 14.9 mg/dL or > 5.4 mmo/L		
D. Blood Counts—Hematology			
White blood cell count (cells mm³)			
All ages	Score = 4		
Else score = 0	< 3,000		
Platelet count (cells/mm³)			
All ages	Score = 2	Score = 4	Score = 5
Else score = 0	100,000-200,000	50,000-99,999	< 50,000
PT or PTT (seconds)			
Neonate	Score = 3		
All other ages	PT > 22 or PTT > 85		
Else score = 0	PT > 22 or PTT > 57		
E. Other factors if any of the following is present		Score = 10	

☐ Nonoperative CV disease ☐ Chromosomal anomaly ☐ Cancer ☐ Previous PICU admission ☐ Pre-ICU CPR.

☐ Post-operative ☐ Acute diabetes (e.g. DKA) ☐ Admission from inpatient unit (exclude post-operative patients).

15. Prothrombin time (PT) or partial thromboplastin time (PTT) (seconds).
16. Presence of underlying disease or preceding events.
    i. Non-operative cardiovascular disease: *yes/no* (includes acute cardiac and vascular conditions as the primary reasons for admission).
    ii. Chromosomal anomaly: *yes/no* and (if yes) *acute/chronic*).
    iii. Cancer: *yes/no* and (if yes) *acute/chronic*.
    iv. Previous PICU admission during this current hospital admission: *yes/no*.
    v. Pre-ICU CPR (must include cardiac massage/chest compression) during this current hospital admission: *yes/no*.
    vi. Post-operative (i.e. within 24 hours of a surgical procedure or a procedure taking place in an operating theater): *Yes/no*.
    vii. Acute diabetes: *yes/no* (includes acute manifestation of diabetes eg. DKA as the primary reason for PICU admission).
    viii. Admission from in-patient unit (excluding post-operative patients): *yes/no* (includes all in-patient location) (Table A21.3).

4. MULTIPLE ORGAN DYSFUNCTION SCORING SYSTEMS

The Multiple Organ Dysfunction Score (MODS)

(By Marshall JC, Cook DJ, Christou NV et al. Crit Care Med. 1995; 23:1638-1652) (See Table)

	Score				
	0	1	2	3	4
Respiratory: PO_2/FIO_2 ratio (mmHg)	>300	226-300	151-225	76-150	<75
Renal- serum creatinine (mg/dl)	< 1.1	1.2-2.3	2.3-4.0	4-5.7	<5.7
Hepatic: serum bilirubin (mg/dl)	< 1.2	1.2 -3.5	3.5-7	7-14	>14
Cardiovascular: PAR	< 10	10.1-15	15.1-20	20.1-30	>30
Hematologic: platelet count ($x10^3/mm^3$	>120	81-120	51-80	21-50	<20
Neurologic: Glasgow Coma Score	15	13-14	10-12	7-9	< 6

* *PAR* = Pressure Adjusted heart rate calculated as the product of the heart rate multiplied by the ratio of the right atrial pressure

5. The Sequential Organ Failure Assessment (SOFA) Score

(By Vincent JL, Moreno R, Takala J et al. Intensive Care Medicine 1996;22:707-710)

Organ system/Variables	0	1	2	3	4
Respiratory: PaO_2/FIO_2(mmHg)	>400	<400	<300	$<200_b$	$<100_b$
Renal: creatinine (mg/dl)or urine output	<1.2 or	1.2-1.9	2.0-3.4	3.5-4.9 or <500 ml/d	>5.0 or 200ml/d
Hepatic: bilirubin (mg/dl)	<1.2	1.2-1.9	2.0-5.9	6.0-11.9	>12.0
Cardiovascular: hypotension	No Hypotension	MAP <70 mmHg	Dopamine < 5 or dobutamine (any dose)	Dopamine >5 or epinephrine <0.1or norepi-nephrine <0.1	Dopamine >15 or epinephrine >0.1 or norepi-nephrine >0.1[a]
Hematologic: platelet count ($x10^3/mm^3$)	>150	<150	<100	<50	<20
Neurologic: Glasgow Coma Score	15	13-14	10-12	6-9	<6

[a] Adrenergic agents administered for at least 1 h (doses given are in mg/kg/him).

[b] With ventilatory support.

Appendix-22

Intracranial Pressure Monitoring (With CODMAN ICP Monitor and Microsensor Transducer)

A catheter connected to a fiberoptic device is placed into an area in the cranium to continuously monitor intracranial pressure. Information obtained may be used to determine cerebral perfusion pressure and cerebral compliance, assess the cerebral hemodynamic response to environmental stimuli and evaluate the effectiveness of therapeutic interventions.

Normal ICP is less than 15 mm Hg. Normal range of CPP is 60 to 100 mm Hg. The brain has the ability to maintain blood flow to the tissue when the CPP is > 60mm Hg. When the CPP is <60 mm Hg, blood flow to the brain is decreased, and the cerebral tissue is deprived of oxygen and nutrients.

Indications

1. GCS 8 or less with abnormal motor posturing or other signs of raised ICP–CNS infections, intracranial bleed, Reye's Syndrome, Hepatic encephalopathy.
2. In Head Injury patient with GCS 8 or less and abnormal CT scan (hematoma, contusion, edema, compressed basal cisterns) or normal CT-scan with abnormal motor posturing or hypotension (systolic BP less than 5th centile).
3. Planned postoperative ventilation following removal of mass lesion.
4. Patients with head injury who require ventilation for any reasons.

Monitoring of ICP enables manipulation of cerebral perfusion pressure, detection of expanding mass lesions such as a delayed extradural hematoma and therapeutic withdrawal of CSF, if a ventricular catheter is used.

Types of ICP Monitoring Systems and Techniques

- Intraventricular catheters (Fig. A22.3)
- Subdural transducer (Fig. A22.2)
- Subarachnoid bolt
- Intraparenchymal monitors (Fig. A22.1)
- Fibreoptic (Camino)
- Strain gauge (Codman).

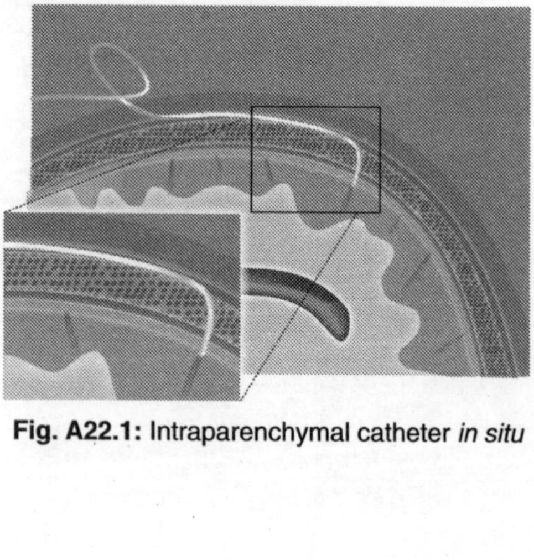

Fig. A22.1: Intraparenchymal catheter *in situ*

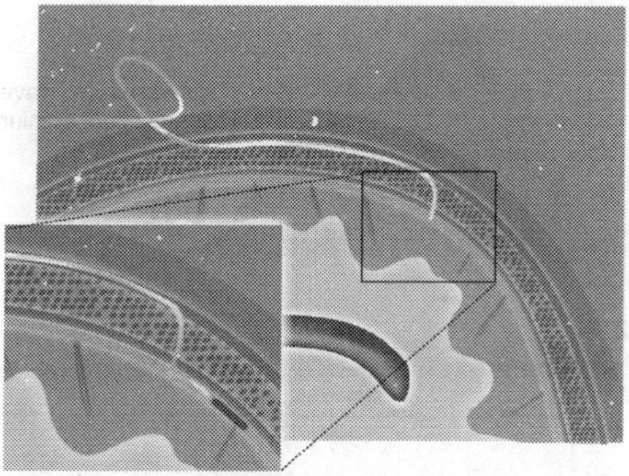

Fig. A22.2: Subdural catheter *in situ*

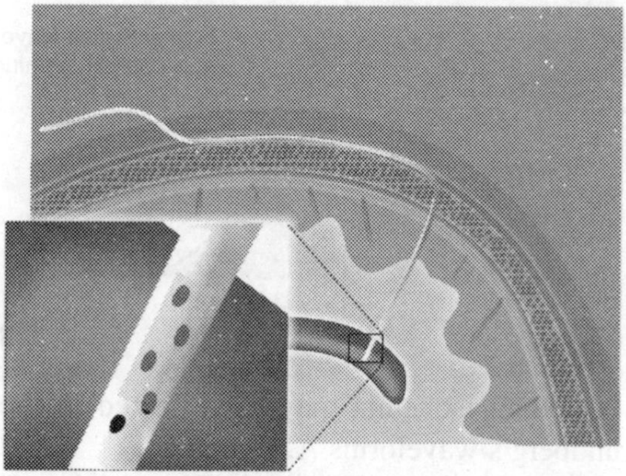

Fig. A22.3: Intraventricular catheter *in situ*

Type of system	*Advantages*	*Disadvantages*
Intraventricular		
A catheter is inserted in the lateral ventricle through a burr hole and then connected to a transducer	Direct and most accurate measurement of pressure . Reliable waveform Allows to drain and sample CSF	Higher risk of infection, Cathether placement more difficult, Occlusion of catheter by blood clots, can cause tissue damage
Intraparenchymal		
A fiberoptic, transducer-tipped catheter is inserted directly	Easy to insert Eliminates the flush system, Accurate ICP values, Sharp and distinct waveforms	Unable to sample or drain CSF, Expensive
Subarachnoid		
A screw is inserted through the skull and dura into the subarachnoid space attached to a closed, fluid-filled system and transducer (a fiberoptic device)	Easy to insert, Ability to obtain pressures	Less reliability and accuracy of waveforms
Subdural		
A catheter is placed in the subdural space and then connected to a closed fiberoptic system	Low risk of infection and hemorrhage	Accuracy and reliability of waveforms and pressures is poor

ICP Waveform

The normal ICP waveform contains three phases (Fig. A22.4):

- P1 (percussion wave) represents arterial pulsations
- P2 (rebound wave) reflects intracranial compliance
- P3 (dichrotic wave) represents venous pulsations

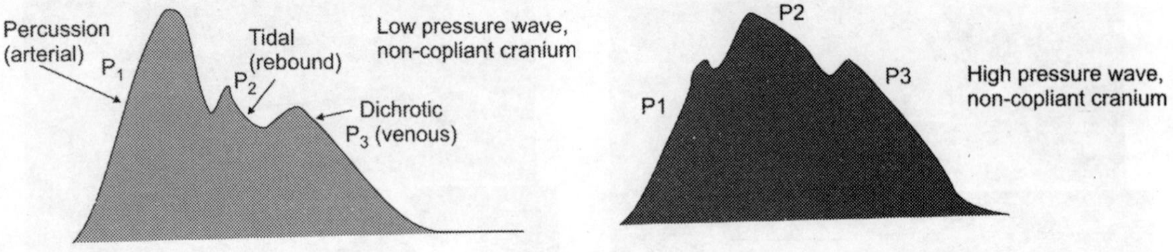

Fig. A22.4

Cerebral ischemia may be reflected in the Lundberg's waveforms A, B, and C.

- A waves are caused by rapid and sustained increases in ICP (>20 mm Hg) that may last 5 to 20 minutes, followed by steep fall to baseline above original level. A waves reflect extreme compromise of compliance and the presence of cerebral ischemia (Fig. A22.5).

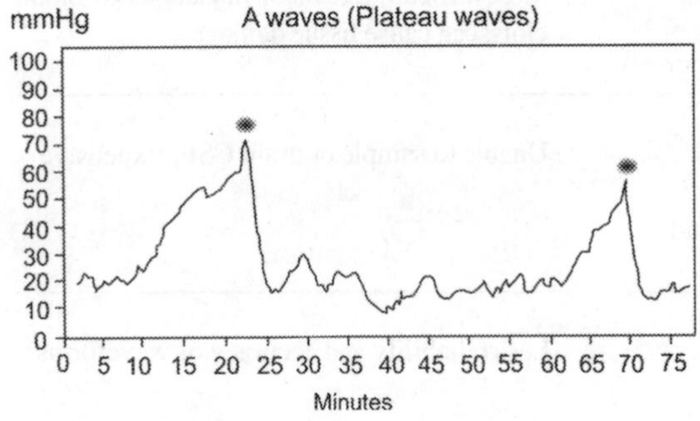

Fig. A22.5: Large A waves on ICP monitor

- B waves are sharp, rhythmic oscillations with a sawtooth appearance that may occur every 0.5 to 2 minutes with ICP elevations up to 20-mm Hg. B waves fluctuate with respiratory patterns and may be affected by arterial pressure. B waves appear more frequently with increasing decompensation and may progress to A waves (Fig. A22.6).
- C waves are small, frequent waves that may occur every 4 to 8 minutes with ICP elevations up to 5 mm Hg. C waves fluctuate with respiration and normal changes in arterial pressure.

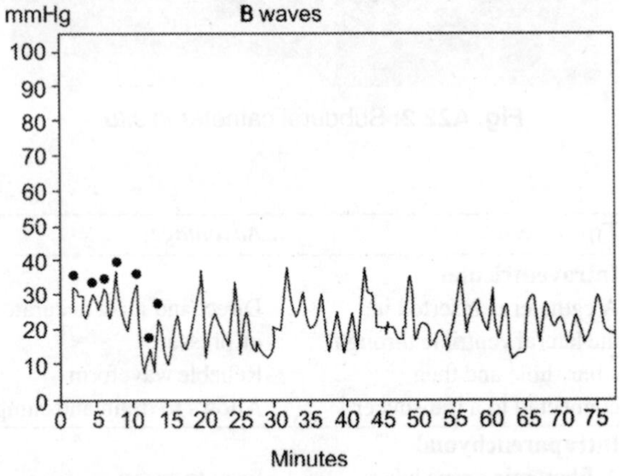

Fig. A22.6: Sawtooth like B waves on ICP monitor

METHOD

A. Zeroing the Transducer

1. Connect the MicroSensor to the Control Unit or ICP Monitor using the appropriate sterile transducer interface cable.
2. Proceed to zero and calibrate the external patient monitor.
3. Prepare to zero the MicroSensor by laying the tip of the transducer in a shallow pool of sterile water or sterile saline. Pour sufficient sterile water to lay at least a 5 cm section of the transducer horizontally just under the surface of the sterile water/sterile saline. Do not submerge the tip of the catheter vertically in a deep pool or cup of sterile water/sterile saline.
4. While keeping the tip of the MicroSensor flat in the sterile water/sterile saline, proceed to

zero the MicroSensor according to the instructions provided with the CODMAN Monitor.

5. Record the three digit zero reference number provided by the MicroSensor Interface Control Unit or Monitor. The number may be marked on the MicroSensor connector housing or patient's chart for reference.

B. Surgical Procedure-Insertion of Transducer

1. Site of insertion: In the frontal region, anterior to the coronal suture, behind the hairline, 2 to 4 cm lateral to the midline.
2. Perform craniotomy and retraction procedures required to expose the skull.
3. Pull the 2.7 mm drill bit into the drill chuck and make a drill hole through the outer table. Proceed gently through the inner table with care to avoid injury to the dura or parenchyma.
4. Carefully bevel the incision site towards the side from which the transducer catheter will exit.
5. Use the Tuohy needle to make a cruciate puncture in the dura.
6. Use the Tuohy needle with stylet in place to tunnel under the scalp from the incision site to the exit site.
7. Remove the stylet and thread the transducer from the tip of the needle until approximately twice the placement length exists from the hub. The inner edges of the Tuohy needle are sharp; exercise caution when threading the catheter through it.
8. Gently remove the needle, and estimate the length of the transducer catheter from the tip to where it will bend upon existing the skull. In a child the catheter is usually inserted to a depth of 4 to 6 cm, and then tunneled to exit at a separate site.
9. Fold the transducer once, completely, at the desired bend site to leave a kink in the catheter (Fig. A22.2).
10. Place the tip of the transducer into the parenchyma through the puncture in the dura until the kink is at the edge of the hole, as shown in (Fig. A22.3).
11. Carefully pull back the excess catheter.
12. Remove the retractor, verify hemostasis in the insertion area
13. Suture the incision site closed.
14. Secure the catheter to the scalp. For additional security, make a small loop with the catheter and tie and loop down.
15. Close and dress the incision site.

Precautions

It is essential to maintain strict sterile technique during transducer placement. All procedures should be performed by a qualified person using standard surgical procedure. This person is responsible for taking appropriate steps and procedures to avoid infections and complications.

Complications

Hemorrhage (risk<1%)may occur at the site of transducer placement from either the skull, cortical or dural areas. Testing of the blood-clotting factor should be conducted on patients before insertion. Assessment about the possibility of subarachnoid, intracerebral or extracerebral hemorrhage at the site of placement must be judged by the intensivists.

Infections (<1%), subcutaneous CSF leakage, and neurological sequelae are potential complications of this procedure.

Index

B

C

G

H

I

K

L

M

N

T

U

V

W

Z